THE ASTHMA EDUCATOR'S HANDBOOK

THE ASTHMA EDUCATOR'S HANDBOOK

Christopher H. Fanta, M.D.

Elisabeth S. Stieb, RN, BSN, AE-C

Elaine L. Carter, RN, BSN, AE-C

Kenan E. Haver, M.D.

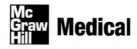
Mc Graw Hill Medical

New York Chicago San Francisco Lisbon London Madrid Mexico City
Milan New Delhi San Juan Seoul Singapore Sydney Toronto

The McGraw·Hill Companies

THE ASTHMA EDUCATOR'S HANDBOOK

1 2 3 4 5 6 7 8 9 0 DOC/DOC 0 9 8 7

ISBN-13: 978-0-0714-4737-9
ISBN-10: 0-0714-4737-7

This book was set in Janson by International Typesetting and Composition.
The editors were Ruth Weinberg and Regina Y. Brown.
The production supervisor was Sherri Souffrance.
The indexer was Susan Hunter.
RR Donnelley was printer and binder.

This book is printed on acid-free paper.

Library of Congress Cataloging-in-Publication Data

The asthma educator's handbook / Christopher H. Fanta ... [et al.].
    p. ; cm.
  Includes index.
  ISBN 0-07-144737-7 (alk. paper)
    1. Asthma—Handbooks, manuals, etc.   2. Asthma in children—
Handbooks, manuals, etc.   3. Asthma—Study and teaching—
Handbooks, manuals, etc.   I. Fanta, Christopher H.
  [DNLM: 1. Asthma—Handbooks.   2. Patient Education—
Handbooks. WF 39 A8525 2007]
RC591.A8181122 2007
616.2'38—dc22   2006046896

CONTENTS

DEDICATION / VII

INTRODUCTION / IX

ACKNOWLEDGMENTS / XV

PART I

THE FUNDAMENTALS / 01

CHAPTER 1

UNDERSTANDING AND EXPLAINING THE MECHANISMS OF ASTHMA / 03

CHAPTER 2

DIAGNOSING AND STAGING THE SEVERITY OF ASTHMA / 47

CHAPTER 3

MEDICATIONS USED TO TREAT ASTHMA / 89

CHAPTER 4

TREATING ASTHMA IN THE AMBULATORY SETTING / 129

CHAPTER 5

SPECIAL CONSIDERATIONS IN CHILDHOOD ASTHMA / 165

PART II

PRACTICAL ASPECTS OF ASTHMA CARE / 205

CHAPTER 6

PULMONARY FUNCTION TESTING AND PEAK FLOW MONITORING / 207

CHAPTER 7

IDENTIFYING ALLERGIC SENSITIVITIES AND PROMOTING ALLERGEN AVOIDANCE / 251

CHAPTER 8

INHALERS AND INHALATIONAL AIDS IN ASTHMA TREATMENT/ 289

CHAPTER 9

MANAGING ASTHMATIC ATTACKS / 329

CHAPTER 10

DEVELOPING AN ASTHMA ACTION PLAN / 363

INDEX / 403

DEDICATION

We dedicate this book

to our patients, who have taught us far more that we could learn just from books or medical journals about what it means to have asthma and how asthma can best be treated;

to our colleagues, whose remarkable abilities inspire us to be better asthma care providers and teachers; and

to our families, whose love and support make it all worthwhile.

INTRODUCTION

Living with asthma can be challenging. And helping a child with asthma grow up active and safe despite his or her asthma can be a daunting task for parents and other caregivers. There are many decisions that need to be made, often on a daily basis. *Should I take my medication today? Which medication? How much? Is it safe to go on this trip away from home? Is this cough with phlegm due to a respiratory infection or my asthma? Should I call my doctor, take more medication, or take my child to the emergency room for evaluation?* The questions and potential uncertainties go on and on.

The outcomes of these decisions matter. With smart decisions, asthma can generally be kept under good control. A child with asthma can go to school, summer camp, sleepovers at friends' homes, and trips to the country without undue limitations. Children and adults can compete in athletic endeavors and sporting competitions unhampered by compromised breathing. On the other hand, poor decisions can lead to canceled vacation plans, days lost from school and work, and unscheduled visits to the doctor's office. Asthma can come to control one's life and the life of one's family. One begins to live in fear of the next terrifying and seemingly unpredictable attack of difficulty breathing.

Like you, we are committed to helping our patients and their families deal effectively with asthma. We believe firmly that a patient armed with the knowledge, skills, and attitudes needed for good asthma care is best prepared to make good decisions about living with asthma. We recognize that what transpires in the doctor's office—making the correct diagnosis and prescribing the most appropriate medications—is only the first step to managing asthma. What good are the right medications if one is uncertain as to the when, how, and why of taking them; if one's fears about medication side-effects or addictive properties have not been answered; if no one has addressed their cost and potential lack of availability? Beyond questions about medications, there are many other topics on the minds of our patients. They range from questions about the role of diet in asthma to the safety of owning "hypoallergenic" pets, from the value of "allergy shots" to the long-term course of the illness: "will my asthma turn into emphysema when I grow old?" There are still other questions that they may not have mentioned but that we think they *should* be asking, such as "what should I do if my child has an asthma attack," and "what's the next step if this initial treatment doesn't lead to prompt improvement?"

In this modern "information age," with seemingly unlimited sources of medical information at our fingertips, it might seem that as healthcare providers our role as asthma educators has become superfluous, but it has not. Our patients and their families are bombarded with information about asthma and its treatment on television and radio advertisements, billboards, magazines, popular medical books, and Internet websites, but how reliable and unbiased is this information? Some of it is superb; some of it is distorted by the desire to sell a product or service; and some of it is sheer nonsense. It remains true today, as it has been for generations, that for many people their most relied upon source of medical information is a trusted (and well-informed) healthcare professional.

As a healthcare provider, you are in the perfect position to provide accurate and useful *knowledge* about asthma, to teach the necessary *skills* of asthma care (whether they be how to use an inhaler properly or how to measure peak flow), and to help cultivate effective *attitudes* about asthma management (such as belief in the value of preventive medication and in the harmful effects of cigarette smoking). Similarly, you are in the best position to guide patients and their families to reliable sources of medical information, whether in print or online. Your word carries special weight simply because you are a nurse, nurse practitioner, physician's assistant, respiratory therapist, physical therapist, case manager, or pharmacist—respected and trusted for your medical knowledge and abilities.

With this respect and trust come, of course, responsibilities. It falls to you to find the time to teach about asthma, to be as well-informed about asthma as possible, and to communicate clearly. With this handbook we hope to help you achieve the latter two tasks. The first task—finding the time in the midst of hurried medical practice to educate about asthma—falls to you.

The goal of this *Asthma Educator's Handbook* is to provide you with the tools to become an effective asthma educator. Both the idea for the book and much of its content derive from a series of one-day continuing education seminars for allied health professionals presented by the Partners Asthma Center's Asthma Educators' Institute, beginning in 2003. Partners Asthma Center is a collaboration among allergists and pulmonologists at five of the major hospitals that participate in the Partners HealthCare System in Massachusetts: Brigham and Women's Hospital, Massachusetts General Hospital, Faulkner Hospital, Newton-Wellesley Hospital, and North Shore Medical Center. Our mission, stated at the founding of our Asthma Center in 1989, is as follows:

> ...to provide optimal medical care for persons with asthma and related diseases; to develop new knowledge about asthma and its management through state-of-the-art medical research; to train medical students and graduate physicians in the specialized skills of asthma care; and to promote improved understanding about asthma and related diseases through educational programs and materials for our patients, for other healthcare providers, and for the community.

In keeping with this mission, we founded the Asthma Educators' Institute to develop and present courses for healthcare workers who want to become more effective asthma educators. To date we have held twelve such courses in and around Boston, attracting more than 1500 registrants. Many Partners Asthma Center physicians and nurses helped to organize and teach these seminars. Also, many health professionals attending the courses shared their ideas for improvement or for new directions of growth. Several asked whether an asthma educator's handbook was available for further study. From these courses and insightful suggestions has emerged this *Asthma Educator's Handbook*.

In a sense it is our patients who have taught us the most about living with asthma. Their stories about asthma and their successes and mistakes in dealing with this chronic condition resonate throughout this book. Like most medical practitioners, we have supplemented our experience-based knowledge with careful and critical reading of the medical literature. The *Asthma Educator's Handbook* is an evidence-based medical text. Throughout the book we have been careful to indicate where, in the absence of strong scientific evidence, we have offered our best clinical judgment in place of proven fact. We have also relied heavily on the asthma practice recommendations of the National Asthma Education and Prevention Program (NAEPP) of the National Institutes of Health. Our recommendations follow closely those published by the NAEPP's Expert Panel II in their 1997 report, *Guidelines for the Diagnosis and Management of Asthma*, and by the Expert Panel's *Update on Selected Topics 2002*.

We have organized the handbook into a two major sections: "The Fundamentals" and "Practical Aspects of Asthma Care." For readers of this book (and for our patients), we consider understanding the theoretical underpinnings of asthma care essential to successful asthma management. It is of limited benefit teaching patients how to actuate their inhalers properly if they don't understand the purpose of the medications they contain or their desired effects. Allergen avoidance only makes sense in the context of understanding the role of allergen exposure in causing asthmatic airway inflammation and triggering asthmatic attacks. In the section on "The Fundamentals" of asthma, we address what asthma is and its relation to allergies; making the diagnosis of asthma; defining the severity of asthma (using the four stages of asthma severity proposed by the NAEPP); the medications used to treat asthma, including their potential side-effects; and the use of these medications in a stepwise approach based on asthma severity. We include a chapter that addresses the special considerations of asthma diagnosis and management in young children.

In the section on "Practical Aspects of Asthma Care," we discuss the many practical details that patients or patients' caregivers need to know about measuring lung function and peak flow; identifying and avoiding allergens in the home, school, or work environments; using metered-dose inhalers, dry-powder inhalers, and inhalational aids (spacers); and developing asthma action plans. We include detailed information about pulmonary function testing as well as discussion of peak flow monitoring. And we include a chapter on hospital-based management of asthmatic attacks as preface to discussing asthma action plans (which are guides to initial, patient-initiated home management of asthmatic attacks). We anticipate that at the end of this section, you will feel fully comfortable teaching someone how to use a metered-dose inhaler, a Diskus, a Turbuhaler, Aerolizer, or Twisthaler. You will be able to advise patients regarding the pros and cons of dust mite covers for mattress and pillows or high-efficiency particulate air (HEPA) filters for their vacuum cleaners. You will be able to demonstrate the use of a peak flow meter and guide patients as to how to make measurements and how to interpret the results obtained. And you will be ready to help patients complete their written asthma action plan or at least to help them to discuss the topic with their principal asthma care provider.

Our goal throughout the book is not only to share information with you but also to help you find effective ways to communicate much of this information to patients and their families. We want you to be not only well-informed but also skilled in teaching others, including those who have no background in health sciences.

This point about talking to patients using language that they can understand bears emphasizing. Remember that if we have asthma (or any other medical problem), those of us in the medical profession—whether doctors or nurses, respiratory therapists, pharmacists, or other healthcare providers—have an enormous advantage in dealing with the challenges of our illness, because of our medical training. We can visualize the anatomy of the bronchi and understand the functioning of the lungs. We know about involuntary muscles and the concept of bronchospasm. Discussion of inflammation of the bronchial tubes conjures up appropriate images of swelling, mucus production, and cellular infiltration of airway walls. The terms "bronchodilators" and "corticosteroids" fit easily into a framework that we have learned from our study of pharmacology.

But what if all of these terms were foreign to you? What if the process of breathing was something taken for granted, like the operation of your car or computer, without thought as to how it works or how it can go wrong? To be effective educators we need to find a common language with which to communicate with our patients, and that language needs to be free of medical jargon. You will need not only to understand the concepts presented in this book but also be prepared to translate them into plain English. That is the charge to any good educator: "know your audience and speak to them in a language that they will understand." We strive to help you achieve this goal by providing useful illustrative materials and patient-friendly explanations throughout the book. We also refer you to additional asthma educational resources available in other publications and online.

Finding adequate time for teaching about asthma (or other major medical problems) is a challenge that we all face. A common refrain in ambulatory medicine is that patient education falls by the wayside because there is no mechanism for receiving financial compensation for the time spent, even though spending that time is widely recognized as important—and enormously appreciated by the recipient. The National Asthma Education Certification Board is one of the groups working to make asthma education (that is provided by certified asthma educators) a billable service.

The National Asthma Education Certification Board makes available a computerized examination (offered at designated testing sites) for official certification as an Asthma Educator. Eligible to take this examination are nurses and nurse practitioners, respiratory therapists, pharmacists, physical and occupational therapists, physicians and physician assistants, social workers, pulmonary function technologists, health educators, or other individuals providing asthma education who have more than 1000 hours of on-the-job experience. One of the motivations for our writing this book is to help those who wish to take this Certification Examination to prepare for the exam and to pass it. Elaine Carter and Elisabeth Stieb, nurse educators in our Partners Asthma Center practices and coauthors of this book, have both completed the examination and received the designation of Asthma Educator—Certified (AE-C). They are familiar with the expectations of the examiners who prepared the Board Examination, and their knowledge of the test has helped to shape the content of this book.

We have created this text as a handbook so that you will have ample opportunity to test your understanding of its content step-by-step throughout, using the *Self-Assessment Questions* and *Discussion of the Answers* sections at the end of each chapter. The material presented in this *Handbook* is the sort of information that you need to know to pass the Board Examination; the questions asked are similar to those that might be posed on the examination. A careful reading of this *Asthma Educator's Handbook* will, we believe, leave you well-prepared to be an asthma educator, and to be officially certified as one.

And if, through your study and teaching, one patient feels newly empowered to care for his or her asthma, one parent again sleeps soundly knowing that his or her child will be safe from asthma, or one potential asthma attack is avoided because of well-timed preventive measures instituted at home, we will have achieved our goals in writing this book.

Christopher H. Fanta, M.D.
Elaine L. Carter, R.N., AE-C
Elisabeth S. Stieb, R.N., AE-C
Kenan E. Haver, M.D.

PARTNERS ASTHMA CENTER
BOSTON, MASSACHUSETTS
JUNE, 2007

ACKNOWLEDGMENTS

The authors wish to thank the other members of our Partners Asthma Center who have taught in the Asthma Educators' Institute courses from which this *Handbook* is derived. They include: Mark Anderson, Dennis Beer, M.D., Christine Blaski, M.D., Fiona Gibbons, M.D., Daniel Hamilos, M.D., Paul Hannaway, M.D., Faysal Hasan, M.D., David Hopper, M.D, Jacob Karas, M.D., Barrett Kitch, M.D., Karen Lahive, M.D., Aidan Long, M.D., James MacLean, M.D., Daniel Muppidi, M.D., Madakolathur Murali, M.D., Walter O'Donnell, M.D., Robert Tarpy, M.D., Elizabeth TePas, M.D., Philip Thielhelm, M.D., and Inna Vernovsky, M.D.

I

THE
FUNDAMENTALS

1

UNDERSTANDING AND EXPLAINING THE MECHANISMS OF ASTHMA

C H A P T E R   O U T L I N E

I.   Begin at the beginning

II. Normal breathing
   a. The tracheobronchial tree

III. Mechanisms of airway narrowing in asthma
   a. Experimental model: allergen challenge and the early and late asthmatic reactions

IV. Things that provoke airway narrowing in asthma
   a. Allergens
   b. Exercise
   c. Respiratory infections
   d. Stress
   e. Medications
   f. Nontriggers of asthma
   g. New triggers of asthma

V.   "Twitchy airways": the concept of bronchial hyperresponsiveness
   a. Bronchial challenge test
   b. "Outgrowing" asthma

VI. What causes airways to become twitchy?
   a. Chronic low-grade airway inflammation
   b. Linking airway inflammation to bronchial hyperresponsiveness

VII. A closer look at "allergic-type inflammation" of the bronchial tubes
   a. Lymphocytes
   b. Immunoglobulin E (IgE antibody)
   c. Mast cells
   d. Chemical mediators of inflammation

CHAPTER   OUTLINE

e. Eosinophils

f. Permanent structural changes in the airway wall ("airway remodeling")

VIII. An expanded definition of asthma

IX. What causes asthma?
a. Occupational asthma: a model for the etiology of asthma

X. The epidemiology of asthma in America
a. Inequalities in the distribution of asthma
b. Rising prevalence of asthma
c. Preventable morbidity and mortality from asthma

BEGIN AT THE BEGINNING

Imagine that you are asked to teach a small group of patients and their families about asthma. You decide to begin with the definition of asthma, and so offer, correctly, that "asthma is a chronic inflammatory disease of the bronchial tubes in which the bronchi narrow excessively and (generally) reversibly in response to a variety of stimuli." You have accurately captured many of the key features of asthma in this succinct definition, but the faces in your audience have a distant, dazed look. One member of the audience bravely raises his or her hand and asks, "What are bronchi?"

And so you are reminded that you didn't always have the words "bronchi" and "inflammatory disease" in your vocabulary. As you think ahead to other topics on your agenda for this educational session, you realize that mucous glands, smooth muscle, bronchospasm, and bronchodilators all fall into this same category: medical terms that we have incorporated into our day-to-day language, no longer viewing them as technical jargon. Yet, to the uninitiated, these terms can be as head-spinning as "tort," "probate," and "jurisprudence" may be to those of us not trained in the legal profession.

For the benefit of your audience, you make a quick recalibration. You will need to rethink your terminology, and begin at the very beginning—normal breathing. It is safe to say that most people have never considered the mechanisms of normal breathing; it is just something that we do. Most of us are guilty in the same way as we go about our lives, driving our car or operating our computer. We rarely stop to consider their functioning other than, perhaps, when things go wrong and they stop working properly. So, too, with breathing. In this case, asthma is the dysfunction that has captured the interest of your audience in how we breathe.

NORMAL BREATHING

When you breathe in, air passes from your nose and mouth through a system of branching tubes that begins with the windpipe (trachea) and divides again and again into smaller and smaller tubes, carrying the air deep into the lungs (Fig. 1-1). The lungs themselves, with a capacity of about 1 1/2 gallons in volume, consist primarily of tiny, microscopic air sacs (alveoli). These air sacs are elastic and highly expandable, enlarging with the entry of air on inhalation and shrinking (sometimes even collapsing closed) with emptying of the lungs on exhalation. It is via these many millions of tiny air sacs that the work of the lungs—transporting oxygen from the air into the bloodstream, and removing carbon dioxide from the blood back into the air—takes place.

The bronchi are the highways for the flow of gas in and out of the air sacs. From the windpipe they branch into left and right main bronchi, then each divides again and again, approximately 23 times in all, until they are microscopic

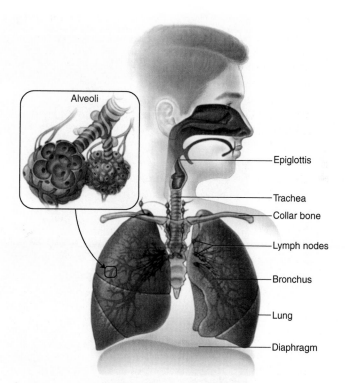

FIGURE 1-1 *This diagram of the respiratory system illustrates the air passageways from nose and mouth, larynx and trachea, into multiple generations of branching bronchi, until finally the air sacs (alveoli) are reached.*

in diameter and give rise to the air sacs that together form the delicate soufflé that is the substance of our lungs. Once the bronchi become very small, less than 1–2 mm in diameter, they are called, appropriately, "small airways," or medically speaking, bronchioles.

The tracheobronchial tree

The image of the system of bronchial tubes, beginning with the windpipe and then branching with each division into bronchi with sequentially narrower diameters, invokes the picture of a tree in winter, beginning with the trunk and dividing into smaller and smaller branches and then twigs; hence the name, the "tracheobronchial tree" (Fig. 1-2). The human tracheobronchial tree is no more an inanimate system of pipes than is a living oak tree. For one thing, lining the inner walls of the bronchial tubes are fine, microscopic hair-like structures, the cilia, that can beat in unison, sweeping mucus (and with it, inhaled dust particles or germs) back toward the throat and mouth, to be expectorated or swallowed.

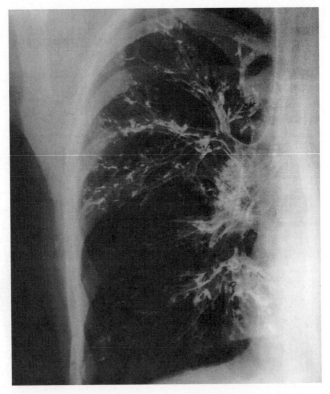

FIGURE 1-2   *In this radiograph the bronchi have been outlined with a radio-opaque oil, an old-fashioned radiographic technique (bronchography) that has been replaced by modern chest imaging using computed tomography (CT).*

For another, mucous glands line the walls of the bronchi, producing the mucus that coats their surface in a very thin layer.

Of particular interest for someone with asthma are the bands of muscle that are distributed in a rim around the bronchial tubes throughout their length, from windpipe to the smallest airways (Fig. 1-3). These muscles are involuntary muscles. Like the muscles that constrict the pupil of your eye in response to strong light or the muscles that move digested food through your intestines, they are not under your direct or voluntary control. Under normal circumstances, when these

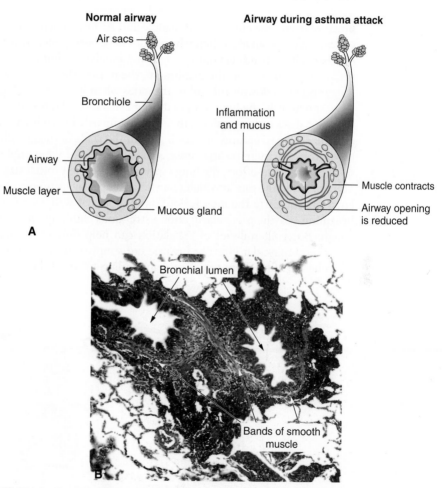

FIGURE 1-3   *Figure (a) depicts airway smooth muscle surrounding the lumen of a normal bronchus and contracting to constrict the airway during an asthmatic attack. Figure (b) depicts the histologic section from the lung of an individual who died of asthma, showing airway smooth muscle surrounding a narrowed small airway.*

muscles contract, the bronchial tubes that they surround narrow a little bit. Exactly what good this function—the ability to narrow temporarily a portion of our tracheobronchial tree—does for us is not entirely clear. Perhaps when one suffers localized lung disease, it can help redirect air to parts of the lung that need it most. In any case, there it is—a widespread system of involuntary muscle positioned in such a way that it can contract to narrow our air passageways somewhat, then relax again to allow them to open normally wide.

As you have already surmised, this brief description of the bronchial tubes brings us to the point where we are ready to consider asthma, a disorder in which generalized narrowing of the breathing tubes can cause difficulty in breathing. But before we proceed, let's take a moment to finish our discussion of how we breathe. To get the air to flow into our lungs through our airways, we need first to expand the chest. By so doing, we create a minor suction—a lower pressure inside the chest than outside—and air flows deep into the lungs and its air sacs, like into an accordion whose sides have been pulled apart. Many muscles contribute to expanding your chest during inhalation, but the most important— the strongest by far—is the diaphragm, the muscle that sits at the bottom of the lungs and pulls downward and to the sides when it contracts (Fig. 1-4).

And how do the lungs empty during exhalation? Here's the interesting part: when we are breathing quietly, they do so primarily by having your muscles relax and the elastic structures of your lungs (in the walls of those millions of air sacs) recoil back to their resting, unstretched position. Like a rubber band pulled open by muscular effort, the lungs spring back to their initial size when released. You can speed the rate at which your lungs empty by using your muscles of exhalation, particularly the muscles of your abdominal wall, as you might do when breathing heavily, particularly after a strenuous climb up a hillside or when you cough. But your muscles of exhalation can help only to a point; beyond that point extra muscular effort to breathe out simply squeezes down on the breathing tubes, causing them to collapse and failing to speed the flow of gas through

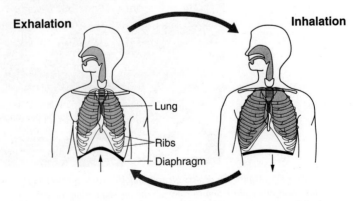

FIGURE 1-4 *Diaphragm contraction contributes importantly to expansion of the lungs and chest wall during inspiration.*

them. Normally, how fast we can breathe *in* is limited only by the capacity of our breathing muscles, whereas how fast we can breathe *out* is limited primarily by the elasticity of our lungs. We will return to these interesting observations about exhalation when we talk more of breathing tests in asthma (measuring how fast air can be exhaled from your lungs), about emphysema (a disease in which the ability to exhale is impaired because the lungs lose their normal elasticity), and about severe flare-ups of asthma (in which exhalation is so severely slowed that breathing *in* becomes difficult!).

MECHANISMS OF AIRWAY NARROWING IN ASTHMA

When asthma causes symptoms, it does so because of extensive narrowing of the bronchial tubes throughout both lungs. If you have asthma, you are likely very familiar with those symptoms: shortness of breath, wheezing, cough, and tightness in the chest. The extra work of breathing as we pull air through narrowed passageways causes us to feel breathless and uncomfortably tight across the chest ("like a too-tight elastic band bound around my chest," "like breathing with a 600-pound gorilla sitting on my chest," "like breathing through a way-too-small cocktail straw"). The whistling sounds that we call wheezing result when air passes through a narrow opening, setting up musical vibrations like the reed of a wind instrument. Bronchial tubes narrowed to a critical diameter generate this sound. Typically in asthma there are many different bronchial tubes—of differing lengths and thicknesses—reaching this critical diameter at the same time and making multiple overlapping musical notes simultaneously. We have had patients tell us that they thought that they heard the sounds of cats or birds somewhere close at hand, only to discover (when they held their breath) that the sounds had been coming from their own chest.

Cough develops in response to stimulation of nerve endings along the inside of the bronchial tubes. Sometimes cough can be helpful, such as when food goes down the wrong pipe and is aspirated into our trachea and bronchial tubes or when we have pneumonia with lots of thick, infected phlegm to be coughed from the lungs. At other times it is just an annoyance, a tiring irritation with no expectoration to show for it. In asthma cough can be some of both. Sometimes it helps to clear excess mucus from our airways, preventing the mucus from plugging up the breathing passages; at other times it is a frustrating, *dry* cough. One potential mechanism for the latter: chemicals released along the bronchial wall as part of the asthmatic reaction can trigger the nerve endings that stimulate a cough reflex. You have probably encountered people, both children and adults, who have been diagnosed with asthma only after months of persistent coughing or after having had a cough that would linger endlessly after every cold.

What causes the bronchi to narrow in asthma? There are two distinct mechanisms: contraction of the muscles that surround the breathing tubes and swelling of the walls of the bronchi themselves, with excess mucus filling up the passageways. Terms that we commonly use to describe the contraction of the (involuntary) bronchial muscles are *bronchospasm* and *bronchoconstriction*. "Inflammation" of the bronchial walls is the very broad term used to describe, among other things, the swelling of the bronchial walls, at times accompanied by stimulation of the mucous glands to produce excess mucus within the bronchial tubes. Sometimes one mechanism predominates, sometimes the other. Often both come into play at the same time. That there are two separate causes of airway narrowing in asthma—bronchial muscle constriction and inflammation—is a key teaching point. For people with asthma to understand their treatments, they need to know of these two different targets of our therapies.

KEY POINT Airway narrowing in asthma can be caused by bronchial muscle contraction, airway wall inflammation with mucus production, or by both mechanisms. These two different processes require different treatments.

Other than by the evidence of coughing up lots of phlegm, it is impossible to distinguish, based on how one feels, airway inflammation from bronchoconstriction. Although you may hear patients speak of feeling that their airways are "inflamed," in fact one cannot sense the inflammation of asthma. It does not cause the inside of one's chest to feel "raw" or like sunburned skin. In terms of the symptoms of cough, shortness of breath, chest tightness, and wheezing, airway narrowing is airway narrowing, regardless of the process that produced it. Besides, both processes often occur together.

Nonetheless, one distinguishing feature worth remembering is the time course over which these processes occur. Contraction of the bronchial muscles can occur over a period of *minutes*, and can likewise reverse (with relief of symptoms) over a similar time frame. Inflammation is a more complex process, involving infiltration of allergy cells into the bronchi, liquid (edema fluid) seeping into the bronchial walls, and stimulation of extra mucus production. It tends to evolve over *hours to days* and regresses, even with treatment, over a comparable period.

Many patients already have some experience with this distinction. Take a quick-acting bronchodilator like albuterol, and asthmatic symptoms begin to abate within 5 minutes. Take a powerful anti-inflammatory steroid like prednisone, and one may experience little or no improvement for several hours and perhaps not until a day or two later. Now, with the help of your explanation, your patients can understand why. We all have prior experience with muscles contracting and relaxing over minutes and with inflammation taking far longer to abate (think of a sunburn or the rash of poison ivy). Your patients can apply this experience to understand their asthma.

Experimental model: allergen challenge and the early and late asthmatic reactions

A clinical experiment that emphasizes the two aspects of airway narrowing in asthma (and that years ago significantly helped to advance our knowledge about the pathogenesis of asthma) is an allergen inhalation challenge in an allergic asthmatic patient. The experiment is quite simple. First, identify a patient with asthma (who now for the purpose of this experiment becomes a research subject) who is allergic to an inhaled allergen, such as dust mite. Then prepare a solution containing the dust mite allergen in it. Measure the subject's pulmonary function. Next have the subject inhale a small amount of an aerosol mist containing the dust mite allergen. Continue to measure the subject's lung function repeatedly over the next 12 hours. The experiment ends here (Fig. 1-5).

In many instances, inhalation of the allergen elicits what is called a "dual asthmatic response," illustrating the dual mechanisms of airway narrowing in asthma. Within minutes of inhaling the allergen, lung function (meaning here the ability to force air rapidly from the lungs during exhalation) decreases. Because it happens so quickly, one can surmise that the dust mite allergen triggered bronchial muscle contraction (bronchoconstriction). The subject likely experiences some chest tightness and cough, perhaps even some wheezing and breathlessness. Over the ensuing hour, without any treatment, the bronchial muscles relax and the breathing test results return to normal or at least close to normal.

But as one continues to observe the subject and monitor pulmonary function, a delayed response begins to emerge. Now some 4–5 hours after inhaling the dust mite allergen, asthmatic symptoms begin to return and lung function again declines. Often, this second episode of airway narrowing is more severe than the first, and it lasts longer. It too resolves spontaneously, but only after

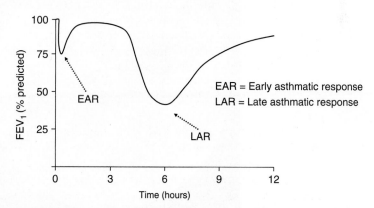

FIGURE 1-5 *Inhalation of allergen to which the subject is sensitive induces not only an immediate reaction, primarily due to bronchial smooth muscle constriction (early asthmatic response), but also a delayed—and often more severe—reaction primarily due to airway inflammation (late asthmatic response).*

several hours. This delayed asthmatic reaction involves not only bronchoconstriction but also, predominantly, airway inflammation. It cannot be made to go
away quickly with a bronchodilator. In fact, if one were to inspect the airways
with a bronchoscope during this period of inflammation, one could directly
visualize the swollen nature of the bronchial tubes and narrowed bronchial ori-
fices, an image of asthmatic inflammation of the airways seen with the naked eye
(macroscopic image) (Fig. 1-6).

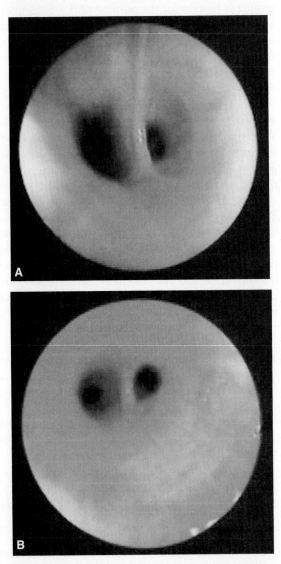

FIGURE 1-6   *Bronchoscopic view of bronchi before (a) and after (b) localized application of
allergen to the airways of an allergen-sensitive asthmatic patient. Modified from Lilly CM, et al.
Eotaxin expression after segmental allergen challenge in subjects with atopic asthma.* American
Journal of Respiratory and Critical Care Medicine 2001; 163:1669–75. *Official journal of the American
Thoracic Society. Copyright American Thoracic Society.*

We will return to other lessons learned from this model of allergic asthma later in this chapter.

KEY POINT   The dual asthmatic response to allergen consists of the "early asthmatic response" that is due to bronchoconstriction and the "late asthmatic response," caused primarily by airway inflammation.

THINGS THAT PROVOKE AIRWAY NARROWING IN ASTHMA

If you or a family member or friend have had asthma for any length of time, you can probably identify at least three or four things that can set off asthmatic symptoms. What comes to mind? Cigarette smoke, respiratory infections, exercising, dusting, stress? In some way, these stimuli can provoke bronchial muscle contraction and/or airway inflammation. We refer to them as "triggers," meaning things that can fire off an asthmatic reaction in your bronchial tubes.

Many asthmatic triggers are inhaled; they reach the bronchi directly via the air we breathe. Some of these inhaled stimuli are simply irritants, chemicals or particles that can cause cough or chest discomfort in anyone, but in a person with asthma provoke airway narrowing and difficulty in breathing. Smoke and air pollutants are examples of such irritants, and if the exposure is sufficiently intense, they function as triggers in all asthmatics. Other triggers are inhaled allergens that stimulate an asthmatic reaction only in those persons with a specific sensitivity to those particular allergens. An asthmatic person allergic to cat allergen will respond with asthmatic symptoms to inhaled cat allergen, but may have no reaction to inhaled dust mite allergen. Similarly, a person with dust mite allergy may develop asthmatic symptoms when dusting but have no reaction to cats, no matter how intense the exposure. Of course, people can have multiple allergies, but one's own pattern of allergies will differ from other people with asthma, who may have no allergies or their own set of allergies, different from one's own.

At this point, let's consider in more detail some of the specific triggers of asthma.

Allergens

Inhaled allergic triggers in asthma—*aeroallergens*—include animals, dust mite, mold, pollen, and cockroaches. The dander (that is, shed skin particles and hair), urine, and saliva of warm-blooded animals contain proteins to which we humans show allergic reactions. Particularly common are allergies to cats, dogs, horses, mice, hamsters, guinea pigs, and rabbits. Recently, latex used to make medical equipment, particularly rubber gloves, has become a potential aeroallergen, especially among healthcare workers. In Chap. 7, "Identifying Allergic Sensitivities and Promoting Allergen Avoidance," we will discuss specific allergens in far greater detail. Also, when we consider occupational asthma, we will make mention of other substances, inhaled in the workplace, that can come to function as allergens, triggering asthma.

Exercise

Exercise is a particularly interesting trigger of asthma. For many years it was noted that some forms of exercise are more likely to provoke asthmatic symptoms than others: swimming was noted to be a particularly good sport for someone with asthma; ice hockey or cross-country skiing especially challenging. But the reason for this distinction was not entirely clear. Joggers and runners with asthma provided a clue: they reported that they could exercise with few symptoms all summer long, but the same activity performed in the cold air of winter triggered symptoms of cough, wheeze, and shortness of breath, which made it impossible to continue running outdoors. Medical researchers confirmed this observation. Run on a treadmill while breathing warm and moist air and a subject with asthma would develop few if any symptoms. Repeat the exercise (same effort and same duration) while breathing cold and dry air and that person now experiences exercise-induced airway narrowing and the associated symptoms of asthma.

Two related experiments provided further insight into the mechanism by which exercise provokes airway narrowing in asthma. First, if a person with asthma sits quietly while breathing cold air, doing no exercise, then little or no reaction is evoked. Second, if a person with asthma breathes cold air rapidly and deeply for 4–5 minutes, doing no exercise other than the rapid breathing (using a special apparatus that prevents the light-headedness associated with hyperventilation by adding carbon dioxide into the inhaled air), airway narrowing results. In fact, if the rate and depth of breathing are the same as would occur while running on a treadmill, then the asthmatic response is the same, even though the subject was simply mimicking the heavy breathing of exercise but not exercising at all.

What can one conclude from these observations? The stimulus for exercise-induced bronchoconstriction is large volumes of air breathed deeply into the bronchial tubes: the more air and the colder and drier the inhaled air, the stronger the provocative stimulus. When large quantities of air are inhaled (such as during exercise), the lining of the bronchial tubes is called upon to give up heat and moisture to warm and humidify that air. You have probably noticed that even on a very cold day, the air that you exhale is warm and moist. When you breathe quietly, the nose, mouth, and pharynx can provide all the necessary heat and moisture to condition the inspired air. However, when you exercise, the air penetrates deep into the tracheobronchial tree before being warmed and humidified. In people with asthma, this process of cooling and drying the surface of the bronchial tubes provokes airway narrowing, primarily due to bronchial muscle contraction. Understanding this mechanism allows us to make sense of the differences observed when exercise is performed in a warmed swimming pool versus on an ice rink. As you can already anticipate, it also leads to certain strategies for minimizing exercise-induced asthmatic symptoms, as we will discuss later.

KEY POINT   The degree to which exercise provokes airway narrowing in asthma is directly related to how hard one breathes during the exercise and to the temperature and humidity of the air that is breathed.

Respiratory infections

Respiratory tract infections, particularly viral infections, are among the most potent triggers of asthmatic symptoms. Even in the age of broadly effective antibiotics (against bacteria), you've heard this familiar story: "It started as a head cold; everyone in my family had one. But they all got better (they don't have asthma). My cold settled right into my chest, and ever since I can't stop coughing or clear the wheezing and congestion from my chest." When people with severe asthmatic flare-ups, those who require emergency treatment or hospitalization because of difficulty in breathing, identify a specific trigger to their exacerbation, they most often point to a respiratory infection.

Stress

Stress and asthma have had a checkered history together. There was a time when asthma itself was mostly or wholly blamed on emotional stresses. "If you could only work out your relationship with your mother" (or sibling or spouse), it was held, you could get rid of your asthma (or ulcers, colitis, and low back pain). An important part of the treatment of asthmatic attacks as recently as the 1970s was to help calm the patient. In the emergency room asthmatic patients would be put in a quiet cubicle—with lights dimmed and curtain pulled—and would sometimes be given a sedative such as diazepam (Valium) to help quiet their anxiety. Now we know better. Anxiety is normal enough when you are struggling to breathe, when it feels as though you may no longer have the strength to take another breath in. And sedatives are risky in this setting, because of their side effect of suppressing the tendency to breathe deeply (depressing ventilatory drive and thereby potentially causing respiratory failure). If you want to help an asthmatic patient feel less anxious during an asthmatic attack, work quickly to restore his or her narrowed airways to normal and offer kind, reassuring words and your presence at the bedside while doing so.

Still, stress may be a trigger of asthma, if not its cause. We know from medical experiments that a stressful situation can provoke mild airway narrowing in asthmatic subjects, and pretreatment with medications can block that response. Certainly many people who have lived with asthma report that in their experiences, stress can set off their asthmatic symptoms. We know that the favorable feeling surrounding a placebo medication can improve lung function somewhat in people with asthma participating in a research study; it is equally plausible that negative feelings can have the opposite effect, although in both instances the impact is relatively minor.

Most recently, additional information about the relation of stress and asthma has emerged from studies that have examined the impact of maternal stress on a child's risk of developing asthma. Very powerful stressors, such as domestic abuse and witnessed physical violence, were assessed; and an increased likelihood of developing asthma was found in the children of mothers who had experienced the highest levels of stress. These observations do not demonstrate cause and effect—they do not prove that the mothers' stress *caused* their children's asthma—but they keep open the possibility of mind-body connections related to the etiology of asthma and further explore the curious relation between stress and asthma.

Not all asthma triggers wreak their havoc via inhalation. Stress is one example of an alternative pathway. In addition, some women report worsening asthmatic symptoms during the few days immediately before and at the onset of their menses. It is likely that hormonal fluctuations are the trigger, but exactly which hormonal change is the key is unknown, as too is the reason why only a minority of women is prone to perimenstrual worsening of asthma.

Medications

Asthmatic symptoms can also be brought on by ingestion of certain medications as well as food additives (for example, sulfites). There are two groups of medications to watch for. One group consists of beta blockers, especially those that are not selective for their heart actions (like the noncardioselective beta blockers propranolol [Inderal] and nadolol [Corgard]). Even the miniscule amounts of medication absorbed into the bloodstream after use of a nonselective beta-blocker eyedrop, such as timolol ophthalmic solution (Timoptic), can provoke an asthmatic attack. Virtually everyone with asthma is susceptible to the bronchoconstricting effects of beta blockers.

The other group of medications consists of aspirin and the nonsteroidal anti-inflammatory drugs (NSAIDs), such as ibuprofen (Motrin, Nuprin) and naproxen (Aleve, Naprosyn). In contrast to the universal sensitivity of asthmatics to nonselective beta blockers, only about 3–5% of adults with asthma will develop a flare-up of their asthma after taking aspirin or one of the NSAIDs. We will discuss more about this unique sensitivity to aspirin and NSAIDs in Chap. 3, "Medications Used to Treat Asthma."

Even less common than aspirin intolerance is sensitivity to sulfiting agents used as food preservatives. You may recall from years ago people experiencing symptoms of their asthma after eating food from the salad bar of a restaurant. Until they were banned from this use in 1986, sulfiting agents such as sulfite, bisulfite, and metabisulfite were commonly sprayed onto fruits and vegetables to keep them looking fresh. Sulfites are reducing agents, which means that they function as antioxidants and delay the withering or rotting of fresh produce. Sulfites are still used in the manufacture of some wines and beers, which may explain why some people with asthma report that drinking alcohol sometimes brings on their asthma. The exact mechanism whereby sulfites trigger asthma is uncertain. Some medical scientists have speculated that chemical reactions in the body form sulfur dioxide from ingested sulfites. Sulfur dioxide is a chemical irritant known capable of causing asthmatic reactions. They argue that enough sulfur dioxide can be released from the stomach to be inhaled, provoking airway narrowing. Sulfites are still used as preservatives in certain prepared foods, as listed in Table 1-1.

Key point   The two groups of medications that can trigger airway narrowing in people with asthma are: 1) beta blockers and 2) aspirin and nonsteroidal anti-inflammatory drugs.

T A B L E   1 - 1

SULFITE-CONTAINING FOODS

Cooked and Processed Foods
Dried and glacéed fruit
Maraschino cherries
Guacamole
Jams
Gravy
Dehydrated, precut, or peeled *fresh* potatoes
Molasses
Shrimp
Soup mixes
Beverages
Beer
Wine
Hard cider
Fruit and vegetable juices
Tea

Nontriggers of asthma

You can imagine how easy it is for people with asthma to form their own ideas about what sets off their symptoms. If it rains for 2 days in a row and you then start to have cough and wheezing, would you not be tempted to blame the weather as the cause of those symptoms? If you eat very hot, spicy food and that night wake with shortness of breath and chest tightness, it is very tempting to blame the hot peppers for your asthma flare-up. But as you know, temporal association is not cause and effect; the two events may be linked only by coincidence. Food allergies, for example, very rarely cause asthma. They can cause other very serious and potentially life-threatening reactions, such as anaphylaxis, but an isolated asthma attack (in the absence of a generalized allergic reaction throughout the body) very rarely occurs.

Many people with asthma describe difficulty in breathing in hot, muggy weather, but (in the absence of high levels of air pollution) heat and humidity do not trigger airway narrowing. They simply make one's breathing feel more labored. Angiotensin converting enzyme inhibitors, such as lisinopril (Zestril, Prinivil), enalapril (Vasotec), and many others, widely used to treat hypertension, heart disease, and diabetic renal dysfunction, can cause a persistent, highly annoying cough, but they do not provoke asthmatic airway narrowing. One other example of what is not an asthma trigger: monosodium glutamate (MSG) was once thought to cause some people to experience asthmatic symptoms. However, when medical researchers tested the effects of MSG in asthma using careful, double-blind scientific techniques (neither the researchers nor the asthmatic subjects knew at the time whether the food the subjects were asked to eat contained MSG or not), no effect on the airways could be found even among people who reported a sensitivity to MSG.

New triggers of asthma

In the end, we do well to keep an open mind when patients report to us about what sets off their asthma. Sometimes they are in error; sometimes we (trained healthcare professionals) are ignorant of the truths of their observations. For instance, the cockroach was not known to be a powerful allergenic trigger for asthma until the 1960s. Before then, if someone had reported that their asthma had been made worse by a cockroach infestation of their apartment, we might well have greeted their presumption with deep skepticism. And what should we make of office workers with asthma who report cough and chest tightness every time they spend time in the copy room, where old photocopy machines run continually in a small, poorly ventilated space? Do they encounter a real or imagined asthmatic trigger there? Only after some careful scientific sleuthing did it become clear that high concentrations of ozone released from photocopy machines can accumulate in such a setting, provoking airway narrowing in susceptible workers (those with asthma). Because with pulmonary function tests we can measure the presence or absence of airway narrowing, we have the ability to test our (and our patients') hypotheses about asthmatic triggers and determine the truth.

TWITCHY AIRWAYS: THE CONCEPT OF BRONCHIAL HYPERRESPONSIVENESS

Asthmatic symptoms come and go. One day you are running 5 miles for your daily exercise, the next day, following exposure to one of your asthmatic triggers, you are struggling to catch your breath walking from room to room. With treatment, your asthmatic attack resolves, your normal breathing is restored, and within a few hours to days you are again able to pursue your usual physical activities without limitation.

A common misconception is that when a person with asthma is feeling well, free of asthmatic symptoms, his asthma has gone away. It is an easy mistake to make. After a difficult winter of frequent chest colds and lots of asthmatic symptoms, your child is finally breathing comfortably again. You are tempted to believe (wishfully) that his or her asthma has disappeared. But in all likelihood, given recurrent exposure to the appropriate trigger, symptoms will recur. The manifestations of asthma—its symptoms of cough, chest congestion, wheezing, and shortness of breath—come and go, but the underlying tendency of the bronchial tubes to narrow in response to certain stimuli remains. Asthmatic symptoms are intermittent and recurrent; sensitivity of the bronchial tubes to asthmatic triggers is chronic. Asthma is a persistent sensitivity of the bronchial tubes—present all day, every day—that manifests as reversible airway narrowing.

This is a critical concept that needs to be communicated to patients with asthma and to their families. It influences not only how we view asthma, but also what makes sense in terms of its treatment. If you were to believe that your asthma went away when you were free of symptoms, you would not consider taking medications except when you had symptoms, just as you wouldn't take an over-the-counter cold remedy except when you had a cold. But if you acknowledge that the vulnerability of your bronchial tubes persists even when you feel well, you are in a better position to understand the need in many cases to take medications on a daily basis to prevent symptoms.

The medical term for this persistent sensitivity of the bronchial tubes to asthmatic triggers, and their tendency to respond abnormally to these triggers with excessive narrowing, is "bronchial hyperresponsiveness." In response to a variety of stimuli, the bronchi narrow too easily and too much. Exposed to the same stimuli, normal airways—the airways of people without asthma—react by narrowing minimally if at all. Asthmatic airways can be described as "twitchy"; they are too readily stimulated to react, and they react (narrow) too much.

KEY POINT   Bronchial hyperresponsiveness or twitchiness of the airways is always present in asthma, even when symptoms are not.

Bronchial challenge test

Bronchial hyperresponsiveness is a fundamental property of asthma. It is easy to demonstrate this tendency in a pulmonary function laboratory. Even when feeling perfectly well, even when lung function is 100% normal, a person with the "twitchy airways" of asthma will react within minutes to an appropriate stimulus (carefully administered in incremental doses to ensure safety) with significant airway narrowing and typical symptoms of asthma. This test, called a bronchoprovocative challenge (or bronchial challenge test), is sometimes used to rule in (or rule out) a diagnosis of asthma. We will review it in greater detail in the next chapter, "Diagnosing and Staging the Severity of Asthma."

The bronchoprovocative challenge teaches us another important lesson about asthma. The degree of bronchial hyperresponsiveness varies from one asthmatic person to another and can vary over time in one person. Some people with asthma have very twitchy airways; they react to even a small dose of a provocative stimulus with profound airway narrowing. Other people with asthma have only mildly twitchy airways; they respond only to a large dose of the same provocative stimulus and even then only with slight airway narrowing. So too, in any given person with asthma, the twitchiness of their airways can vary. For example, it can intensify during their allergy season, then lessen out of allergy season. It can increase when a new kitten is brought home, then decrease again when another home is found for the cat. We will return to this subject of the variability of bronchial hyperresponsiveness when we discuss the treatment of asthma, because some treatments are designed to lessen the twitchiness of asthmatic airways. In a sense, they are designed to make asthmatic airways less asthmatic.

"Outgrowing" asthma

"But isn't it true," you are asked, "that asthma can sometimes just go away? Don't people sometimes outgrow their asthma?" The answer is "yes." As many as 30–50% of children with asthma, especially those with mild asthma, will have their asthma disappear before adulthood. Typically, when children outgrow their asthma, their symptoms abate in early adolescence, often around the time of puberty. For unknown reasons, they lose their bronchial hyperresponsiveness and never again experience symptoms of asthma.

In some cases, however, asthmatic symptoms resolve in late childhood only to recur in early adulthood. We frequently encounter young adults with asthma who report having been symptom-free for 5–10 years or more, only to experience a recurrence of their asthma in their 20s or 30s. Still other adults are newly diagnosed with asthma, but in retrospect can identify symptoms of asthma in their childhood—a lingering cough all winter, cough and wheezing when playing outside in cold weather—that were never diagnosed as such. For these adults with asthma, it is likely that their bronchial hyperresponsiveness lessened in late childhood and now has worsened again as an adult. Their underlying asthmatic tendency probably never fully went away.

Adults with asthma rarely experience a remission of their disease. More than 90% of the time, adults with asthma can expect to live their entire lives with twitchy airways and the vulnerability of those airways to develop abnormal narrowing.

WHAT CAUSES AIRWAYS TO BECOME TWITCHY?

A fair question and one that has likely occurred to you already is the following: Why in people with asthma do the bronchial tubes react to asthmatic triggers in the way that they do, when the very same stimuli have no effect on the airways of someone without asthma? For those without asthma, exercise, stress, beta blockers, and cat dander, for example, are totally harmless when it comes to our breathing. What is it that makes asthmatic airways respond abnormally to some or all of these triggers? What causes bronchial hyperresponsiveness? What perpetuates the twitchiness of asthmatic airways even when breathing is normal and one feels fine?

The easiest, most truthful, and least satisfying answer is that we don't exactly know. Some evidence points to abnormal growth and behavior of the bronchial muscles that surround the bronchial tubes; lots of evidence documents a role for inflammation in the walls of the bronchi; and these two mechanisms are potentially related (inflammation of a certain type can foster increased growth of the bronchial muscles). Still other possibilities exist, such as an imbalance of nervous system input to the bronchi, favoring a tendency toward contraction of bronchial muscles over their relaxation.

Lack of a definitive answer does not mean that we do not already know a great deal about the disease of the bronchial tubes that we recognize as asthma. For many decades we have known what the bronchial tubes look like in fatal asthma. Autopsy specimens from people who died with overwhelmingly severe asthmatic attacks provided this information about asthma at one extreme of severity. In most instances, what was found was severe inflammation of the walls of the bronchi and bronchioles throughout both lungs, characterized by edema, infiltration by inflammatory cells (especially the allergy cells, eosinophils), and excess mucus production. Often gelatinous mucus would fill most of the airways, totally blocking the path for air to flow. The bronchial muscles were larger and more plentiful than normal, but their role in the fatal episode was hard to discern (because muscle contraction releases in death).

Chronic low-grade airway inflammation

It was only approximately 20 years ago that direct observations began to be made about the condition of the bronchial tubes at the other extreme of asthma. With these groundbreaking studies, researchers discovered that it is safe to perform bronchoscopy in people with asthma who are feeling well and have normal or near normal lung function. What do the bronchi look like when a person with asthma feels well, has normal lung function, and perhaps is even able to compete in the

Olympics or professional sports? Can a clue be found there as to what causes the abnormal behavior of bronchial tubes in asthma, what perpetuates bronchial hyperresponsiveness in the absence of any signs or symptoms of asthma? The answer, as it turned out, is a resounding "yes." Bronchoscopic biopsies of the airway walls provided remarkable insight into asthma as a *chronic* disorder, with demonstrable abnormalities of the bronchi even when one feels entirely well.

To a large extent, these abnormalities are of the same sort as found in autopsy studies of fatal asthma, just far milder. The bronchi of someone with asthma do not become normal when that person feels normal and has normal breathing capacity. They continue to exhibit some degree of persistent inflammation, and that inflammation—different from that seen in a long-term cigarette smoker (chronic bronchitis) and different from what occurs in a lower respiratory tract infection (acute bronchitis)—has the appearance that we associate with allergic reactions. A persistent, allergic-type inflammation of the bronchi lingers in the airways. Almost certainly, this chronic, allergic-type inflammation contributes importantly to the always-present twitchiness of the airways.

KEY POINT   Some allergic-type inflammation exists in the airways of people with asthma at all times, even when they are free of symptoms. This chronic inflammation of the airways contributes to the twitchiness of asthmatic airways, even when it isn't sufficiently severe to cause airway narrowing and related symptoms.

Before proceeding with more details about this unique bronchial inflammation that is asthma, we need to make an important distinction. We have used the term "inflammation" to describe one of the ways that the airways can narrow (swollen, mucus-filled tubes), and now we are using the same term to describe the abnormalities in the bronchial walls that contribute to bronchial hyperresponsiveness, even in the absence of airway narrowing. The term "inflammation" is applicable in both circumstances, and to a great extent the difference is one of degree. A very mild degree of inflammation exists in the bronchial tubes of asthmatics at all times, without causing any symptoms or airway narrowing. When that swelling intensifies, it can reach the point that the passageway for air within the bronchi (bronchial lumen) is reduced in diameter, causing impaired breathing.

Still, as we use the term "inflammation" in conversation with our patients, the potential for confusion is high. When our patients are having an asthma attack, we discourage them from relying on treatment with a bronchodilator only. We tell them that they need also to treat the inflammatory portion of their disease, usually with anti-inflammatory steroids, not just treat the bronchial muscle constriction. At the same time, we may tell our patient with frequently recurrent asthmatic symptoms who is currently feeling perfectly fine that he or she should use an anti-inflammatory medication (for instance, an inhaled steroid) every day in order to suppress asthmatic inflammation and prevent asthmatic symptoms and asthmatic attacks. Yes, even though you are feeling well, your bronchial tubes remain inflamed and twitchy, making you vulnerable to recurrent symptoms were your airways to narrow again.

Perhaps we have to remind ourselves, too, that the high-school athlete with asthma, who only needs his or her bronchodilator prior to work-outs and competitions and who has been diagnosed with "exercise-induced asthma," has this same allergic-type inflammation present in his or her bronchi. This chronic inflammation of the airways is present all the time in everyone with asthma. Only sometimes does it flare up to the point that it causes airway narrowing, together with cough, chest congestion, and shortness of breath that do not go away with bronchodilator treatment only.

It might be better—for the sake of clarity—if we had two expressions to describe the inflammation of the bronchial tubes: one that referred to the "minimal," "baseline," or "essential" inflammation that is found at all times in asthma; another that described the "excess," "flared-up," or "constrictive" inflammation that can be part of the airway narrowing that causes the symptoms of asthma. For the time being, we have no such distinction in our medical vocabularies. We can only try to be clear in our thinking and in our explanations to our patients.

Linking airway inflammation to bronchial hyperresponsiveness

Recall our experiment in which we gave an asthmatic subject an allergen to inhale, one to which we knew him to be allergic. He experienced, as some people with asthma do, both early and late asthmatic reactions. (In this experimental circumstance, some subjects with asthma will have only an early reaction and others only a late response; our subject experienced a "dual response.") The early asthmatic reaction was due to bronchial muscle contraction and the late asthmatic reaction due to both muscle constriction and an acute increase in the inflammatory swelling in the walls of the bronchial tubes. Here's an interesting observation about the late (inflammatory) asthmatic reaction; it is accompanied by an increase in twitchiness of the airways. On the other hand, those subjects who react to the inhaled allergen with only an early asthmatic reaction do not experience a transient increase in bronchial reactivity. So here is an experiment— one of many different types of investigations on this topic—that points to the role of allergic-type inflammation of the airways in causing, or at least enhancing, the property of twitchy airways in asthma.

There is also an important practical lesson for our patients that can be learned from this experiment. It turns out that the heightened bronchial reactivity that occurs after allergen-induced late asthmatic reactions can last for up to several days. So the cat-allergic patient with asthma gets a "double whammy" after spending the night with the pet cat curled up on the pillow next to him. Not only does he awake the next morning with cough, wheezing, and some labored breathing, but for a time he will become more sensitive to any and all of his asthmatic triggers. During this period of increased twitchiness of his airways, he will find himself more sensitive to second-hand smoke, to the exercise-induced effects on his breathing of snow-shoveling, and to his other allergic triggers, like mold exposure.

Some triggers of asthma, such as exercise, do not provoke significant airway inflammation and therefore do not induce a period of heightened bronchial responsiveness (when the twitchiness of the airways increases above its usual amount). Other triggers, such as allergens and viral respiratory tract infections, are capable of inciting this type of inflammation and its associated shift in the sensitivity of the airways. These latter are both *triggers* of asthmatic symptoms and *inciters* of worsened asthmatic inflammation—and worse asthma control. As we shall see, the inciters of asthmatic inflammation may play a role in the initial development of asthma in genetically predisposed individuals.

KEY POINT Allergens and viral respiratory tract infections can incite airway inflammation that is associated with a period, lasting up to several days, of heightened bronchial hyperresponsiveness.

A CLOSER LOOK AT ALLERGIC-TYPE INFLAMMATION OF THE BRONCHIAL TUBES

Although our patients probably do not need to know all of the details about the cellular and molecular constituents of inflamed airways in asthma in order to deal effectively with their illness, you probably want to learn some more about them. Here are a couple of good reasons to probe deeper into this topic (and to continue reading this chapter!). (1) As you talk to your patients about medications used to treat asthma, you may have occasion to speak with them about leukotriene blockers (such as Singulair and Accolate) and anti-IgE antibody therapy (Xolair). It would be helpful if you understood and could explain what leukotrienes and IgE antibodies are and what role they play in asthma. (2) If you plan to take the asthma educators' certification examination of the National Asthma Educators Certification Board, you may be asked questions on this topic. So please read on.

If you have ever seen a person with hives or observed a person with hay fever in their allergy season, tissues in hand, with red, watery eyes and drippy nose, you have witnessed the manifestations of allergic-type inflammation firsthand. Imagine that you could examine this reaction more closely, using a microscope to inspect the skin in a person with hives, or the lining of the eyes (conjunctivae) and mucous membranes of the nose in a person with hay fever (more properly called, seasonal allergic rhinitis and conjunctivitis). You would see the following shared features: swollen blood vessels, edema fluid leaked from those blood vessels into the surrounding tissues, and an accumulation in those tissues of inflammatory cells of a particular kind, specifically lymphocytes, eosinophils, and mast cells. All of these findings pertain to the bronchial tubes of someone with asthma, whether or not they have known allergies, whether or not they have been diagnosed with allergic asthma. The same blood vessel dilation, edema fluid formation, and cellular infiltration occur within the walls of the bronchial tubes throughout the tracheobronchial tree.

Lymphocytes

Lymphocytes are a type of white blood cell that are formed in the bone marrow, circulate through the blood, and migrate in and out of various organs throughout the body. They are the "masters and commanders" of the immune system, playing a crucial role in regulating our immune responses to the world around us. You may know that there are different types of lymphocytes in the body, functioning in different ways. When one characterizes the lymphocytes in the bronchial tubes of a person with asthma (or in the skin of a person with hives or nasal passageways of someone with hay fever), one finds predominantly the type of thymus-derived or T lymphocyte called helper T lymphocytes, and specifically the type-2 helper-type T lymphocytes. Scientists can distinguish types of lymphocytes from one another based on the molecules found on their cell surfaces and by the chemicals that they produce.

So already we can see that the inflammation found in the bronchial tubes of someone with asthma looks different under the microscope from the inflammation found, for example, in someone who has smoked a pack of cigarettes each day for 30 years. In the cigarette smoker, instead of eosinophils and mast cells, we find predominantly neutrophils and macrophages in the airways, along with different types of lymphocytes. The type of inflammation found in the airways of persons with asthma is unique to asthma and different from other inflammatory diseases involving the airways and lungs. It looks similar, however, to the pattern of allergic reactions found in other parts of the body. And it looks generally the same in all people with asthma, whether they are thought to have allergic or nonallergic asthma.

Lymphocytes are great communicators. They send chemical signals to other cells, regulating their behavior. These cell-to-cell chemical signals are called cytokines, and lymphocytes of the sort found in asthmatic airways, type-2 helper T lymphocytes, make a distinctive group of cytokines, different from those manufactured by other types of lymphocytes. An important group of these cytokines bears the name interleukins (meaning "between leukocytes" or white blood cells).

You now have the vocabulary to begin to dissect the fascinating process by which the human body makes allergic reactions. Imagine that you are programmed by your genes to make allergic reactions to dust mites. When you breathe in the dust mite allergen, the type-2 helper T lymphocytes in your bronchial tubes send out the word, using the chemical signal interleukin 4, instructing other lymphocytes—specifically, the antibody-producing lymphocytes called B-lymphocytes—to start manufacturing antibodies that will recognize and bind the dust mite allergen. (This reaction would make good sense were the dust mite allergen a harmful microbe to be fought off by the immune system; in allergy it is an immune system mistake, in that the allergen is a harmless piece of protein.)

Immunoglobulin E (IgE antibody)

The B lymphocytes obey this signal and synthesize a particular kind of antibody to "fight off" this dust mite allergen, called an immunoglobulin E or IgE antibody. These newly formed, specially designed IgE molecules will at one end be able to bind only dust mite allergens. At their other end, like all IgE antibodies, they have a site along their surface that specifically recognizes and binds to their docking station, the IgE receptor molecule. In fact there are a number of different types of IgE receptors found on a variety of cells, but the receptors with the greatest *stickiness* for the IgE antibodies, called the high-affinity IgE receptors, are found primarily on mast cells.

KEY POINT   People with allergies make IgE antibodies directed at specific allergens. The IgE antibodies attach to the surface of mast cells like sentinels, awaiting the next encounter with these allergens.

Mast cells

So now, enter the mast cell. Mast cells are found wherever allergic diseases of this sort (atopic diseases such as hay fever, eczema, or hives) take place. In asthma, mast cells are found in the walls of the bronchi and also along their inner surfaces, perfectly situated to greet any allergens that may be inhaled. Because the outside cell wall of mast cells is rich in the high-affinity IgE receptors, our IgE antibody formed to recognize dust mite allergen has bound to the outside surface of the mast cell. There it sits, a sentinel on guard for the next exposure to dust mite allergen.

And as you shuffle along the carpeting of your bedroom and collapse onto the mattress of your bed, you release into the air a fresh supply of this allergen. You breathe it into your lungs, and along the surface of your bronchi the IgE molecules, adherent to the surface of mast cells, bind the allergen that comes near them. For the mast cell, the reaction between allergen and antibody on its surface is a powerful signal, and within minutes a dramatic response takes place. The mast cell, filled with packets of inflammatory chemicals, releases these chemicals into the surrounding cellular environment of the bronchial wall. It is a remarkable and rapid explosion of the mast cell in response to this allergic trigger (Fig. 1-7). If you want to see it in action, watch the skin of an allergic patient when a skin test is performed. The skin test puts a small amount of antigen superficially into the surface of the skin. The hive and surrounding erythema (wheal and flare) that develops within a few minutes is the expression of this process we have just described: antigen-IgE antibody interaction and mast cell release of potent inflammatory chemicals into the skin.

Chemical mediators of inflammation

You already know the names of some of these inflammatory chemicals made by mast cells: histamine is one, the leukotrienes are another; and there are many others. They are called the "mediators" of allergic inflammation. They cause small blood

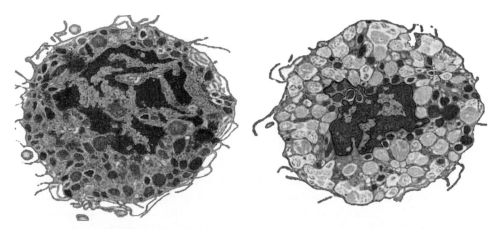

FIGURE 1-7   *Upon activation of mast cells, chemical mediators important in the allergic response are released into the surrounding cellular tissues. This figure depicts a mast cell before (left) and after (right) activation.*

vessels to dilate and leak edema fluid; they cause bronchial muscles to constrict; they stimulate mucous glands along the bronchial tubes to make more mucus; and they stimulate nerve endings along the airways, triggering cough. You can see how they bring about (or mediate) many of the features of an asthmatic reaction.

The chemical signals released by type-2 helper T lymphocytes and the chemical mediators released by mast cells have another important effect. They summon reinforcements for this battle against the allergens. In particular, they are powerful attractants for the white blood cells called eosinophils. Eosinophils are drawn out of the bloodstream and into the site of the allergic reaction (here, the bronchial tubes) by these chemical signals (including interleukins 4, 5, and 13 made by type-2 helper T lymphocytes and leukotrienes and eotaxin made by mast cells). Like mast cells, eosinophils contain packets (granules) within their cytoplasm, each loaded with inflammatory chemicals. (The proteins in these granules take up the stain called eosin used when studying tissue under the microscope, turning the granules bright red and lending the cells their name, meaning eosin lovers!)

Eosinophils

Eosinophils are found wherever there is an allergic disease of this (atopic) type, and they are present throughout the bronchial tubes of persons with asthma. They are effective fighters of disease-causing parasites, like the worms called strongyloides and ascaris, but it remains somewhat a matter of debate as to what their role is in allergic reactions to harmless allergens. Still, their potential for causing more damage is striking. Like mast cells, they make chemical mediators of inflammation, like the leukotrienes. They also make many other chemicals, including some enzymes with the potential to injure the lining cells of the bronchial tubes, a characteristic finding in asthma. In some studies of asthma, the greater the number of eosinophils found in the bronchial tubes (via bronchoscopy), the more severe the symptoms of asthma. One recent series of investigations has suggested that we should monitor the concentration of eosinophils in induced sputum from our patients with asthma to assess how well we are controlling airway inflammation with our anti-inflammatory medications.

You have now met many of the important players needed to understand the basic mechanisms of allergy and asthma. You are equipped to read more about the science of asthma and to consider novel treatments for asthma, like the medication designed to remove IgE antibodies from the blood of people with allergic asthma (called omalizumab or Xolair). You can also help your patients understand that there are different types of allergies. We use the term *atopic diseases* to describe allergic reactions involving IgE antibodies, mast cells, and eosinophils, as just described. Atopy is the inherited tendency to make these types of allergic reactions. Other allergies, like medication allergy (for example, to penicillin) may not involve IgE antibodies, are unrelated to this group of allergic diseases, and are no more common in someone with asthma than in someone without asthma.

There is one additional concept that we wish to discuss before leaving the subject of allergic-type inflammation of the bronchial tubes. It is a *hot topic* in recent asthma literature—airway remodeling.

Permanent structural changes in the airway wall ("airway remodeling")

Remember that the inflammation of the bronchial tubes is chronic; it is present to some degree day-in and day-out, week after week and year after year. You might wonder whether this persistent inflammatory reaction ever leads to scarring—as happens with different types of inflammation in other parts of the body. Is it possible that the bronchial tubes might become permanently narrowed after years of unchecked allergic-type inflammation of the airways? The answer is "yes, occasionally."

Perhaps you know someone with long-standing asthma who has impaired lung function, even at his or her best, when feeling well and free of asthmatic symptoms. Such a patient is, fortunately, the exception rather than the rule. Most people with asthma continue to have normal lung function when at their best. A minority—and we can't be any more precise as to exactly what percent of patients—develops irreversible narrowing in their bronchial tubes, mimicking the problem in the cigarette-smoking related chronic obstructive lung diseases, chronic bronchitis and emphysema.

KEY POINT   Sometimes people with asthma develop airway narrowing that is permanent and irreversible. It is as if they had developed chronic obstructive pulmonary disease (COPD) without ever having smoked cigarettes.

Airway remodeling refers to the permanent structural changes in the bronchi that accompany and presumably result from long-standing allergic-type inflammation. A superficial cut of the skin typically heals without a trace. A deep wound heals with deposition of dense bands of fibrous tissue, made up of collagen fibers, the substance of scars. And as you know, scars last forever. In the airways, we find collagen fibers being deposited beneath the lining (epithelial) cells, in what used to be referred to during microscopic inspection of asthmatic bronchi as "thickened basement membrane." This area of collagen deposition is universal in asthma, but perhaps in some people it progresses, forming circumferential bands of fibrous tissue within the walls of the bronchi. It is likely that scar tissue of this sort is part of the airway remodeling that takes place in some people with asthma, permanently altering the architecture of the airway walls and restricting the diameter of the bronchi.

At what age does airway remodeling most often take place, in whom is it mostly likely to occur, and how can it be prevented are important but unanswered questions at the forefront of the science of asthma. Many scientists believe that the early institution of effective anti-inflammatory therapy may prevent airway remodeling (and the associated loss of lung function over time), but the jury is still out on this hypothesis.

AN EXPANDED DEFINITION OF ASTHMA

With this brief discussion of airway remodeling, we have in place all the elements for a comprehensive definition of asthma. Here is one such definition, modified from the National Asthma Education and Prevention Program (1997):

> *Asthma is a chronic inflammatory disorder of the airways in which many cells and cellular elements play a role. In susceptible individuals, this inflammation causes recurrent episodes of wheezing, breathlessness, chest tightness, and cough. These episodes are associated with widespread but variable airway narrowing that is often reversible either spontaneously or with treatment. Inflammation also causes an associated increase in the existing bronchial hyperresponsiveness to a variety of stimuli. In some patients with asthma, reversibility of airway narrowing may be incomplete.*

All the key features of asthma, with which you are now familiar, are included in this definition: reversible airways obstruction (bronchoconstriction), airway inflammation, twitchy airways (bronchial hyperresponsiveness), and the possibility of airway remodeling with permanent airway narrowing.

WHAT CAUSES ASTHMA?

It is likely that someday the definition of asthma will include information about the specific genes that cause or predispose to asthma. There will be not one gene but several genes, whose interaction—under the right environmental circumstances—leads to the development of asthma. These genes will likely be closely linked to and overlap with the genes that cause other atopic diseases, like hay fever, atopic dermatitis (eczema), hives, and food allergies. In research laboratories all across the world, the hunt is on for the asthma genes. We know that a tendency to develop asthma is inherited. If one parent, particularly your mother, has asthma, you are more likely to develop asthma than if neither parent had asthma. If both parents have asthma, your risk of developing asthma increases further. Still, we know that even an exact duplicate set of genes (as in identical twins) does not guarantee that both people will develop asthma. Some set of encounters in our environment—possibly allergens, viruses, bacterial proteins, or other yet-to-be-identified precipitants—is required for asthma to develop in a genetically predisposed individual.

Occupational asthma: a model for the etiology of asthma

Asthma that develops in the workplace (occupational asthma) is a good model with which to consider this interplay of genes and environment. Here's a typical scenario. A 45-year-old woman without any history of asthma begins to work in a crab-processing factory. After several months on the job, she notes that towards the end of the workweek, she develops a cough and chest tightness that resolve during her weekends away from work. Pretty soon her symptoms begin to bother her throughout the week at work and include wheezing and some shortness of breath. She finds that she now has difficulty jogging, particularly in cold weather, because it brings on cough and wheezing. Before long, her symptoms are present weekdays and weekends alike. She has become sensitive to second-hand smoke and strong perfumes; viral infections quickly settle in her chest, causing severe wheezing and difficulty breathing. In brief, she has developed asthma. Repetitive exposure to allergens released into the air as part of crab processing caused allergic sensitization of her airways, mediated by type-2 helper T lymphocytes, IgE antibodies, mast cells, and eosinophils. Not only did she become allergic to inhaled crab antigen, but as a consequence of the resultant allergic-type inflammation in her airways, she developed nonspecific bronchial hyperresponsiveness or twitchy airways to multiple different stimuli.

If diagnosed early enough, her occupational asthma may go away when she stops working at the crab-processing plant. However, at some point the airway inflammation can become self-sustaining, and her asthma may persist despite never again inhaling crab antigen. In some studies, as many as half of the people who develop occupational asthma continue to have asthma even after they leave their workplace environments.

KEY POINT Some people with occupational asthma continue to have asthma even in the absence of further exposure to the sensitizing substance that caused their disease in the first place. Their airway inflammation becomes self-perpetuating and their asthma permanent.

Despite apparently identical antigenic exposure for the same length of time or even longer, most of her coworkers do not develop occupational asthma. It seems likely that something about her genetic make-up predisposed her but not the others to make this unique immune response to her environment that we recognize as asthma.

In this example, and other examples of occupational asthma, it is a specific sensitizing substance released into the air at the workplace that incites the asthmatic immune response. More than 250 such chemicals have been identified, with new ones added to the list each year (Table 1-2). But what if one substitutes a 3-year-old child instead of an employee, what if the environmental exposure occurs in the home rather than the workplace, and what if the sensitizing agent is not crab antigen but house dust mites? Might not the mechanism for the development of asthma be identical? Repetitive exposure to an appropriate allergen in a genetically susceptible individual over time leads to self-sustaining airway inflammation, which manifests as asthma.

One long-term follow-up study of children at risk for allergic reactions has lent credence to this proposed explanation for why some people develop asthma. Children with at least one atopic parent were entered into this study. Investigators measured the concentration of dust mite antigen in the homes (and specifically, in the bedrooms) of these children when they were one year old. They then kept track of these families and reported how many of the children went on to develop asthma at age 11. They found a direct correlation between the likelihood of developing asthma in adolescence and the amount of dust mite antigen exposure at age 1. Sensitization to allergens followed by continued intense exposure to those same allergens—in someone with an inherited predisposition—seems to be at least one prescription for the development of asthma.

THE EPIDEMIOLOGY OF ASTHMA IN AMERICA

It is estimated that approximately 16 million Americans have asthma, 5.5% of the population. Asthma is the most common chronic illness of childhood, affecting an estimated 3.7 million children under the age of 15. If you ask Americans, have they or their children had an episode or attack of asthma within the last 12 months, approximately 14 million say yes. If the question is phrased, have you ever in your lives been given a medical diagnosis of asthma, the number swells to 28 million who respond affirmatively. These numbers are enormous, and they translate into huge impacts on individuals and their families, as well as tremendous societal costs: an average of 4 days per asthmatic child missed from school each year and 2.5 days per adult missed from work; 11 million outpatient medical visits; 2 million emergency room visits; nearly 500,000 hospitalizations for asthma; and approximately 5000 deaths annually (Fig. 1-8).

These numbers paint a portrait of asthma in America with broad strokes, like a photo taken from an airplane at 35,000 feet altitude. They capture the enormity of the problem, but not its toll on individuals and their families—including quite possibly, you or a family member or close friend. It is often

TABLE 1-2

SELECTED CAUSES OF OCCUPATIONAL ASTHMA[*]

High Molecular Weight Compounds		AGENTS	OCCUPATIONS

AGENTS	*OCCUPATIONS*	ANHYDRIDES:
		Phthallic anhydrates
		Trimellitic
		  anhydrates
			*Epoxy resin and
			  plastics workers*

ANIMAL PRODUCTS: Dander, Excreta Serum, Secretions	*Animal handlers Laboratory workers Veterinarians*	WOOD DUST: Oak Mahogany California redwood Western red cedar	*Carpenters Sawmill workers Furniture makers*

PLANTS:
Grain
Tea
Flour
Tobacco
Hops
Dust
	*Grain handlers
	Tea workers
	Bakers
	Natural oil manu-
	  facturing workers
	Tobacco and food
	processing workers
	Healthcare workers*
		METALS:
		Platinum
		Nickel
		Chromium
		Cobalt
		Vanadium
		Tungsten carbide
			*Platinum- and
			  nickel-refining
			  workers
			Hard-metal workers*

ENZYMES: *B. subtilis* Pancreatic extracts Papain Trypsin Fungal amylase	*Bakers Detergent, pharma- ceutical, and plastic industry workers*	SOLDERING FLUXES	*Solderers*

VEGETABLE:
Gum acacia
Gum tragacanth
	*Printers
	Gum manufacturing
	  workers*
		DRUGS:
		Penicillin
		Methyldopa
		Tetracyclines
		Cephalosporins
		Psyllium
			*Pharmaceutical and
			  healthcare industry
			  workers*

OTHER:
Crab, Prawn
	*Crab and prawn
	  processors*
		OTHER ORGANIC
		CHEMICALS:
		Urea formaldehyde
		Dyes, Formalin
		Azodicarbonamide
		Hexachloroethylene
		  diamine
		Dimethyl
		  ethanolamine
		
		Polyvinyl chloride
		  pyrolysates
			*Chemical, plastic,
			  and rubber industry
			  workers
			Hospital workers
			Laboratory workers
			Foam insulation
			  manufacturing
			  workers
			Food wrapping
			  workers
			Spray painter*

Low Molecular Weight Compounds			

DIISOCYANATES:
 	
Toluene diiso-
  cyanate (TDI)
Methylene
  diphenyl diiso-
  cyanate (MDI)
	*Polyurethane industry
	  workers
	Plastics workers
	Workers using varnish
	Foundry workers*		

[*]Mechanism believed to be IgE-mediated for high molecular weight compounds and for some low molecular weight compounds. The immunologic mechanism for many low molecular weight substances remains undefined. Adapted from: Chan-Yeung M, et al. *Am Rev Respir Dis* 1986; 133:686.

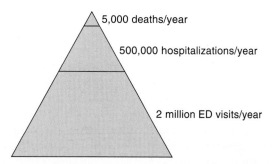

FIGURE 1-8   *Asthmatic deaths represent the extreme of severe asthmatic attacks, those resulting in fatal hypoxemia. They are the tip of the iceberg of asthmatic exacerbations requiring medical attention.*

easier to relate to the image of a single child struggling to breathe, gasping for each breath, looking with imploring eyes for your help, than to the abstract statistics about asthma attacks. Imagine how one feels when vacation plans are canceled (again) because of needing to deal with a flare of asthma; when your job security is threatened by another work absence due to asthma; when your athletic child is limited in her ability to participate in sports because of her asthma; or when the unspeakable tragedy occurs—a loved one suffocates to death because of a severe asthma attack.

Inequalities in the distribution of asthma

Nonetheless, we can learn a lot of useful information from epidemiologic data about asthma. Two specific observations are worth emphasizing. First, the burden of asthma is not uniformly born across our society. Look closely at the frequency of hospitalizations and deaths from asthma—indicators of the most severe attacks of asthma—and one finds the urban areas like New York City, Chicago, and Los Angeles have particularly high rates. Look more closely still, at neighborhoods within these cities, and one finds that these markers of severe asthma vary widely between one neighborhood and the next, even though they may be located within just a few miles of one another. The explanation? Poverty and racial minority status.

KEY POINT   In general, asthma is more severe among people of color, people living in our inner cities, and people living in poverty.

Neighborhoods with low average family incomes and high percentages of minorities have significantly more asthma hospitalization and fatality rates than wealthier and predominantly white neighborhoods. It is not certain whether there are racial differences in the prevalence of asthma (that is, the percentage of the population having the disease), but there are definite differences in disease severity. In this country, minority status and poverty are closely linked. In our inner cities people of color on average have significantly higher rates of poverty. And it is perfectly plausible that poverty contributes to more severe asthma. More exposure to the inciters and triggers of asthma, less ability to modify these exposures, multiple barriers to good medical care, and a higher rate of comorbid illnesses are just a few of the many likely factors linking poverty and asthma severity. Across the nation, the rates of asthma-related emergency department visits, hospitalizations, and deaths are three to four times greater among blacks and other minorities than among whites. Asthma is one of many diseases in this country where social inequity translates directly to greater disease morbidity and mortality.

Rising prevalence of asthma

The second lesson of the epidemiologic study of asthma is that asthma prevalence is on the rise. Here's a sobering statistic: between 1980 and 1996, in the United States the number of people who reported having asthma within the previous 12 months (or having a child with asthma in that same time period) increased by 74%. Similar increases have occurred in other westernized countries around the world, including Western Europe, Australia, New Zealand, and Japan. In an era when we are triumphing over many infectious and cardiovascular diseases, why is it that asthma and allergies are on the rise? Why are we, as some have voiced, in the midst of an "asthma epidemic?" As an asthma educator, you will likely be asked at some point, why it is that asthma has become so common, why every other child on the school playground seems to be carrying an asthma inhaler.

The simple but unhelpful answer is that no one knows for sure. Despite what one might think, air pollution does not seem to be the answer. One interesting study points away from air pollution as the explanation. When the Berlin wall came down in 1989 and the people of Germany were united again, researchers investigated the prevalence of asthma in the old East and West Germanies, where the genetic make-up of the two populations is relatively homogeneous. If air pollution were a major contributor to new cases of asthma, one might predict that industrialized and heavily polluted East Germany would have a higher rate of asthma than West Germany, but just the opposite was found. Likewise, in the United States, while over recent decades asthma prevalence has been rising, there has been a trend toward improving air quality.

Some would argue that increased exposure to the allergens that incite asthmatic inflammation is the answer. As a nation we spend more time indoors (at our televisions, computers, and video games), and our homes have become more airtight, in an effort to conserve energy costs for heating and air conditioning. Perhaps the explanation for our asthma epidemic is more time spent breathing in the indoor allergens of dust mites, cockroaches, cats, mice, and mold. In rural communities, where people tend to spend more time outdoors, the incidence of asthma tends to be lower.

An alternative theory offered to explain the rising prevalence of asthma is called the "hygiene hypothesis." It suggests not that our immune systems are being driven more and more to make allergic reactions but that they are being stimulated less and less to fight germs. In a sense, without the need to fight bacteria, viruses, and bacterial toxins as much as in years gone by, the immune system has the leisure to be redirected toward allergic reactions. Consider the following pieces of evidence supporting the idea that the rise in asthma and allergies in the westernized countries of the world results from our exposure to fewer germs. If you have had tuberculous infection or vaccination against tuberculosis (as practiced in many countries of the world), you are less likely to develop asthma. If you have had hepatitis A or measles, you are less likely to have asthma. If you have an older sibling or go to daycare (and by either means encounter more germs at a younger age), you are less likely to develop asthma. If you live on a farm in close proximity to farm animals and their droppings (and your exposure to animal droppings is documented by the concentration of bacterial endotoxin from animal feces isolated from your mattress), you are less likely to have asthma—in direct relationship to the concentration of endotoxin exposure. Perhaps if the immune system is engaged in reacting to germs and their byproducts, it is less likely also to expend its efforts on fighting allergens.

There is an immune basis for this hypothesis. It suggests that helper T lymphocytes can be of two types: type-1 (infection-fighting) and type-2 (allergy-producing). There is a dynamic ying-yang interrelation between these cells, and stimulation of the type-1 helper T lymphocytes by bacterial endotoxin or viral infections can lead to decreased expression of the type-2 T lymphocytes—and so less allergy and asthma. It makes one think that if we knew how to stimulate the type-1 helper T lymphocytes safely, at the right age, for the right duration, and with the right intensity, perhaps we could stay the rising tide of asthma cases. This approach remains at present purely speculative, but it represents an avenue for research into the primary prevention of asthma.

Preventable morbidity and mortality from asthma

We wish to end this chapter on understanding and explaining asthma with a positive note. We have noted that asthma is common, and it causes considerable morbidity and mortality. But asthma can be controlled, and asthmatic attacks can be prevented. In fact, asthma has been identified as one of the most common causes of *preventable* hospitalizations. In many practice models, preventing asthmatic attacks that require emergency room utilization and hospitalization is used as a yardstick of quality care.

KEY POINT Hospitalizations for asthma are considered, to a large extent, to be preventable.

Consider here the goals of asthma care proposed by the National Asthma Education and Prevention Program:

- Prevent persistent and troublesome symptoms (for example, coughing or breathlessness in the night, in the early morning, or after exertion);
- Maintain normal or near-normal lung function;
- Maintain normal activity levels (including exercise and other physical activity);
- Prevent recurrent exacerbations of asthma and minimize the need for emergency department visits or hospitalizations;
- Provide optimal pharmacotherapy with minimal or no adverse effects; and
- Satisfy patients' and families' expectations of asthma care.

In most instances, these are realistic and achievable goals. We have at our disposal the scientific knowledge and the medical therapies necessary to make these goals a reality. As asthma care providers and asthma educators, we are committed to achieve these outcomes for all of our patients, regardless of their level of education, race, or income. In this chapter we have outlined the magnitude of the problem. With your study to become an effective asthma educator, you become part of the solution.

Self-Assessment Questions

QUESTION 1

You are asked to explain to a group of sixth graders what causes wheezing in asthma. You tell them:

1. Inflammation of the bronchial tubes
2. Rapid, deep breathing, such as during exercise
3. Air passing through narrowed air passageways in the lungs, setting up vibrations like the musical instrument, the recorder
4. Bronchospasm
5. Throat tightening

QUESTION 2

*Which of the following is **not** considered a trigger of asthma?*

1. House dust
2. Hot, spicy food
3. Exercise
4. Viral infections
5. Emotional stress

QUESTION 3

A middle-aged woman with asthma and multiple other medical problems wonders whether any of her medications might be causing her asthma to be more difficult to control. You review her list of medications and indicate the one that you think might be causing her trouble.

1. Acetaminophen (Tylenol) with codeine for her back pain
2. Enalapril (Vasotec) for her hypertension
3. Metformin (Glucophage) for her diabetes
4. Celecoxib (Celebrex) for her arthritis
5. Timolol (Timoptic) eye drops for her glaucoma

QUESTION 4

An 18-year-old college freshman with asthma reports to you that she no longer has asthma. She had the onset of asthmatic symptoms at age 5 and was treated with theophylline for many years. As recently as 6 months ago she had an acute asthmatic attack triggered by a visit to the house of her boyfriend's parents, who have two cats and a dog. However, this week she saw an internist for the first time. The doctor reported that her chest was entirely clear and her breathing tests entirely normal. You indicate that in spite of this good news, you think that she still has:

1. Small airway disease
2. Bronchial hyperresponsiveness (twitchy airways)
3. Occult airway narrowing
4. Susceptibility to hypoxemia, especially at high altitude
5. Exercise limitations

QUESTION 5

If a person with asthma and allergic sensitivity to mold is subjected to an allergen challenge with a carefully controlled, dilute concentration of mold to inhale, he may experience both an early reaction with cough and chest tightness and a late reaction several hours after allergen inhalation with similar asthmatic symptoms. The late asthmatic response is thought due to both bronchoconstriction and increased airway inflammation. In subjects who experience the late asthmatic reaction, you might also expect to find at approximately that same time:

1. Nasal congestion and a watery nasal discharge
2. Abdominal discomfort and gaseousness
3. An erythematous, pruritic rash over the face and extremities
4. Red, itchy eyes with increased tearing
5. Increased airway sensitivity to exercising in cold air

QUESTION 6

Immunoglobulin E (IgE) is a type of antibody made by B lymphocytes. It is important in asthma because:

1. It binds to the surface of mast cells and can activate them when a specific allergen attaches to it.
2. It has the ability to bind to allergens, helping mast cells digest them and remove them from the airways.
3. It binds to bacteria, helping mast cells and lymphocytes fight respiratory infections more effectively.
4. It can be used as a diagnostic test for asthma.
5. It is a powerful chemoattractant, drawing eosinophils into the airways.

QUESTION 7

Mast cells and eosinophils make chemicals that promote inflammation in the airways. These chemical mediators of inflammation, which can cause contraction of bronchial muscles, leakage of edema fluid into the airways, and excess mucus production include which of the following:

1. Alpha-1 antitrypsin
2. Nitric oxide (NO)
3. Leukotrienes
4. Ozone
5. Sulfites

QUESTION 8

The term "airway remodeling" is used to describe which of the following?

1. Mucous gland enlargement with excess mucus production
2. Permanent scarring of the airways due to long-term cigarette smoking
3. Irreversible dilation of airways with susceptibility to chronic bacterial infections
4. Permanent scarring of the airways due to long-term allergic inflammation
5. New growth of airways after severe inhalational injury

QUESTION 9

You are asked to comment on the genetic basis of asthma. You indicate that:

1. The genes that cause asthma have recently been identified.
2. The children of mothers with asthma are more likely to develop asthma than the children of mothers without asthma.
3. If one member of an identical twin pair has asthma, the other member will always develop asthma as well.
4. Changes in our genes help to explain why asthma has become more common in the past few decades.
5. Asthma develops because of intense environmental exposures, such as to allergens, and cannot be blamed on any genetic predisposition.

QUESTION 10

You are speaking with one of the asthmatic women for whom you have been caring. She has a 45-year-old brother who has been working for the past year in the baking industry, where he has lots of exposure to flour dust. In the last few weeks he has developed a troublesome cough, particularly toward the end of each work week. She wonders whether he too may be developing asthma. You indicate that:

1. It would be very unusual for asthma to begin at age 45.
2. He won't develop work-related asthma unless he has a strong prior history of allergies or cigarette-smoking.

3. He is safe in the absence of exposure to asbestos or silica.

4. It shouldn't be a problem for him if he wears a surgical face mask, which you offer to provide.

5. He is at risk for occupational asthma and should be tested for asthma.

QUESTION 11

Imagine that you begin to work at an inner-city neighborhood health center in a large city. You are struck by how often your patients require emergency department care or hospitalization for their asthma. Your family wonders why this might be true, knowing the excellent medical care that you and your colleagues provide. You suggest the following explanation:

1. Patients use the emergency department to get free medications for their asthma.

2. Your patients are forced to work in jobs with a higher rate of occupational asthma.

3. Inner-city residents tend to keep more pet cats to help with mouse control.

4. Poverty has an impact on allergen exposures in the home and your patients' ability to comply with recommended treatments.

5. Most asthmatic attacks occur at night and in the early morning hours, when your health center is closed.

QUESTION 12

A tired-looking mother of two asthmatic children comes to see you for advice about the care of her children. She has recently heard of the "hygiene hypothesis" about asthma and has been carefully bathing her young children at least once daily. She finds it difficult to get them to keep their hands clean. You applaud her efforts at cleanliness but gently suggest that:

1. The hygiene hypothesis is a theory about the cause of the rising incidence of allergies and asthma and does not relate to the care of individuals with asthma.

2. The hygiene hypothesis relates only to cockroaches, mice, and rats, not personal hygiene.

3. Only potent antibacterial soaps are effective in reducing the sorts of germs that colonize her children's skin.

4. The hygiene hypothesis relates to efforts at reducing childhood ear and respiratory tract infections, not asthma.

5. The hygiene hypothesis suggests that *more* germs would be good for her children's asthma, not less.

Answers to Self-Assessment Questions

ANSWER TO QUESTION 1 (DEFINING ASTHMA IN LAY TERMS)

The correct answer is #3. Inflammation of the bronchial tubes (answer #1) and bronchospasm (tightening of the bronchial muscles that surround the airways) (answer #4) are both potential causes of airway narrowing and wheezing, but there are two problems with these answers. First, sixth graders are not likely to understand exactly what you mean if you use the terms "inflammation" or "bronchospasm." Second, each answer is half the story: in asthma it is most often some combination of both swelling of the walls of the bronchial tubes, secretions accumulating in the bronchial tubes, and constriction of the bronchial smooth (involuntary) muscles that causes airway narrowing. When that narrowing reaches a critical diameter, air passing through the narrowed opening generates a whistling sound, wheezing. The airway narrowing that comes on with prolonged exercise (answer #2), or often after a short period of exercise, is only one of many instances when a child with asthma may experience wheezing. Throat tightening (answer #5) is not part of asthma; it may occur in a child with food allergies and is a medical emergency. The loud, inspiratory sound that results from critical narrowing of the upper airway is called stridor.

ANSWER TO QUESTION 2 (TRIGGERS OF ASTHMA)

The correct answer is #2. Hot, spicy food may cause indigestion, but it does not provoke airway narrowing in asthma. All of the other choices are potential triggers of airway narrowing in someone with susceptible airways, that is, asthma. House dust (answer #1) contains the allergen, house dust mites, to which many children and adults with asthma are allergic. Exercise (answer #3) provokes airway narrowing as a result of cooling and drying of the airways during exercise. The mechanisms by which viral respiratory tract infections (answer #4) and emotional stress (answer #5) can provoke airway narrowing in asthma are not understood in great detail, but these are common and widely recognized *provocateurs* of asthma.

ANSWER TO QUESTION 3 (MEDICATIONS THAT CAN WORSEN ASTHMA)

The correct answer is #5. People with asthma are highly sensitive to the effects of beta-blocker medications, such as propranolol (Inderal) and timolol (Timoptic Ophthalmic Solution and Blocadren). It seems that without the bronchodilator effect of beta-adrenergic stimulation, the airways can narrow dramatically in asthma. Even the miniscule amounts of medication that are systemically absorbed after administration of beta-blocker eyedrops can provoke bronchoconstriction and sometimes even life-threatening airway narrowing. Beta blockers that are selective for the beta receptors in the heart (selective beta-1 blockers) have less effect than the nonselective beta blockers such as propranolol and timolol. Angiotensin converting enzyme inhibitors such as enalapril (Vasotec) (answer #2) can cause cough in persons with or without asthma, but they do not aggravate asthma. Some people with asthma (approximately 3–5%) are aspirin sensitive and will develop an asthmatic exacerbation if they ingest aspirin or any of the nonsteroidal anti-inflammatory drugs. However, the selective cyclooxygenase-2 (COX-2) inhibitor celecoxib (Celebrex) (answer #4) appears to be safe in this patient group. Antidiabetic medications such as metformin (Glucophage) (answer #3) and analgesics such as acetaminophen and codeine (answer #1) have no effect on asthma.

ANSWER TO QUESTION 4 (PERSISTENCE OF BRONCHIAL HYPERRESPONSIVE-NESS IN ASTHMA)

The correct answer is #2. Bronchial hyperresponsiveness (twitchy airways) is a fundamental property of asthmatic airways. It does not go away even when the symptoms of asthma do and when lung function returns to normal. It is important for patients to remember that this vulnerability to bronchial narrowing persists even when they feel well. Her normal pulmonary function tests are reasonable evidence that she does not at this time have small airway disease (answer #1) or any significant airway narrowing at all (answer #3). If her asthma remains in good control (normal lung function), her blood oxygen will be normal and fall no more than normal at high altitude (answer #4). Because she has normal lung function, she should be able to exercise without limitation (answer #5). Although exercise may bring on airway narrowing, it is generally preventable and treatable and should not cause any restriction to her exercising (as you know from the successes of many renowned athletes who have asthma).

ANSWER TO QUESTION 5 (ASSOCIATION OF THE LATE ASTHMATIC RESPONSE AND HEIGHTENED BRONCHIAL HYPERRESPONSIVENESS)

The correct answer is #5. The late asthmatic reaction to inhaled allergen illustrates that airway narrowing can be caused by both bronchial constriction and inflammation (swelling and cellular infiltration) of the airway walls. It also illustrates the association between airway wall inflammation and bronchial hyperresponsiveness. In subjects who experience the late asthmatic response (but not in those who have only an early asthmatic reaction, due to bronchosconstriction without an inflammatory reaction), there is a period lasting many hours to days of heightened bronchial responsiveness. This means that during this period, asthmatic subjects will be more sensitive to any of their asthmatic triggers—their airways will have a heightened sensitivity to any and all asthmatic stimuli. An antigen inhalation challenge causes a local reaction within the airways only. It does not cause a nasal response (answer #1), abdominal symptoms (answer #2), skin rash (answer #3), or conjunctivitis (answer #4).

ANSWER TO QUESTION 6 (THE ROLE OF IMMUNOGLOBULIN E [IGE] IN ASTHMA)

The correct answer is #1. When IgE antibody molecules bind to the specific allergen that they were designed to recognize, they activate the mast cells on which they sit and thereby initiate the allergic inflammatory reaction. This reaction is important not only in asthma but in other allergic diseases that share this common mechanism, referred to as atopic diseases (allergic rhinitis and conjunctivitis [hay fever], atopic dermatitis [eczema], hives, and anaphylaxis). Allergens are not digested by mast cells (answer #2). Immunoglobulin G and other immunoglobulins help neutrophils fight bacterial infections (answer #3). It is true that elevated levels of IgE may be found in the blood of some people with allergic asthma (answer #4), but this finding is not specific for asthma (for example, it may be found in someone with eczema who does not have asthma), and normal blood levels of IgE do not exclude a diagnosis of asthma. Certain chemicals released by lymphocytes and mast cells attract eosinophils into the airways as part of the allergic reaction, but not IgE (answer #5).

ANSWER TO QUESTION 7 (CHEMICAL MEDIATORS OF INFLAMMATION IN ASTHMA)

The correct answer is #3. Leukotrienes are synthesized by mast cells and eosinophils when these cells are activated, such as during an allergic reaction. Histamine, leukotrienes, and numerous other chemicals act to promote the effects in the airways that we recognize as asthma. A deficiency of alpha-1 antitrypsin protein (answer #1), which is made in the liver, can cause emphysema. Nitric oxide (answer #2) is synthesized by epithelial lining cells along the bronchial tubes. It is a potential marker of asthmatic inflammation, as will be discussed in the next chapter. Ozone (answer #4) is a constituent of air pollution; high ambient concentrations can act as an irritant to worsen asthma. Sulfites (answer #5) are additives used in food processing that can occasionally worsen asthma in sulfite-sensitive asthmatic patients.

ANSWER TO QUESTION 8 (DEFINING AIRWAY REMODELING IN ASTHMA)

The correct answer is #4. The mechanism by which lifelong nonsmokers with asthma may develop permanent, irreversible narrowing of their airways is referred to as airway remodeling. Although the exact pathology is unknown, formation of scar below the layer of lining cells (subepithelial fibrosis) is thought to play an important role. Mucous gland enlargement with excess mucus production (answer #1) can occur in asthma, but it is thought to be a reversible feature of the disease. Permanent scarring of the airways due to long-term cigarette smoking (answer #2) is one of the causes of COPD. Irreversible dilation of airways with susceptibility to chronic bacterial infections (answer #3) occurs in bronchiectasis, such as in patients with cystic fibrosis. New growth of airways after severe inhalational injury (answer #5) does not occur. Growth of the tracheobronchial tree is complete at birth.

ANSWER TO QUESTION 9 (GENETICS OF ASTHMA)

The correct answer is #2. If one parent has asthma, the chance of a child developing asthma is increased compared to when neither parent has asthma. When only the mother has asthma, the risk for the child to develop asthma is greater than when only the father has asthma. Genes that are closely linked to asthma are being sought, and some potential "candidate genes" have been identified, but we are still far from identifying all of the genes that interact to cause asthma (answer #1). If one member of an identical twin pair has asthma (answer #3), the chance that the other member will also develop asthma (despite an exact duplicate set of genes) is only about one third. The changes in our genes (answer #4) that occur gradually over time (evolution) take many thousands of years to occur. They cannot explain the increases in asthma prevalence that we have witnessed over the past 20–30 years. Asthma may be caused by intense environmental exposures (answer #5) *in a genetically susceptible individual*. The same intense exposures in a person with a different genetic makeup will not lead to development of asthma.

ANSWER TO QUESTION 10 (OCCUPATIONAL ASTHMA)

The correct answer is #5. Flour dust can be a sensitizing agent in the workplace. In susceptible individuals it can lead to the development of asthma. This form of occupational asthma has been dubbed "bakers' asthma." While it is true that adult-onset asthma is less common than childhood asthma (answer #1), occupational asthma is one of the settings in which the new onset of asthma routinely occurs among adults. Occupational asthma is not restricted to those with a prior history of allergies or cigarette-smoking (answer #2). Long-term asbestos or silica dust exposure can cause serious lung disease (the inflammatory and scarring lung diseases called asbestosis or silicosis), but they do not cause asthma (answer #3). A surgical face mask is inadequate protection from work-related exposures of this sort (answer #4). Sometimes a regulation respirator with canister filters can help, but the most certain treatment for someone with documented occupational asthma is removal from that particular work environment.

ANSWER TO QUESTION 11 (POTENTIAL CAUSES FOR THE SEVERITY OF INNER-CITY ASTHMA)

The correct answer is #4. Low socioeconomic status is strongly associated with emergency department utilization and hospitalizations for asthma. There are many potential reasons for this association, of which cockroach and other allergen exposure in the home environment is one. Emergency departments are not a reliable source of free medications for asthma (answer #1). Occupational asthma (answer #2) is not more prevalent among inner-city residents, and it accounts for only a small percentage of all asthma cases. Pet cat ownership (answer #3) is not more common in the inner cities. Although it is true that many asthmatic attacks occur overnight (answer #5), this observation pertains to those living in suburban and rural locations as much as to inner-city residents. It does not adequately account for differences in emergency department utilization.

ANSWER TO QUESTION 12 ("HYGIENE HYPOTHESIS" TO EXPLAIN THE RISING INCIDENCE OF ASTHMA)

The correct answer is #1. The hygiene hypothesis is a theory, not fact. It suggests that perhaps the reason for the increasing prevalence of allergies and asthma in our westernized societies is a decrease in our exposure to germs, both human infections and the germs found in animal droppings. According to the theory, with fewer germs to drive our immune systems to fight infections, the immune responses are more likely to shift to the allergic type. The theory pertains to the new onset of asthma and allergies. It does not relate to already established asthma (answer #5); it is not meant to help reduce childhood infections (answer #4); it has nothing to do with insect and rodent infestations (answer #2); and it does not pertain to bacteria that live on our skin (answer #3).

CHAPTER

2

DIAGNOSING AND STAGING THE SEVERITY OF ASTHMA

CHAPTER OUTLINE

I.   A typical history for asthma
     a. Characteristic symptoms
     b. Typical triggers
     c. Age of onset
     d. Common associated illnesses

II. Physical examination
     a. Characteristic wheezing of asthma
     b. Other types of wheezing
     c. Physical findings in associated allergic diseases

III. Diagnostic tests
     a. Pulmonary function testing
     b. Therapeutic trial
     c. Peak flow monitoring
     d. Bronchoprovocative challenge
     e. Exhaled nitric oxide concentration
     f. Other tests that may be helpful but are not conclusive

IV. Excluding alternative diagnoses
     a. In children
     b. In adults

V.   Staging the severity of asthma
     a. Origins of the national "Guidelines for the Diagnosis and Management of Asthma"
     b. Criteria for judging asthma severity
     c. Step 1: mild intermittent asthma
     d. Step 2: mild persistent asthma
     e. Step 3: moderate persistent asthma
     f. Step 4: severe persistent asthma

CHAPTER OUTLINE

g. Applying the stepwise criteria
h. Limitations of the staging system

VI. Case examples

VII. An overview of asthma severity in the United States

It is true that as an asthma educator, you are most often called upon to help people whose diagnosis of asthma has already been established, rather than to make a diagnosis of asthma yourself. Nonetheless, we think that it is good to consider how a diagnosis of asthma is made for two simple reasons: some people who carry a diagnosis of asthma do not have the disease, and other people who do have asthma have never been given the diagnosis. Said in another way, we find that asthma can be both overdiagnosed and underdiagnosed. One day you may have the opportunity to advise a patient to consider the possibility that his or her symptoms are due to an illness other than asthma; and alternatively, you may be the first one to suggest that a person's recurrent cough and shortness of breath are due to asthma, not just frequent colds.

A TYPICAL HISTORY FOR ASTHMA

Sometimes, making a diagnosis of asthma is incredibly easy. Consider the following example. You are told of a 5-year-old boy who develops persistent coughing and noisy, whistling breathing every time that he goes out to play in the cold air or whenever he goes into the barn and is around horses. Your diagnosis: asthma. His mother, aunt, and school teacher all came to the same conclusion as well!

Characteristic symptoms

In this example the diagnosis of asthma is easy because there are several highly characteristic features to his story. First, his symptoms are typical of asthma: cough and wheezing. Coughing is probably the most common symptom of childhood asthma, although it is not at all specific for asthma. Wheezing certainly makes one think of asthma. Although it may be heard in a variety of other lung conditions, the number of possible causes is relatively small, and it is helpful in that it points to a condition involving the airways. Other characteristic symptoms of asthma, as you know, are chest tightness and shortness of breath. Sometimes, people with asthma may report an itch or tickle under their chin, and you may find them rubbing this area to relieve the symptom.

Second, the symptoms are intermittent. For days or weeks at a time, the boy feels perfectly well. At other times he feels miserable because of his symptoms of cough and wheeze. Intermittent symptoms are typical of asthma and would not be expected in many other chronic lung conditions in which symptoms, although they may vary in severity, tend to be present every day. Because symptoms in asthma are generally episodic, people are often fooled into thinking that they have had multiple bouts of an acute, self-limited illness, such as viral respiratory tract illnesses. What parent wouldn't prefer to think that his or her child has had a "bad winter" with many lingering colds rather than to ascribe the child's recurrent and lingering respiratory symptoms to asthma?

Typical triggers

The third feature of this history that makes you suspect a diagnosis of asthma is the nature of the things that provoke his symptoms. Exercise in cold air and animal exposure are typical triggers of asthma. Intense exercise can make anyone have labored breathing, but typical of the bronchoconstriction brought on by exercise is its timing and duration. It generally begins within a few minutes *after* a brief run, and once it occurs it tends to last for up to 30–60 minutes. This duration is very different from the brief period of recovery (1–3 minutes) that a child without asthma might need to "catch his breath" before starting to run again. Allergic exposures, such as barn dust and horses, would very rarely cause the abrupt onset of respiratory symptoms in the absence of allergic sensitivity of the airways (that is, asthma).

Other triggers can be equally irritating to persons with asthma and to other people with many different lung diseases: for example, walking outdoors in very hot, humid weather; intense exposure to second-hand smoke in a crowded bar; or a bout of bronchitis. Their mention in a history of "what makes your breathing worse" is nonspecific. A child with cystic fibrosis or an adult with chronic obstructive pulmonary disease might well report that these circumstances cause him or her to develop worsened chest symptoms in the same way that they bother a person with asthma.

Age of onset

Finally, the age of onset of symptoms is helpful. Approximately three quarters of all cases of asthma begin before age 9 years (Fig. 2-1). Asthma can begin at any age, but in people who are 50 years or older, we look hard and long for an alternative explanation for asthma-like symptoms before settling on a diagnosis of asthma. Respiratory symptoms such as cough and wheezing that begin in middle age or older are far more often due to some other etiology, such as chronic obstructive pulmonary disease (COPD), bronchiectasis, or congestive heart failure, than to the new onset of asthma. On the other hand, in a 5-year-old boy, the most common cause would be asthma.

It is not uncommon for asthma to be newly diagnosed in young adulthood. In such patients we often hear a story of symptoms in childhood that might have

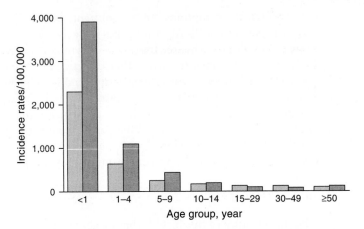

FIGURE 2-1 *This study of the new onset of asthma among residents of Rochester, Minnesota demonstrates that asthma typically begins in early childhood. Most cases of asthma have their onset before age 4. Lighter bars = females; darker bars = males. Reproduced with permission from Yunginger JW, et al., A community-based study of the epidemiology of asthma.* American Review of Respiratory Disease *1992; 146:888–94. Official Journal of the American Thoracic Society. Copyright American Lung Association.*

been due to asthma, such as a lingering cough throughout the winter months, or recurrent bronchitis occurring much more frequently than among other children, or a cough that would linger for months after each cold. Perhaps no diagnosis of asthma was made at the time, or the person was thought to have asthma that he or she then *outgrew*. Other patients with the new onset of asthma in early adulthood have a strong history of allergies, such as eczema as a young child, troublesome seasonal allergies each spring and fall, and multiple positive results on allergy skin testing. It is on this atopic background that asthma newly emerges.

KEY POINT   The diagnosis of asthma is easy when typical symptoms occur intermittently, are brought on by characteristic triggers, and begin at a young age.

Common associated illnesses

Because they share a common allergic immune mechanism (involving IgE anti-bodies, mast cells, type-2 helper T lymphocytes, and eosinophils), atopic dis-eases commonly occur together. In some people their allergies manifest in their nose and eyes as allergic rhinitis and conjunctivitis (hay fever); in other people they localize to their skin as atopic dermatitis (eczema) or as hives; in still oth-ers they appear as food allergies involving the digestive tract anywhere from lips to intestines. A severe allergic reaction that takes place in the bloodstream can

TABLE 2-1

ATOPIC DISEASES BY ORGAN OF INVOLVEMENT

Organ	Disorder
Skin	Hives, Atopic dermatitis (eczema)
Nose	Allergic rhinitis
Eyes	Allergic conjunctivitis
Bronchi	Asthma
Gastrointestinal tract	Food allergies
Systemic	Anaphylaxis

cause life-threatening low blood pressure due to vasodilation: anaphylaxis. Also, long-standing allergic inflammation in the nose is one pathway to the formation of nasal polyps (Table 2-1).

It is possible to have nonatopic asthma and no identifiable allergies. It is also possible to have atopic (allergic) asthma but no other allergic diseases. However, quite commonly, atopic asthma is accompanied by one or more of the atopic diseases mentioned above. Their presence in a child with intermittent cough, shortness of breath, and wheezing favors a diagnosis of asthma—although of course it does not prove it.

As an aside, we remind you of the now-outdated terminology of "extrinsic" and "intrinsic" asthma. Extrinsic was the term used to describe asthma for which external allergic triggers could be identified; intrinsic asthma referred to the absence of such identifiable allergic triggers, making a presumption that some internal stimulus in the body must be driving the asthmatic reactions. The concepts have not totally been discarded: we still speak of atopic and nonatopic asthma or, more simply—and more appropriately for discussions with our patients—allergic and nonallergic asthma.

Among children asthma is almost always associated with some allergic sensitivities. As many as 80–90% of school-age children have documentable allergies. Among adults, the number of persons with asthma having allergies (atopic asthma) probably falls to 50–60%. One might wonder: are we talking about two different diseases here? Most evidence suggests that we are not: all patients with asthma—with or without allergies—have identical symptoms, identical airway narrowing, identical bronchial hyperresponsiveness, and identical pathologic findings on bronchial biopsy or bronchoalveolar lavage.

KEY POINT   The atopic diseases of hay fever, eczema, hives, and asthma commonly occur together in various combinations in families and in individuals.

PHYSICAL EXAMINATION

Most of the time, the chest examination of a person with asthma is normal. In the absence of significant airway narrowing, one does not expect to encounter abnormal chest findings. Abnormal physical findings, like asthmatic symptoms, are generally intermittent and may not be present at the moment that you apply your stethoscope to the chest.

Characteristic wheezing of asthma

On the other hand, when you examine a *symptomatic* child or adult with asthma, you may hear characteristic wheezing. The wheezing of asthma has the following features: it can be heard in all lung fields (posterior, anterior, and lateral); it is almost always heard during exhalation and sometimes during both exhalation and inhalation; it is usually heard throughout exhalation (not just toward the very end of exhalation); and it has a high-pitched, musical quality—multiple overlapping notes of varying pitch and varying duration. Consider the origin of each note: a bronchus whose internal opening (lumen) has been narrowed to the point of generating a vibration like a musical instrument. In asthma, many different bronchi throughout the tracheobronchial tree reach this critical diameter at the same time, but because the length and diameter of these bronchi vary, the notes that they produce differ from one another. With time (or treatment), different bronchi in different locations in the lung become narrowed to this critical diameter, and the musical wheezing changes somewhat. Add to this the low-pitched sounds (often called rhonchi) generated when air passes through mucus-filled central airways, and you can see why chest auscultation in asthma can sound orchestral!

KEY POINT   The wheezes of asthma have distinctive features that help you distinguish asthma from other causes of wheezing.

Other types of wheezing

A truism of asthma diagnosis is that "not all that wheezes is asthma." If you listen carefully, you will be able to distinguish different types of wheezing and to recognize wheezing that is not due to asthma. Here are four examples. First, *upper airway stridor* is a low-pitched, harsh, inspiratory wheeze that is loudest in the neck area and may be softly transmitted to the chest or may be inaudible to auscultation there. Swelling of the epiglottis caused by an infection (epiglottitis) can cause upper airway stridor in children and, less often, in adults. Vocal cord dysfunction is a functional abnormality of normal-appearing vocal cords that can bring the cords too close during inhalation, causing stridor.

Second, a *focal wheeze*, localized to one area of the chest, suggests narrowing of one major bronchus. The further you move your stethoscope from that particular area, the fainter the wheeze becomes. Typically, the sound that is generated represents just one note (monophonic), and it sounds exactly the same breath after breath. Partial bronchial obstruction caused by an aspirated foreign body may be the cause; or a lung cancer originating within the wall of the bronchus (hence the name, bronchogenic carcinoma) may obstruct or compress the bronchial lumen.

Third, you may be able to distinguish the *end-expiratory, polyphonic wheezes* of emphysema from asthmatic wheezing. Most often the chest auscultation in advanced COPD is remarkable for distant-sounding breath sounds. With chest percussion you may also detect signs of overinflation of the lungs: hyperinflation (low-lying diaphragms) and hyperresonance (very easily elicited resonant note on percussion). Sometimes, you also hear wheezing. Bronchi progressively narrow throughout exhalation; in severe COPD, toward the end of exhalation, bronchi of similar diameter throughout the lungs reach that critical diameter at which a wheeze is generated. With each breath, throughout the lungs you hear the same wheezing sound at almost the identical point in time during exhalation. As you might expect, there are generally many other clues that help you to distinguish severe COPD from asthma!

Finally, *low-pitched wheezing (rhonchi or one rhonchus)* is created when air passes through large, centrally located bronchi that are partially blocked by mucus or blood within their lumens. The sound is said to be similar to the sound that you make when, trying to get the very last of your drink to come up through a straw, you suck in both liquid and air. Have the patient make a deep cough to clear secretions, then listen again. The rhonchi will likely change and may well go away altogether. If you have worked in an intensive care unit, you may have encountered rhonchi in intubated patients receiving mechanical ventilation who are unable to cough effectively. Suction secretions from their airways, and the rhonchi will change or clear completely. Lay your hand firmly on the patient's chest wall, and you can *feel* these vibrations; the sensation is called tactile fremitus. (Try that one on your colleagues one morning during rounds!)

The point that we hope to emphasize is that there are a variety of types of wheezing, just as there are a variety of types of heart murmurs. The wheezing of asthma is distinctive and often readily distinguishable from other types of wheezing. It is probably the most common type of wheezing that we encounter in our practices, but "common" should not be confused with "only," because—to reiterate—"not all that wheezes is asthma."

Physical findings in associated allergic diseases

Perhaps our patient (the 5-year-old boy who has cough and wheezing when he spends time in the barn) has a normal chest exam at the time of his visit with us. We are unable to confirm our suspicion of asthma at that moment, but we may be able to find other signs of associated allergic diseases. Like a history of other atopic diseases, these physical findings will be circumstantial evidence, but not proof, that his respiratory symptoms are due to what one might call "atopic bronchitis" or asthma.

We will want to look in his nose to see if the membranes are pale and swollen, with a clear watery nasal discharge. Perhaps we will catch the child making the "allergic salute," that is, rubbing the tip of his itchy nose with the palm of his hand in an upward sweeping motion (Fig. 2-2). In an adult, we may find glistening, rounded growths of tissue plugging up the nasal passageways. These cannot be cleared, even when the patient vigorously blows his nose. They are nasal polyps, sometimes seen in association with long-standing nasal allergies (Fig. 2-3).

Here's a diagnostic pearl worth remembering. Nasal polyps in a child should make you think of cystic fibrosis, not asthma. Nasal polyps due to asthma tend not to develop before age 18 years or later.

As we look in the back of his throat, we may see mucus draining from above along the posterior pharyngeal wall, and in response to chronic irritation we may see a bumpy, *cobblestoned* appearance to that mucosal surface. Dark circles around the eyes are referred to as "allergic shiners." Bright red, prominent blood vessels in the white linings of the eyes, with tearing or a clear, watery discharge at the corners of the eyes, indicate allergic conjunctivitis.

We'll examine the child for an erythematous rash with fine superficial scaling along skin fold creases, particularly at the elbows and behind the knees, to look for signs of eczema. And hives we'll readily recognize as red, raised-up papules, sharply demarcated at their edges, often appearing in groups. Eczema and hives tend both to be terribly itchy, so be prepared for signs of lots of scratching.

To be clear, let us reiterate that the presence of these physical findings indicative of atopic diseases outside of the chest does not prove that our patient

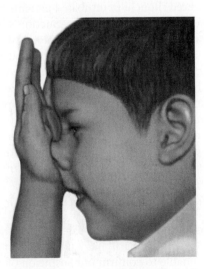

FIGURE 2-2 *The "allergic salute" is a common sign of nasal allergies in children. Children often rub their itchy, watery nose with an upward motion of the palms of their hands.*

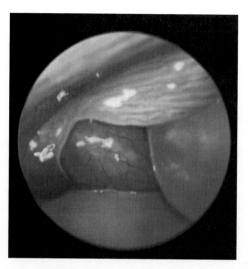

FIGURE 2-3   *Nasal polyps are fleshy growths of tissue originating along the membranes of the nasal mucosa. As here, they often have a silvery, glistening surface. They can frequently be visualized in the medical office with an otoscope and nasal speculum.*

has asthma. It is certainly possible for a 5-year-old boy with seasonal rhinitis and conjunctivitis, eczema, and/or hives to develop bronchopneumonia, aspirate a foreign body, or have severe gastroesophageal reflux with aspiration. However, among the various possibilities, these findings weigh the probabilities more in favor of asthma as the likely diagnosis. We cannot ignore them in our thinking.

KEY POINT   Besides examining the chest, you will want to look for other signs of allergic diseases, particularly in the nose, eyes, throat, and skin.

DIAGNOSTIC TESTS

As you know, patients often present with medical histories that are not as clear-cut as that of our 5-year-old boy with intermittent cough and wheezing. One patient has shortness of breath when playing soccer and wonders whether asthma is the cause. Another wakes at night with cough; you consider asthma but also gastroesophageal reflux disease and postnasal drip. Still another patient describes frequent bouts of cough and chest congestion this winter. Is the reason asthma or perhaps frequent respiratory tract infections?

Perhaps the patient has diffuse musical wheezing on physical examination to suggest asthma, but perhaps not. It is possible to have airway narrowing due to asthma without wheezing; and because airway narrowing in asthma is intermittent, it is possible that the patient's wheezes have resolved by the time that you apply your stethoscope to his chest. You would like to make a definite, not just a presumptive diagnosis of asthma. What diagnostic tests can help you—not only in establishing a diagnosis of asthma but also in assessing its severity? The answer is pulmonary function testing.

Pulmonary function testing

You may or may not be familiar with pulmonary function testing. Its mention may summon bad memories of a confusing alphabet soup of abbreviations and a jumbled list of numbers on a breathing test report. If you've worked near a pulmonary function laboratory in a hospital, your memory may be of the words of encouragement offered by the pulmonary function technician during the testing: "push, push, push...."

For asthma specialists like the authors of this book, pulmonary function testing is an essential tool of our trade. We find it incredibly valuable in understanding a patient's symptoms, assessing the severity of disease, and making correct diagnoses. We incorporate pulmonary function testing into our daily practices, and terms like "FVC" and "FEV_1" have become part of our routine medical vocabulary. With this book we would like to help you to become equally comfortable with the basics of pulmonary testing. We believe that you will find the concepts of pulmonary function testing remarkably easy and the results of pulmonary testing strikingly useful in your care of patients with asthma and other lung diseases. Understanding pulmonary function tests will help you interpret for your patients the significance of their test results, and if you pursue certification as an Asthma Educator, it will help you pass the examination.

Later in this book (Chap. 6, "Pulmonary Function Testing and Peak Flow Monitoring"), we devote a full chapter to spirometry, flow-volume curves, and peak flow measurements. We will review in detail the concepts, the testing, and interpretation of the results. For now, as we discuss the role of pulmonary function testing in establishing (or excluding) a diagnosis of asthma, we need only make the following general observation: pulmonary function testing (specifically spirometry) can measure how fast air can be forced from the lungs. If the bronchial tubes narrow throughout the lungs (as in asthma), air empties more slowly than when the bronchial tubes are wide open. The most useful test to assess for the airway narrowing of asthma is to have a person try to force air from the lungs as fast as possible. If air empties from the lungs at a normal speed (compared with people known to be healthy), there is no significant airway narrowing present. If air empties slower than normal—that is, if there is obstruction to the flow of air during exhalation, or *airflow obstruction*—one has evidence for airway narrowing.* The forced expiratory volume in one second or FEV_1 is the most widely used measure of expiratory airflow derived from spirometry.

---

*Another possible cause for slowing of air exiting from the lungs can be loss of the springiness of the lungs, as occurs in emphysema, but we will get to the fine points later.

Pulmonary function testing (spirometry) allows you to detect and quantify the presence of airway narrowing, a key feature of asthma.

Pulmonary function testing requires a cooperative patient giving a maximal effort on the test. In general, children before the age of approximately 6–7 years old find the procedure too difficult to complete reliably. In older children and adults, the test results are enormously useful. Consider a 13-year-old girl with breathlessness when playing basketball. At the time of her medical appointment, she has a dry cough but no wheezing. You suspect that she might have asthma, but you wonder too whether she might be breathless simply because she is not used to this level of strenuous physical exertion—whether she is just "out of shape." She undergoes pulmonary function testing, which reveals mild airflow obstruction during the forced expiratory maneuver of spirometry. And there, pretty much, is our diagnosis. An otherwise perfectly healthy young person with evidence for airway narrowing on pulmonary function testing and an appropriate medical history most likely has asthma.

True, there are other lung diseases that can cause this pattern of airflow obstruction on pulmonary function testing, such as bronchiectasis (as in cystic fibrosis) or a viral bronchiolitis, but far and away the most common cause is asthma. One feature that tends to distinguish asthma from other diseases characterized by airflow obstruction (called collectively the obstructive lung diseases) is the variability of the obstruction in asthma. At one point in time the bronchial tubes in asthma are constricted and swollen; at another moment they are wide open and normal in diameter. One can test for this reversibility of airway narrowing in the pulmonary function laboratory by administering a quick-acting bronchodilator. To the extent that constriction of the bronchial muscles is contributing to the airflow obstruction, the bronchodilator will cause the muscles to relax and the airways to open within just a few minutes. Repeat the pulmonary test, and now there is a large improvement in expiratory airflow. The airflow obstruction has lessened and perhaps totally disappeared. We have secured our diagnosis of asthma.

Airflow obstruction on spirometry that reverses within minutes in response to a quick-acting inhaled bronchodilator is indicative of asthma.

On the other hand, what if the spirometry on our 13-year-old basketball player is normal? Have we ruled out asthma as her diagnosis? Probably not. As she would point out to you, she feels fine now, sitting in the medical office or having her breathing measured on pulmonary function testing. It is only when she runs hard on the basketball court that she has her problem. Come measure my breathing then, she suggests! Although asthma is present all the time (meaning there is persistence of some degree of airway inflammation and bronchial hyper-responsiveness), airflow obstruction in asthma comes and goes. What if, at this moment, it happens to be gone, making the pulmonary function test normal?

The medical practitioner has a number of options at this point to pursue a possible diagnosis of asthma in the presence of initially normal pulmonary function tests. You can have the patient come back at a time when he or she is having symptoms, explaining, by analogy, that it is easier to diagnosis the knocking sound in the car engine when the engine is actively making the sound. This approach scores high on the inconvenience and lack of satisfaction scales. Nonetheless, if over time you can document airflow obstruction on some pulmonary function tests and none on others, you have secured a diagnosis of asthma. Incidentally, a bout of bronchitis (a chest cold) usually does not cause airflow obstruction on a breathing test.

Therapeutic trial

Another approach is to give a therapeutic trial of an inhaled bronchodilator. Use the medication whenever you have your coughing, wheezing, or shortness of breath, and let me know at your next visit whether it is helpful in relieving your symptoms. This method of diagnosis is simple and inexpensive, but it has significant potential for error. When the patient returns reporting no benefit, can we conclude that this is not asthma, or might it be that she failed to take the medication properly or that the medication was not sufficiently strong? Conversely, if she reports improvement with the inhaled bronchodilator, are we certain of the diagnosis of asthma, or could there be a placebo effect making our patient feel better? And if she returns to report that the inhaler helped some, but "only a little," we are totally in limbo. The therapeutic trial is commonly practiced and often informative, but it is not without its pitfalls.

Peak flow monitoring

What if we could make multiple measurements of lung function over time, morning and night and whenever symptoms are present, wherever the patient is located? We would obtain a dynamic record of airway patency over time. Decreases in expiratory flow rates that correlated with respiratory symptoms would indicate asthma; unchanging results day in and day out would argue against asthma. Are we talking about a mobile pulmonary function laboratory? No. We are referring to the use of a portable peak flow meter to monitor lung function over time and thereby to evaluate for asthma in the person with normal lung function at the time of initial evaluation.

Peak flow meters are inexpensive ($20 or less) and simple to use (Fig. 2-4). They measure the maximal rate at which air can be forced from the lungs, and therefore peak flow is a reflection of airways diameter. Narrowing of airways in asthma causes the peak expiratory flow to fall. In fact, many other conditions can cause the peak flow to fall, including conditions that are not obstructive lung diseases (as explained in Chap. 6), so peak flow measurements cannot substitute

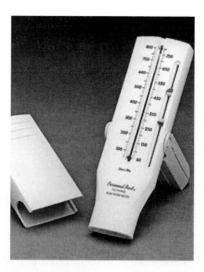

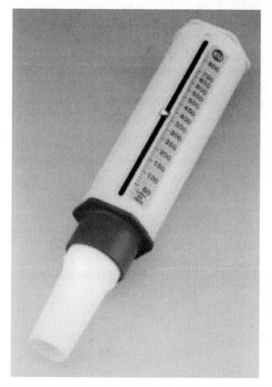

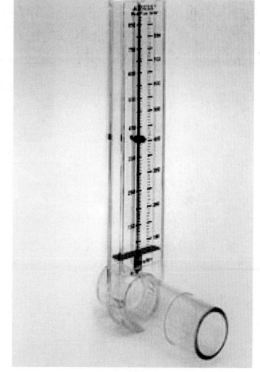

FIGURE 2-4 *Peak flow meters.*

fully for spirometry. Still, when your suspicion for asthma is high, variable peak flow measurements can provide strong supportive evidence. On the other hand, if a patient reports the presence of his symptoms of cough, shortness of breath, or chest tightness but the peak flow remains stable throughout, the diagnosis of asthma is unlikely.

Combine the therapeutic trial of a quick-acting bronchodilator with peak flow monitoring, and you have a particularly effective means to test for reversible airway narrowing (that is, asthma). We tell our patients to check their peak flow when they experience their respiratory symptoms, then use their quick-acting bronchodilator (such as albuterol). Five to ten minutes later, repeat the peak flow measurement. In Chap. 1 we spoke of asthma as "variable airway narrowing that is often reversible either spontaneously or with treatment." With a peak flow meter, our patients can test for airway narrowing that improves with the passage of time or in response to bronchodilator treatment (Fig. 2-5).

This diagnostic approach is inexpensive and usually very informative for the patient. It has the disadvantage of relying on the accuracy of measurements and record-keeping made by the patient. Even with the best of intentions, some patients will be unable to generate reliable data. With inaccurate information, the clinician is at risk for reaching erroneous conclusions about the presence or absence of asthma.

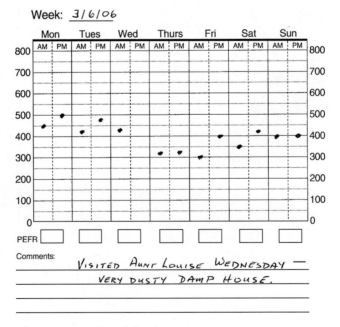

FIGURE 2-5   *Sample peak flow diary.*

In subsequent chapters, we will discuss the role of home peak flow meters to monitor the course of asthma (once the diagnosis has been established) and to assess the severity of asthmatic attacks. In this section we are considering peak flow meters as a tool for the diagnosis of asthma by recording expiratory flow at multiple points in time.

Bronchoprovocative challenge

In medical centers with extensive pulmonary function testing capabilities, a testing procedure may be available for persons suspected of asthma whose initial pulmonary function tests are normal. The concept is simple: if we suspect underlying bronchial hyperresponsiveness but find normal expiratory flow, we can try to provoke airway narrowing using a provocative stimulus, an asthma trigger. Pick a stimulus to which those with asthma react, whereas those without asthma do not, such as an allergen to which our patient is sensitive, exercise, or deep breathing of cold air. Measure lung function (spirometry) before and after the stimulus is administered. If the stimulus brings out airway narrowing (often with associated cough and chest tightness), we have demonstrated "twitchy airways" and probable asthma. If the stimulus causes no significant change in expiratory flow, the patient has normal bronchial responsiveness and a diagnosis of asthma is excluded.

The bronchoprovative challenge test is similar to the cardiac stress test in a person suspected of having coronary artery disease. This patient reports chest pains, but the electrocardiogram at the time of his office visit is normal. To pursue a possible diagnosis of angina, you arrange for an exercise stress test. Exercise is used to provoke myocardial ischemia, and with exercise you now find typical electrocardiographic changes of ischemic heart disease. By analogy, the bronchoprovocative challenge brings out airflow obstruction on pulmonary function testing in someone with asthma.

The provocative stimulus most widely used in pulmonary laboratories across the country is methacholine. Methacholine is a chemical substance closely related to the neurotransmitter, acetylcholine. It stimulates bronchial muscle contraction in all people, but those with asthma react to smaller doses and react with greater degrees of bronchial constriction. You may have misgivings about causing someone to have an asthma attack, but the test is done with great care. It begins with inhalation of a miniscule amount of methacholine, then measurement of lung function. If there is no significant decline in expiratory flow, the next largest concentration of methacholine is given and spirometry repeated. This sequence continues until expiratory flow decreases by 20% (a positive result) or until the largest dose of methacholine has been administered without a 20% decline in expiratory flow (a negative result). Severe airflow obstruction is very rarely precipitated by this test, and it can be reversed quickly by administration of bronchodilators.

A negative bronchoprovocative challenge test—indicative of normal bronchial responsiveness—excludes a diagnosis of asthma with greater than 95% certainty. A diagnostic answer is obtained immediately, and it does not rely on the precision of measurements made by the patient himself. The shortcomings of the test are: its expense (several hundred dollars); its lack of routine availability; and the fact that a positive result—indicative of bronchial hyperresponsiveness—is not definitive for asthma. A mild degree of bronchial hyperresponsiveness can be found in people with hay fever who do not have asthma and in a small percentage of normal people. On the other hand, a great degree of bronchial hyperresponsiveness (that is, when airflow obstruction develops after just a small dose of methacholine) is diagnostic of asthma.

KEY POINT   A negative methacholine bronchoprovocative challenge test reliably excludes a diagnosis of asthma.

To review, the best confirmatory test for asthma is the pulmonary function test called spirometry. The demonstration of airflow obstruction on exhalation that reverses to normal following a bronchodilator is diagnostic of asthma. This test requires a cooperative patient (usually 6–7 years of age or older) and may not identify asthma in an asthmatic person who at the time of testing has normal lung function. In this latter circumstance, other strategies include a therapeutic trial of antiasthmatic medication; home peak flow monitoring; and bronchoprovocative challenge testing. Each of these approaches has its own shortcomings. It would be helpful if we had a simpler, more reliable method for diagnosing asthma, including in young children. One exciting experimental prospect is measurement of exhaled nitric oxide.

Exhaled nitric oxide concentration

With spirometry or peak flow measurements, one can measure the reversible airways narrowing of asthma. With a methacholine challenge, one can test for the bronchial hyperresponsiveness of asthma. Wouldn't it be nice if we had a test that would assess for the bronchial inflammation of asthma—short of bronchial biopsies? Recently, there has been great interest in the possibility of measuring in the air one breathes out some marker that would distinguish airways with asthmatic inflammation from normal airways. Currently, the leading candidate is the gas, nitric oxide. Nitric oxide (NO) is formed by the superficial lining cells of the bronchi in larger amounts among people with asthma than among those without asthma. For tens of thousands of dollars, you can purchase a nitric oxide analyzer that will measure—in parts per billion quantities—the exhaled nitric oxide concentration of your patient. A high value points to a diagnosis of asthma; a low value is normal and argues against asthma. This new and exciting test is still experimental and is available in only a few very specialized asthma centers. Someday it may revolutionize how we diagnose asthma. (In the meantime, it is a topic not likely to be included on a standardized examination about asthma education.)

Other tests that may be helpful but are not conclusive

A 45-year-old baker has cough and shortness of breath, particularly at the end of the workday. She has heard about occupational asthma caused by exposure to flour dusts ("bakers' asthma") and is concerned that she may be developing asthma. Her doctor has ordered pulmonary function testing, but she asks you whether there isn't some other type of test that she can take to check for asthma. A blood test? CT scan? MRI? Allergy tests?

In fact, the answer is "no," she is on the right track with pulmonary function testing. Other tests may be useful to assess for allergic sensitivities and to exclude other diagnoses, but they won't answer the question of whether or not she has asthma.

For instance, it would be reasonable to obtain a chest x-ray to evaluate the new onset of cough and shortness of breath in a 45-year-old woman, but its purpose is to exclude a variety of other lung diseases, like pneumonia, pulmonary fibrosis, sarcoidosis, or lung cancer. The chest x-ray in asthma is usually normal. Even high-resolution computed tomographic (CT) scans cannot routinely detect the abnormalities of the airway walls that characterize asthma. To repeat, with rare exceptions (such as during severe asthmatic attacks or when there are unusual complicating illnesses), the chest x-ray in asthma is normal.

KEY POINT   The chest x-ray in asthma is almost always normal.

Allergy testing (by blood tests or allergy skin tests) may be useful in characterizing a patient's asthma. Perhaps we could test for allergy to flour dust in our patient, the baker. But the results will not tell us whether or not our patient has asthma. It is possible to be allergic to flour dust (or cats or dust mites), but not have asthma; and it is possible to have asthma and not to have allergies. As we will discuss in more detail in Chap. 7, "Identifying Allergic Sensitivities and Promoting Allergen Avoidance," allergy testing is often useful in the management of asthma, but it is not a diagnostic test to establish the presence or absence of asthma. In the same way, measurement of blood eosinophils or immunoglobulin E (IgE) concentrations can give you a sense of the patient's tendency to allergic reactions, but allergies cannot be equated with asthma. Many people with atopy (including hay fever and eczema) do not have asthma; and many people with asthma do not have allergies.

EXCLUDING ALTERNATIVE DIAGNOSES

We have considered here in some detail ways to establish (or exclude) a diagnosis of asthma with certainty. Perhaps you are thinking to yourself: "Well, what else could it be? The child or adult with wheezing, cough, and shortness of breath that come and go are almost always going to have asthma, aren't they?" As specialists in asthma care, we can assure you that misdiagnosis of asthma is common—in both directions. We encounter patients who have had some of the symptoms of asthma for years but failed to receive a correct diagnosis of asthma; and we have had patients labeled with a diagnosis of asthma who in fact had a different cause for their respiratory symptoms. The underdiagnosis and over-diagnosis of asthma are not rare. And we remind you that for you or your patient, the correct diagnosis is critical. You are less interested in what this constellation of findings usually means than in knowing, for you, exactly what is the diagnosis.

In children

In Chap. 5, "Special Considerations in Childhood Asthma," we will consider more extensively the special diagnostic challenges in children, particularly children too young to perform pulmonary function testing. Very young children (under age 4 years) are prone to wheezing with viral respiratory tract infections. Some have only wheezing-associated respiratory tract illness and grow out of these symptoms as they get older, others have asthma. The term, "reactive airways disease," has been widely used to describe this intermittent airway narrowing in small children (with their small airways) when a diagnosis of asthma remains in doubt.

Two other major considerations are worth mentioning here. One is cystic fibrosis, an inherited disease in which the bronchial tubes are affected by thickened mucus and chronic infection. Cough, wheeze, and shortness of breath are symptoms of cystic fibrosis as well, but the cause is chronic infection involving permanently damaged airways (bronchiectasis), not allergic-type inflammation. Potential clues to the diagnosis of cystic fibrosis include a family history of cystic fibrosis, sputum that is thick and discolored, bacteria often found on culture of the sputum, and findings outside of the chest: nasal polyps and recurrent sinus infections, chronic diarrhea, and impaired weight gain. Over time, the chest x-ray becomes abnormal in cystic fibrosis due to extensive inflammation surrounding the bronchial tubes. Once a doctor considers the possibility of cystic fibrosis, reliable diagnostic tests are available, including the sweat chloride test (to test for an abnormally high concentration of chloride in the child's sweat) and now a blood test for genetic typing.

The other alternative diagnosis important not to miss in young children is an aspirated foreign body. In this circumstance, airway narrowing is focal, the consequence of some solid material having been inadvertently inhaled into the bronchial tubes. A child's cough and wheezing may begin simultaneously with disappearance of a small plastic toy or toy part. The astute clinician may detect on examination that the child's wheezing is localized rather than widespread throughout the thorax as in asthma. A chest x-ray will reveal the foreign body only if it is metal (and therefore denser than all of the surrounding tissue), but it may suggest the presence of an aspirated foreign body because of a section of collapsed (unaerated) lung distal to the bronchial obstruction. Bronchoscopy can usually extract the foreign body, and—more than once—the procedure has *cured* a case of misdiagnosed asthma.

KEY POINT   Two important alternative diagnoses to consider in young children are cystic fibrosis and aspirated foreign bodies.

In adults

In middle-aged and older adults the cigarette-smoking related lung diseases, chronic bronchitis and emphysema, can be—and often are—confused with asthma (Table 2-2). Chronic bronchitis is a chronic inflammation of the bronchial tubes from the irritant effects of cigarette smoke. Mucus glands along the bronchial walls enlarge, leading to excess sputum production. The hallmark of chronic bronchitis is the "smoker's cough," daily expectoration of whitish sputum, especially first thing in the morning. The small airways can also become inflamed and narrowed, leading to breathlessness, particularly on exertion. The bronchial inflammation of chronic bronchitis looks different to the pathologist than the inflammation of asthma. Instead of mast cells and eosinophils, the white blood cells called polymorphonuclear leukocytes (also called *polys* or neutrophils) dominate in the inflammatory response.

Children and adults who have had frequent bouts of bronchitis (that is, frequent chest colds) have sometimes been labeled as having "chronic bronchitis." The truth is that they have recurrent bronchitis, and in between chest infections they are perfectly normal. The chronic bronchitis of cigarette smokers is present day in and day out, everyday.

By contrast, emphysema is not a disease primarily involving the bronchial tubes. In emphysema the inflammatory reaction to cigarette smoking attacks and degrades the walls of the airsacs (alveoli). Because the elastic substance of the lungs normally resides in those alveolar walls, emphysema leads to loss of the elastic springiness of the lungs. As mentioned in Chap. 1, in emphysema air

TABLE   2 - 2

DIFFERENCES BETWEEN ASTHMA AND COPD

Feature	Asthma	COPD
Age of onset	Childhood	Middle-age
Related to allergies	Yes, often	No
Due to cigarette smoking	No	Yes
Improvement following bronchodilator	Large	Small or none
Progressive decline in lung function	Rarely	Usually, with continued cigarette smoking

enters the lungs without difficulty, but the elastic force needed to drive air from the lungs on exhalation is lost. In addition, this same elasticity of the lungs normally helps to hold bronchial tubes open during exhalation. In its absence, even normal bronchial tubes have a tendency to collapse more readily than normal. As a consequence, emphysema causes the very same slowing of air emptying from the lungs on exhalation that is found in asthma and chronic bronchitis, even though emphysema is a disease of the alveolar walls, not the air tubes.

In susceptible individuals, long-term cigarette smoking (typically at least 1 pack of cigarettes per day for at least 20 years) can cause some degree of both chronic bronchitis and emphysema. When a cigarette smoker complains of cough and dyspnea, it is difficult for the clinician to sort out how much of the patient's symptoms can be attributed to chronic bronchitis and how much to emphysema. It has proven most useful to discuss these two lung diseases caused by cigarette smoking under the single heading of chronic obstructive pulmonary disease or COPD. (Others have preferred the label of chronic obstructive lung disease or COLD). COPD refers to chronic bronchitis and emphysema without any attempt to differentiate or quantify the contribution of the individual components.

On pulmonary function testing (spirometry), COPD causes obstruction to expiratory flow that is identical to the pattern seen in asthma. However, unlike in asthma, the obstruction does not tend to go away after administration of a quick-acting bronchodilator. An increase in expiratory flow of 15% or more following two puffs of albuterol is typical of asthma; a smaller or absent increase in expiratory flow following bronchodilator is characteristic of chronic bronchitis and emphysema. With smoking cessation, the daily cough and sputum production of chronic bronchitis often resolves. However, the airflow obstruction improves minimally or not at all. The scarring of the small airways (chronic bronchitis) and loss of lung elasticity (emphysema) are permanent.

KEY POINT   The pattern of airflow obstruction on spirometry is identical in persons with asthma and those with COPD. The distinction is made by assessing the reversibility of airflow obstruction after inhalation of a quick-acting bronchodilator.

With rare exceptions, COPD develops as a consequence of cigarette smoking. In a lifelong nonsmoker this diagnosis is unlikely. On the other hand, cigarette smokers can develop asthma, and, sadly, teenagers and adults with asthma often smoke cigarettes. And as we mentioned in Chap. 1, occasionally persons with long-standing asthma develop permanent airway narrowing, referred to as *airway remodeling*, and have features that mimic COPD. At times, distinguishing these entities can be tricky.

As a result, perhaps you won't be surprised by the results of a study published some years ago that found a gender bias in the diagnosis of asthma among adults. These researchers found that when cigarette-smoking patients came to their doctors complaining of cough and dyspnea on exertion, more often women were given a diagnosis of asthma whereas men were diagnosed with COPD. The perception at the time was that COPD was mostly a disease of men. Nowadays, as cigarette smoking has become an "equal-opportunity addiction," a diagnostic distinction based on gender seems less common. Still, we often encounter long-term cigarette smokers with COPD who come to us believing that they have asthma. Doctors would rather tell a patient—and patients would rather hear—of a diagnosis of asthma than of emphysema. The latter carries in the minds of many a frightening sense of inevitability, with progression to wheelchair dependence, need for chronic supplemental oxygen, and death. In fact, this inexorable progression is common in those people with COPD who continue to smoke cigarettes but is uncommon in those who are able to quit smoking.

It may catch you by surprise to learn that another common illness among adults, congestive heart failure, is also sometimes mistaken for asthma. We don't usually think of congestive heart failure as one of the obstructive lung diseases, but sometimes heart failure does cause wheezing. Perhaps you have heard of the expression "cardiac asthma," used to describe wheezing caused by congestive heart failure. And it certainly won't surprise you to think of heart failure as a chronic condition characterized by intermittent bouts of increased shortness of breath and coughing, much like asthma. Nighttime worsening of symptoms is also common in both conditions.

As you know, we have excellent tests to diagnose congestive heart failure, beginning with physical examination, a chest x-ray, and a new blood test (brain natriuretic peptide or BNP). What is necessary is for the clinician to consider the possibility of congestive heart failure as the cause of the patient's symptoms. Too often, we have found that among older individuals inhaled bronchodilators are prescribed for intermittent shortness of breath, without further consideration as to the etiology of symptoms.

STAGING THE SEVERITY OF ASTHMA

If you or your child were to be diagnosed with asthma, probably one of the first questions that would come to mind is: "How bad is my asthma?" The question acknowledges that the severity of asthma varies widely among different people. Some people with asthma seem to have quite severe disease, continuously troubled by their symptoms, requiring daily medications, and plagued with frequent attacks that are quite frightening. At the other extreme, some people seem to have mild disease with rare symptoms. They use their bronchodilator inhaler infrequently and remain fully active—as competitive athletes, sports people, and routine exercisers. "Where do I fit on this continuum?" your patient wonders.

Categorizing the severity of asthma is useful in ways other than satisfying your patient's natural curiosity about how he or she compares with other asthmatics. For one thing, it helps caregivers to match their treatments to the severity of the problem. Not all people with asthma require the same therapy. If we adjust the intensity of treatment according to the severity of asthma, it is best if we can clearly define that severity for all who are involved in the patient's care. On a broader scope, national guidelines have been developed that contain recommendations for asthma treatment across the entire spectrum of severities. Which treatment is most appropriate for my patient? The answer depends on what stage of severity you consider your patient to have.

One other example of the usefulness of categorizing asthma severity in a standardized way: when conducting medical research studies, it proves very helpful to enroll patients with similar degrees of asthma severity. For example, research subjects who receive a new drug for asthma should be matched in terms of disease severity with the subjects who receive placebo. And when it comes time to interpret the results of the study, the outcome can be applied to other patients with a similar degree of severity. Otherwise, the findings in subjects with mild asthma may not pertain to patients with severe asthma, or vice versa.

KEY POINT   A systematic approach to categorizing the severity of asthma helps in choosing the appropriate treatment for an individual patient, in disseminating recommendations for asthma treatment, and in designing medical experiments involving patients with asthma.

Origins of the national "Guidelines for the Diagnosis and Management of Asthma"

In 1990 the federal government through its National Institutes of Health organized a National Asthma Education Program (NAEP). It followed similar highly successful national education programs that had focused attention on the health hazards of high blood pressure and high cholesterol levels and that set standards for their treatment. The 1980s had seen a dramatic rise in the morbidity and mortality of asthma in the United States. The medical community rightly saw the need for an organized, multifaceted approach to this rising problem. The NAEP committed to raise public awareness about asthma as a potentially serious illness and to help care providers to deliver appropriate treatment.

The NAEP brought together many different groups to collaborate in this project, including medical societies, patient advocacy groups, and federal institutes, such as the National Heart, Lung, and Blood Institute and the National Institute of Allergy and Infectious Diseases. As part of their work, they assembled an "Expert Panel" to draft guidelines for assessing and treating asthma. The chairperson of this first Expert Panel was Dr. Albert Sheffer, a founding member of our Partners Asthma Center. The panel was broadly inclusive in its make-up, including physicians (both specialists and generalists), nurses, and health educators. The result of their deliberations was widely disseminated as a document called the *Guidelines for the Diagnosis and Management of Asthma*—often referred to simply as "the Asthma Guidelines."

The first version of the *Guidelines* was released in 1991. For many, it became the bible of asthma assessment and treatment in this country. Thereafter, the program was renamed as the National Asthma Education and Prevention Program, and in 1997 a reconstituted Expert Panel released its updated report: *Expert Panel Report 2: Guidelines for the Diagnosis and Management of Asthma* (NIH Publication No. 98-4051). This document is available online at the website of the National Heart, Lung and Blood Institute: www.nhlbi.nih.gov/guidelines/asthma/. As of this writing, the most recent update to these national guidelines was published in 2002. *Expert Panel Report: Guidelines for the Diagnosis and Management of Asthma—Update on Selected Topics 2002* (NIH Publication No. 02-5074) is accessible as both full report and quick reference summary at the same website cited above. Expert Panel Report 3 is currently in preparation as this book goes to press.

As an editorial aside, we recommend these documents to you as invaluable references about asthma and its treatment. They contain detailed information about the diagnosis, assessment, and treatment of asthma in children and adults in the ambulatory, emergency department, and inpatient settings. They represent the current consensus on how best to manage asthma, and they include useful patient educational materials. One other virtue: it is unlikely that a question asked on the National Asthma Educators Certification Board examination will not have its answer contained in these books.

Beginning in 1997 the Expert Panel members of the NAEPP have recommended that asthma severity be categorized into four steps. This recommendation is in accord with the guidelines prepared by an international group of asthma specialists assembled under the auspices of the Global Initiative for Asthma (*Global Strategy for Asthma Management and Prevention*, NIH Publication No. 02-3659; www.ginasthma.com). In brief, this system of categorizing asthma severity is now accepted worldwide.

Criteria for judging asthma severity

There are three key criteria used to assign patients to one of these four steps of asthma severity: daytime symptoms, nighttime symptoms, and lung function. The system is best applied when patients are newly diagnosed and have only a quick-acting bronchodilator to use for relief of symptoms. We begin by asking how often the patient experiences asthma symptoms (troublesome cough, bouts of wheezing, shortness of breath, or chest tightness). If he or she uses a quick-acting bronchodilator to relieve the symptoms, it is easy to ask: how often do you use your inhaled bronchodilator medication? Another way to ask the same question is to inquire how long on average does one canister of albuterol last—knowing that there are 200 puffs in each canister. We also ask how often do you have to interrupt what you are doing because of asthma. That is, how often do you find that an asthma attack interrupts your normal activities?

The second criterion is based on nighttime symptoms of asthma and assumes a normal cycle of wakefulness during the day and sleep during the night. We make it a part of our routine asthma history: How often does asthma wake you from your sleep at night? Asthma often worsens during the nighttime hours. You will perhaps be amazed to find how often people with asthma are woken from their sleep by chest symptoms, use their inhaler for relief, then go back to sleep. Many asthmatics routinely sleep with their bronchodilator inhaler tucked under their pillow or carefully placed on the nearby bedside table, so that it can be easily located when sleep is disturbed by coughing or chest discomfort. Those who can readily fall back to sleep may think nothing of it: waking with asthmatic symptoms has become a routine part of their lives. Unless you specifically ask about nighttime symptoms, they may fail to mention them to you.

The third criterion is lung function and specifically, expiratory airflow based on spirometry (FEV_1) or peak flow measurement (PEFR). It makes sense that in responding to a question of "how bad is my asthma," one would want to measure the degree of airway narrowing. The more narrowed the airways, the slower the flow of air from the chest even with maximal effort, and the worse the asthma.

KEY POINT   To categorize a patient's asthma according to severity, ask about daytime and nighttime symptoms and make a measurement of lung function.

For any given patient, what should the expiratory flow be? What is normal for that individual? There are two ways to answer that question. We will use the example of peak flow, because it is the measurement most commonly made. One way is to look up on a published table what the average peak flow value should be for a person of that particular gender, age, and height. That value is his predicted normal peak flow, and his test result can be expressed as a percentage of that predicted normal value. For instance, using Table 2-3, as a 5-foot-tall, 40-year-old woman, your predicted peak flow is 402 L/min. If you check your peak flow and find the measured value to be 300 L/min, at that moment your peak flow is 75% of the predicted average normal value, or, in brief, 75% of predicted.

A second way to determine your target peak flow is to measure your peak flow repeatedly at a time when you are feeling perfectly well. In this way you can determine your *personal best* peak flow—the best value that you have recorded over a few weeks of monitoring. Although this value should be close to the value predicted as normal for you in a table of normal values, it may not be exactly the same. For one thing, not all normal people of the same age, height, and gender have the exact same peak flow. There is a range of normal values (±100 L/min in men; ±80 L/min in women), and you need to find where within that range you lie. For another, it is possible that as a result of airway remodeling you have developed some amount of permanent scarring of your airways. Even at your best, your peak flow is less than normal. In judging your asthma severity, we will assess your peak flow with respect to your personal best when feeling entirely well, even if that best value is less than normal.

We are ready now to review the criteria for each of the four steps of asthma severity (Table 2-4).

TABLE 2-3

NORMAL PEAK FLOW TABLES

	Women (Height)						Men (Height)				
Age	55"	60"	65"	70"	75"	Age	60"	65"	70"	75"	80"
20	390	423	460	496	529	20	554	602	649	693	740
25	385	418	454	490	523	25	543	590	636	679	725
30	380	413	448	483	516	30	532	577	622	664	710
35	375	408	442	476	509	35	521	565	609	651	695
40	370	402	436	470	502	40	509	552	596	636	680
45	365	397	430	464	495	45	498	540	583	622	665
50	360	391	424	457	488	50	486	527	569	607	649
55	355	386	418	451	482	55	475	515	556	593	634
60	350	380	412	445	475	60	463	502	542	578	618
65	345	375	406	439	468	65	452	490	529	564	603
70	340	369	400	432	461	70	440	477	515	550	587

Adapted from: National Asthma Education Program Expert Panel Report, Guidelines for the Diagnosis and Management of Asthma. 1991.

STEP 1: MILD INTERMITTENT ASTHMA

Beginning in 1997, members of the Expert Panel of the NAEPP suggested that patients with mild asthma be divided into two separate steps: mild intermittent asthma and mild persistent asthma. The thinking behind this recommendation was the belief that some asthmatic patients whose lung function remained normal or near-normal should receive regular preventive medications—and others

TABLE 2-4

STEPS OF ASTHMA SEVERITY

Step	Daytime Symptoms	Nighttime Symptoms	Lung Function (FEV$_1$ or PEFR)	Peak Flow Variability
Mild intermittent	≤2 days/wk	≤2 nights/mo.	≥80	≤20%
Mild persistent	3–6 days/wk	3–4 nights/mo.	≥80	20–30%
Moderate persistent	Daily	≥5 nights/mo.	>60–<80%	>30%
Severe persistent	Continual	Frequent	≤60%	>30%

Adapted from: National Asthma Education and Prevention Program Expert Panel Report II, Guidelines for the Diagnosis and Management of Asthma. 1997.

not—based primarily on the frequency of their symptoms. Those with relatively frequent symptoms would feel better if they took preventive medication every day; those with more infrequent symptoms could treat those symptoms with quick-relief medications on an as-needed basis. The dividing line between the two steps is, of necessity, somewhat arbitrary. It reflects the consensus of the Expert Panel about what level of symptomatic discomfort from asthma is unacceptable and should be prevented by daily medication use.

Step 1, mild intermittent asthma, identifies those patients whose asthma is deemed sufficiently mild not to warrant daily preventive (anti-inflammatory) medication. These patients on average have symptoms of their asthma (cough, chest tightness, wheeze, or breathlessness) no more than two times per week, and they are awakened from their sleep by asthmatic symptoms no more than two times per month. When you (or they) check their lung function, their expiratory flow (FEV_1 or PEFR) is 80% of normal or greater. If they check their peak flow when symptomatic, their peak flow dips by no more than 20% below their best values. They rarely experience asthmatic attacks.

Perhaps in order to judge the severity of her asthma, you have asked your patient how often in a typical week she uses her quick-acting bronchodilator inhaler, such as albuterol. She responds that she uses it every day before exercising at the gym to prevent exercise-induced symptoms, but she almost never needs it at any other time. Does this daily use of a bronchodilator medication make her asthma more severe than mild intermittent? We don't think so. The goal of therapy is prevention of asthmatic symptoms. If use of a quick-acting bronchodilator prior to exercise reliably achieves that goal, no additional medication is needed. If the bronchodilator is needed to *alleviate* asthmatic symptoms more than twice per week, then her asthma step is no longer mild intermittent asthma.

A quick reminder: even patients with mild intermittent asthma have underlying chronic, persistent airway inflammation and "twitchy airways," as discussed in Chap. 1. Symptoms of asthma may be infrequent and intermittent; the basic asthmatic inflammation of the airways is present all the time, every day.

STEP 2: MILD PERSISTENT ASTHMA

Imagine that you counsel a young woman about her asthma. When you see her in a medical facility, she looks entirely well and very fit. Her chest examination is free of wheezes. Her peak flow measured with your peak flow meter is 100% of normal. She has a quick-acting inhaled bronchodilator that she uses whenever she experiences her asthmatic symptoms, generally achieving quick relief. On the surface, all seems well.

What the national asthma guidelines have taught us is that we need to probe deeper before categorizing the severity of her asthma. We need to ask exactly how often she needs to use her inhaled bronchodilator for relief of symptoms; how often she awakens from sleep because of her asthma; and how often she experiences asthmatic attacks. Has she ever checked her peak flow when suffering an asthmatic exacerbation? How low did the peak flow fall?

If she indicates that she uses her inhaled bronchodilator to relieve symptoms more than twice per week but less than once daily, she is considered to have mild persistent asthma. If she wakes from sleep because of asthma more than twice monthly (but not more than once weekly), she has mild persistent asthma. An asthmatic exacerbation should occur less than twice weekly and may affect her activity. If her peak flow falls no more than 30% below her best values with these exacerbations, she has mild persistent asthma.

When you ask these probing questions about asthma symptoms and frequency of bronchodilator use, you will be amazed how much asthma lies just below the surface of apparent well-being. Remember that when your patient sees you at the medical facility, it may be her best time of the day (or week). The environment is clean, the temperature comfortable, she is at rest, and her daytime lung function is typically better than nighttime. Only by inquiring further do we learn about her asthma severity in the context of her daily home/work/school environments and activities, including sleep.

KEY POINT By asking questions about the frequency of asthmatic symptoms, including nighttime symptoms, you will often uncover information about the severity of asthma not evident at the moment of a daytime medical office visit.

STEP 3: MODERATE PERSISTENT ASTHMA

Consider this scenario: a mother brings her 8-year-old child to see you for advice about his asthma. She is frustrated because he seems always sick. He has episodes of cough and wheezing every day. Two or three times each week he is up at night, coughing and laboring to breathe. His albuterol inhaler runs out before the next refill, which is due to be filled at the pharmacy at the end of each month. When he was seen by the doctor, his peak flow was only 70% of what a boy his age should have. When his asthma acts up—as it does a couple of times each week—he can't continue to play with the other children but needs to rest quietly for the remainder of the day.

This child has moderate persistent asthma. The criteria for this step of asthma severity are: daily symptoms; daily use of an inhaled quick-acting bronchodilator for relief of symptoms; nighttime awakenings more than once weekly; measured expiratory flow (FEV_1 or PEFR) greater than 60% of normal (or personal best) but less than 80%; and asthmatic exacerbations that occur two or more times per week and limit normal activities.

These set of symptoms—daytime, nighttime, and with activity—and level of lung function are grouped together with the thought that they are features of asthma of a certain intensity (moderate persistent). When airway inflammation and bronchial hyperresponsiveness are present to this degree, it is thought that one will see symptoms of this severity and airway narrowing in this range. But of course not every patient fits perfectly into this portrait of moderate persistent asthma. For example, some patients have some symptoms of asthma every day but rarely wake from their sleep with asthma; others have reduced lung function (60–80% of normal) but relatively infrequent asthmatic symptoms. The national guidelines indicate that if *any* feature of the patient's asthma is this severe, the patient should be designated as having moderate persistent asthma.

STEP 4: SEVERE PERSISTENT ASTHMA

Other than for the level of lung function, the distinction between moderate persistent asthma and severe persistent asthma is somewhat fuzzy. Symptomatic patients with an FEV_1 or PEFR less than 60% of normal (or of their personal best value) have severe persistent asthma. Patients with symptoms even worse than those described for moderate persistent asthma have severe disease. Thus, a patient with asthmatic symptoms most all of the time, with frequent nocturnal awakenings due to asthma (many nights per week and often more than once per night), with exacerbations that prevent work or school or normal activities of daily living and that occur frequently—that patient has severe persistent asthma.

Applying the stepwise criteria

The Expert Panel members offered three footnotes or clarifications about applying the asthma steps to specific patients, and we add a fourth reminder here.

1. As we have already noted, not every patient will have all of the features of a particular step. Symptoms may be mild but peak flow markedly reduced. Nighttime symptoms may be frequent, but during the day the patient feels well. How should one categorize a patient's asthma severity when some features are appropriate to one step and other features are appropriate to a different step? The guidelines are clear on this point: choose the most severe category. Here's an example: a patient reports to you that her asthma is doing well. She has an albuterol inhaler but rarely uses it. Her sleep is rarely if ever disturbed by asthmatic symptoms. She admits to living a very sedentary life. When you check her lung function, her expiratory flow (FEV_1 or PEFR) is only 65% of normal. She has moderate persistent asthma—based on the most severe aspect of her disease, her low lung function.

2. The severity of a patient's asthma can vary over time. The child who leaves home and escapes a house full of pets may note improvement in his asthma. The category to which he is assigned should be changed, with the understanding that his treatment should also be adjusted appropriately. Some people will have features of moderate persistent asthma during their allergy seasons (for example, spring and fall), with mild persistent asthma the rest of the year. The implication is that as their asthma improves or intensifies, their preventive treatment should be adjusted accordingly. From our understanding of asthma pathophysiology, as discussed in Chap. 1, this

variation makes sense. Fuel the fire of asthmatic inflammation with inhaled allergens, and it burns more intensely—and more treatment is needed to extinguish it. Withdraw those inciters of inflammation, and usually the swelling and sensitivity of the airways lessen—and treatment can be decreased accordingly.

3. Patients with any degree of asthma severity are susceptible to exacerbations of their asthma, including severe asthmatic attacks. In the words of the Expert Panel: "Patients with any level of severity can have mild, moderate, or severe exacerbations. Some patients with intermittent asthma experience severe and life-threatening exacerbations separated by long periods of normal lung function and no symptoms." The take-home point here is that even patients with mild asthma need to be aware of the possibility of asthmatic attacks. As asthma educators we need to help prepare all of our asthmatic patients for dealing with such attacks.

KEY POINT   Patients with any degree of asthma severity can suffer asthmatic exacerbations, including severe, life-threatening attacks.

4. "How often do you use your albuterol inhaler?" is often used as an alternative version for inquiring about how often a patient has symptoms of cough, wheeze, chest tightness, or shortness of breath. As discussed earlier, a patient who needs to use a quick-acting bronchodilator every day for relief of asthmatic symptoms has moderate persistent asthma. We simply caution you here that some patients use their quick-acting bronchodilator as part of their daily medication routine or as a *reflex* or habit under certain circumstances (for example, "whenever I go out in the cold"). Some patients will have been told in the past to use their bronchodilator inhaler four times a daily on a regular basis and continue to do so. This pattern of use does not necessarily indicate severe persistent asthma. In applying the steps of asthma severity, frequency of bronchodilator use is meant to equate with frequency of troubling asthmatic symptoms requiring quick relief.

Limitations of the staging system

The staging of asthma into four categories or steps is the foundation for recommendations by the Expert Panel members of the NAEPP for asthma treatment tailored to disease severity. (We will review this step-care approach to asthma treatment in Chap. 4, "Treating Asthma in the Ambulatory Setting"). Their purpose has been to help clinicians choose an intensity of treatment matched to the severity of disease. As a result, their recommendations are based on the premise that patients initially have only a short-acting bronchodilator to use for quick relief of symptoms; additional treatment is guided by how severe asthma symptoms are and the level of lung function. However, as you know, many of the patients whom you encounter are already taking one or more medications for their asthma on a regular basis. How then can one stage the severity of their disease? How do you compare the severity of asthma among two people: one has daily symptoms on a low-intensity treatment regimen, such as a low-dose of an inhaled steroid; and the other has symptoms only once or twice a week but requires a high-intensity treatment program, including daily oral steroids for control?

The published guidelines are vague on this subject. In our opinions, a reasonable approach is to increase the step of asthma severity by one category when symptoms or low lung function occurs despite appropriate preventive treatment for asthma (prescribed and taken appropriately). Our recommendation is supported by the set of guidelines issued by the international committee of experts who prepared the recommendations of the Global Initiative for Asthma, called the GINA guidelines.

KEY POINT Increase the step of asthma severity if a patient's symptoms of asthma and reduced peak flow occur despite taking optimal daily preventive medication.

For instance, a patient with cough and chest tightness four to five times per week and nocturnal awakenings three to four times per month due to cough and wheeze (manifestations of mild persistent asthma) who is already taking a daily inhaled corticosteroid (recommended treatment for mild persistent asthma) should be considered to have moderate persistent asthma. In the step-care management of asthma, this patient will need treatment appropriate for moderate persistent asthma to achieve good control of his or her symptoms. If this same patient had signs and symptoms of moderate persistent asthma (daily symptoms and frequent nocturnal awakenings; peak flow 60–80% of normal or of personal best) despite daily preventive medication, then the appropriate category would be severe persistent asthma. Any patient who is being treated with daily or alternate-day oral steroids (prednisone or methylprednisolone) for asthma should be considered to have severe persistent asthma.

The asthma guidelines note that even patients with mild intermittent asthma can on occasion suffer serious asthmatic exacerbations. They do not specify how one should categorize a patient with mild intermittent asthma who has just required emergency medical treatment for a severe asthmatic attack. Since evidence is clear that regular preventive asthma medication reduces the risk of subsequent asthmatic attacks requiring emergency department care, we would argue that such patients be considered to have persistent asthma and be treated with daily preventive medication. If the trigger for the exacerbation is identifiable and avoidable, perhaps the preventive medication can be stopped after a period of a few months and the patient is considered again to have mild intermittent asthma.

CASE EXAMPLES

Here are three case examples of people with asthma for you to evaluate and to apply the four-step system of asthma severity. If you are preparing to take the National Asthma Educators Certification Board examination, remember that multiple-choice examinations need to avoid ambiguity and controversy; the cases provided as part of the examination will be clear-cut.

▶ ▶ ▶ CASE 1

Peter is a 10-year-old boy brought by his mother for a general medical check-up. He was diagnosed with asthma at age 3 and has been using an albuterol inhaler for the last 3 years. His pediatrician asks you, as asthma educator, to spend some time with him and his mom to review his asthma.

You inquire how often he experiences his asthma symptoms, such as coughing, tightness in his chest, or difficulty with his breathing. He relates to you that approximately two to three times a week he finds it difficult to breathe and needs to find the school nurse so that he can be given his bronchodilator medication. Sometimes running with his friends brings on his symptoms; sometimes they come on even when he is sitting quietly in class.

When you ask him and his mother about his sleeping, they agree that he awakens with cough and chest congestion more often than either would like. They find it hard to say precisely how often this happens, but estimate approximately once every one to two weeks.

They do not have a peak flow meter at home. You measure his peak flow in the office, and find it to be 100% of normal for a boy of his height. His mother inquires: "How bad do you think Peter's asthma is?"

What category of severity does he have?

Peter has *mild persistent asthma*. He has daytime symptoms of asthma more than twice per week (but less than daily); he has nighttime symptoms of asthma more than twice per month (but not more than once weekly). As we will discuss in Chap. 4, the implication of this categorization of his asthma is the understanding that he should be begun at this time on regular preventive medication for his asthma. Even though he looks perfectly healthy, even though his expiratory flow is perfectly normal at the time of his office visit, he is troubled by relatively frequent asthmatic symptoms—which can be prevented. With daily preventive medication he will rarely need to interrupt his school day because of asthma symptoms, and he (and his mother) will be able to sleep the night through without disturbance due to asthma. By placing his asthma severity at the correct step, you help direct his therapy to the appropriate intensity.

▶ ▶ ▶ CASE 2

A 27-year-old investment banker wonders if she should be doing something more to treat her asthma. She had troublesome symptoms as an adolescent, but after approximately age 18 her asthma seemed to abate. For years she felt that her asthma had gone away. However, in the last two years she has again begun to experience asthmatic symptoms. She obtained an over-the-counter bronchodilator (Primatene Mist) and uses it whenever she feels that her symptoms flare up.

She doesn't need her bronchodilator medication often. If she goes for a long run on a winter day, she might need it at the end of the run. Also, when she visits her in-laws' home (and their pet cat) on holidays, she develops wheezing and a runny nose and uses her inhaler then. She mostly sleeps well without chest symptoms, although she recalls waking once last month because of cough and wheezing. On that occasion she got out of bed, made herself some tea, and then gradually felt better over the ensuing hour or so.

She brings a diary of peak flow measurements that she has made over the last several months. Her peak flow at home has been consistently between 400 and 450 L/min (normal for her age and height). On the night when her asthma woke her from sleep, she recorded her peak flow at 350 L/min. In the office today she has had spirometry performed; her FEV_1 was 92% of predicted.

How would you classify her asthma?

She has *mild intermittent asthma*. Her daytime symptoms occur two or fewer times per week; her nighttime symptoms bother her two or fewer times per month. Her lung function has been consistently within the normal range. When she is symptomatic, her peak flow falls by less than 20% from her usual value when she feels well (her personal best). These are the features of mild intermittent asthma.

Based on this assessment, it will be recommended that her treatment remain intermittent use of her bronchodilator on an as-needed basis. In Chap. 4, we will discuss some helpful suggestions that you might offer her, including use of prescription rather than over-the-counter bronchodilator and preventive use of her bronchodilator *prior to* exercise.

▶ ▶ ▶ CASE 3

Charles A. Davis is a 60-year-old high-school teacher. He is referred to see you for discussion of his asthma, which has been interfering with his work lately. He was first diagnosed with asthma two years ago, when he began experiencing episodic shortness of breath, particularly when walking fast or climbing stairs. Sometimes he would waken from sleep, sit up quickly, and find himself gasping for his air. He was given a quick-acting bronchodilator to use whenever he experienced these symptoms, and he found it somewhat helpful.

Six months ago he moved into a new home. It is a nineteenth century farmhouse with attached barn. He and his wife greatly enjoy their new home, but he has found that his breathing has worsened. Almost every day he uses his bronchodilator inhaler, sometimes two or three times each day. It is embarrassing for him to have to leave his students in his class to step outside and use his medication. He finds it difficult climbing the one flight of stairs up to the faculty lounge during school breaks. Although his sleeping has been better, he still wakes up with shortness of breath and tightness in his chest at least once every month.

He appears quite comfortable in the office today. His chest exam is normal, and his peak flow is likewise 95% of the normal predicted value. He is pleased with the result and wonders out loud: "maybe it is all in my head."

How would you categorize his asthma?

Mr. Davis appears to have *moderate persistent asthma*. His symptoms occur virtually every day and interfere with his routine daily activities. He needs to use his bronchodilator medication daily. These are features of moderate persistent asthma. Even though his nighttime awakenings are fewer than three times per month (as in mild intermittent asthma) and his lung function is normal (as in mild intermittent asthma and mild persistent asthma), he should be classified according to the feature that indicates the most severe disease (the highest step). It is predicted that treatment appropriate to the category of moderate persistent asthma will be needed to bring his symptoms under control.

KEY POINT   When not all aspects of a patient's condition fit into one asthma category, stage the severity according to the feature of the disease that puts the patient in the most severe category (highest step).

You receive *extra credit* if besides concluding that this patient has moderate persistent asthma, you wonder whether indeed he has asthma at all. Perhaps he has "adult-onset asthma," but at your visit with him today you cannot confirm the presence of asthma. On chest exam, he has none of the typical wheezing of asthma, and his expiratory flow is normal. His symptoms of exertional dyspnea and nighttime awakening with chest tightness might be due to another common disease of middle-aged men: coronary artery disease with congestive heart failure. The fact that his initials are C.A.D. might make you doubly suspicious!

AN OVERVIEW OF ASTHMA SEVERITY IN THE UNITED STATES

In 1998 a large nationwide telephone survey was conducted in the United States in an attempt to characterize the severity of asthma using the four-step system designed by the Expert Panel of the NAEPP. Adults with asthma were interviewed about their symptoms; parents provided information for children less than 16 years of age. No lung function data were available. To identify people with asthma, the surveyors systematically screened a national sample of 42,022 households. Information on just over 2500 people with asthma was collected, giving a snapshot of asthma in America at that time. The findings of this study are available on-line at www.asthmainamerica.com.

Overall, approximately 40% of those interviewed reported symptoms consistent with mild intermittent asthma, and the other categories (mild persistent,

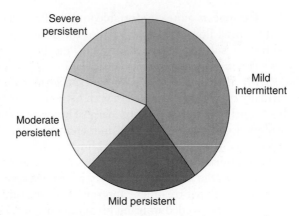

FIGURE 2-6   *Conducted in 1998, the Asthma in America telephone survey of 42,000 households across the United States provided information about the severity of asthma among 2500 persons with this condition. From: www.asthmainamerica.com.*

moderate persistent, and severe persistent) each held 20% of the total population. Comparing adults with children, more adults fit the description of moderate persistent and severe persistent; more children were considered to have mild intermittent asthma (Fig. 2-6).

These same data were subsequently reanalyzed by researchers at Brigham and Women's Hospital and elsewhere, who made two additional observations of interest. For their analysis, these researchers studied only the telephone responses of the adult patients, and they combined the categories of moderate persistent and severe persistent into one. First, they found strong associations between the stage of asthma and measures of asthma morbidity (besides daytime and nighttime symptoms). Compared to those with mild intermittent asthma, persons with moderate-to-severe persistent asthma over the preceding year had four times as many hospitalizations for their asthma, required urgent care twice as often, and missed more than 5 days of work four times more often.

Second, these investigators found that categorizing asthma based only on daytime and nighttime symptoms may have underestimated the burden of disease. If they included in their analysis a measure of the functional impact of asthma, the picture changed considerably. Two-thirds of those interviewed indicated that asthma had *some* or *a lot* of impact on their physical activity. Incorporating these responses into their staging schema, they found that 77% of respondents had moderate or severe persistent asthma and only 10% truly had mild intermittent disease.

The inescapable conclusion from these and other studies is that we, as asthma educators, have our work cut out for us. The burden of asthma is huge, and we are falling short—by far—of our ambitious goals for asthma care, which include infrequent asthmatic symptoms and unimpeded exercise capacity. Add to this the observations that fewer than 30% of the adult respondents to the telephone survey had used controller medications within the 4 weeks prior and more than 30% had active or passive cigarette smoke exposure in their homes, and you can see the great need for intensive asthma education.

Self-Assessment Questions

QUESTION 1

Which of the following historical features would be atypical of asthma?

1. Intermittent wheezing
2. Cough with white or clear phlegm
3. Episodes of tightness in the chest
4. Pleuritic pain under both sides of the rib cage anteriorly
5. Shortness of breath immediately following exercise

QUESTION 2

The presence of other atopic diseases may support your suspicion that a patient's symptoms are due to asthma. Which of the following is not considered an atopic disease?

1. Penicillin allergy
2. Hives
3. Seasonal allergic rhinitis (hay fever)
4. Perennial allergic rhinitis
5. Eczema

QUESTION 3

Which of the following physical findings is characteristic of asthma?

1. Nasal polyps
2. Musical expiratory wheezes heard throughout the chest
3. Expiratory wheezing heard loudest over the trachea
4. Wheezing of a single musical note heard best over the left anterior chest
5. Bilateral symmetric wheezing heard on each breath beginning near the end of exhalation

QUESTION 4

Based on a history of persistent cough of 3–4 months' duration, you suspect a possible diagnosis of asthma. Pulmonary function testing is likely to provide the most reliable information in which of the following patients?

1. A 4-year-old boy accompanied by his mother
2. A 9-year-old girl with braces on her teeth
3. A young man with profound mental retardation
4. A young woman with recent rib fracture
5. A middle-aged man sedated for alcohol withdrawal symptoms

QUESTION 5

Which of the following test results points most strongly to a diagnosis of asthma?

1. Multiple positive allergy skin tests, including to dust mite, cats, dogs, and mold
2. An elevated blood eosinophil count
3. An elevated blood immunoglobulin E (IgE) level
4. Hyperinflation on chest x-ray
5. A reduced expiratory flow on spirometry that reverses following bronchodilator

QUESTION 6

A 30-year-old woman complains of cough and chest tightness that she finds most troublesome during the daytime when she is at her work as a baker. While at the doctor's office, she feels well. Her chest exam and spirometry are normal. Which of the following tests might be useful to assess further the possibility of asthma?

1. Chest computed tomography (CT scan)
2. Oxygen saturation (by pulse oximetry) at rest and with exercise
3. Peak flow monitoring before and after her work shift
4. Skin testing for allergy to wheat
5. A detailed family history for asthma and allergies

QUESTION 7

Which of the following statements about methacholine bronchoprovocative challenges is true?

1. The test can be safely performed regardless of the degree of airflow obstruction noted on initial pulmonary function testing.
2. For safety reasons, the test requires overnight hospitalization.
3. Only persons with asthma develop airflow obstruction in response to methacholine.
4. The test is contraindicated in children (<18 years of age).
5. Persons who do not develop airflow obstruction in response to methacholine almost always do not have asthma.

QUESTION 8

A 16-year-old high-school senior comes to see you prior to the start of football season. He reports having had asthma for 10–12 years and uses an albuterol inhaler (Ventolin) whenever he experiences symptoms of his asthma. Which of the following questions would not be helpful as you assess what step of severity best describes his asthma?

1. How often do you use your albuterol (Ventolin) inhaler?

2. How often do you wake at night with symptoms of your asthma?

3. How often do you experience asthmatic attacks?

4. How many flights of stairs can you climb before needing to stop to catch your breath?

5. What number do you get when you check your peak flow at home?

QUESTION 9

Which of the following statements about the stage (or step) of asthma severity is correct?

1. Like asthma itself, the stage of asthma severity is inherited.

2. Assign a patient to that stage to which the *majority* of his or her signs and symptoms apply.

3. The stage of asthma severity can vary with the seasons.

4. A patient requiring inhaled steroids every day for treatment of asthma is automatically assigned to the severe persistent category.

5. Not every patient with asthma can be assigned to one of the four proposed categories of asthma severity.

For Questions 10–12: *To what step of asthma severity would you assign the following patient?*

QUESTION 10 (CASE EXAMPLE 1)

A 12-year-old girl is brought to the school infirmary because of shortness of breath. She was playing soccer earlier today, a cold October morning, and developed wheezing and shortness of breath. Her coach said that she had been gasping for her air and for a brief while could not speak at all. She used her albuterol inhaler, taking four puffs in rapid succession, and now is beginning to feel better.

She reports that in general she rarely needs her albuterol. She last used it sometime in the Spring. She never wakes from her sleep due to asthma and has never had a severe attack requiring emergency department treatment or hospitalization. After she has sat in the office for a while, you check her peak flow. It is 350 L/min, a normal value for a girl of her height.

1. Mild intermittent asthma

2. Mild persistent asthma

3. Moderate persistent asthma

4. Severe persistent asthma

QUESTION 11 (CASE EXAMPLE 2)

A mother brings her 6-year-old son to their neighborhood health center for treatment of his asthma. She is clearly frustrated by his health problems. He has missed school 10 days in the last 3 months because of his asthma. Nearly every night over the last several months, he has been waking with cough and sounds of chest congestion. Although normally active during the day, he prefers to play inside. She has given him cough drops, Robitussin cough syrup, and warm tea with milk to help control his symptoms. At night she will sometimes take him into the bathroom and turn on the shower with very hot water to create a warm mist for him to breathe.

On your inspection, he appears to be a healthy young boy. His height and weight are normal for his age. His chest examination reveals bilateral musical wheezes on exhalation. The remainder of his examination is normal.

1. Mild intermittent asthma
2. Mild persistent asthma
3. Moderate persistent asthma
4. Severe persistent asthma

QUESTION 12 (CASE EXAMPLE 3)

A 21-year-old college student presents to the health services office complaining of a severe head cold. In speaking with her about her symptoms, it comes out that she has asthma. She reports that she has never had a severe attack of asthma and manages with intermittent use of her bronchodilator inhaler, albuterol. She uses her albuterol whenever she develops shortness of breath or tightness in her chest, generally three to four times per week. At night she always makes sure that her inhaler is placed close at hand on her bedside table. If she wakes at night with cough or chest congestion—as she does approximately once every 1–2 weeks—she takes two inhalations from her inhaler and generally can fall back to sleep within 10–15 minutes.

On examination, she is afebrile; her throat is mildly erythematous; and her chest is entirely clear to auscultation. You measure her peak expiratory flow; it is 400 L/min, a normal value of a woman of her age and height.

1. Mild intermittent asthma
2. Mild persistent asthma
3. Moderate persistent asthma
4. Severe persistent asthma

Answers to Self-Assessment Questions

ANSWER TO QUESTION 1 (THE MEDICAL HISTORY IN ASTHMA)

The correct answer is #4; pleuritic pain implies pleural irritation, which is not a feature of asthma. You probably recognize the other answers as representing typical symptoms of asthma: intermittent wheezing (answer #1); cough with clear or white phlegm (answer #2); episodic chest tightness (answer #3); and shortness of breath brought on by exercising (answer #5). Occasionally, expectorated phlegm in asthma may be yellow, made yellow not by bacterial infection but by the accumulation of eosinophils in the sputum. In describing their chest discomfort, patients with asthma will sometimes use words similar to those used to describe angina: "tightness," a "weight on my chest," a "tight band around my chest."

ANSWER TO QUESTION 2 (IDENTIFYING ATOPIC DISEASES)

The correct answer is #1; penicillin allergy may not mediated by immunoglobulin E, mast cells, and eosinophils and does not occur more commonly in people with asthma than in those without asthma. The other answers—hives (answer #2); seasonal allergic rhinitis (answer #3); perennial allergic rhinitis (answer #4); and eczema (answer #5)—are all illnesses that are associated with asthma. Like asthma, they share features of the same allergic-type immune mechanism, involving immunoglobulin E, mast cells, and chemical mediators of inflammation like histamine. Their presence increases the likelihood that a patient's respiratory symptoms may be due to asthma.

ANSWER TO QUESTION 3 (PHYSICAL FINDINGS IN ASTHMA)

The correct answer is #2 (musical expiratory wheezes heard throughout the chest). Often the physical examination of a person with asthma is entirely normal. However, a common and characteristic abnormal finding in the presence of airway narrowing due to asthma is musical wheezing, most often present on exhalation, and sometimes present on both inspiration and expiration. Nasal polyps (answer #1) are found in a small minority of patients with asthma (and in some patients with cystic fibrosis). Expiratory wheezing heard loudest over the trachea (answer #3) suggests upper airway narrowing, not the widespread intrathoracic airway narrowing of asthma. A localized wheeze (answer #4) is heard in people with focal airway narrowing, as may occur with aspirated foreign bodies or endobronchial tumors. Some people with emphysema will have wheezing that occurs late in exhalation, at the same point during exhalation with each breath, and continues until the end of exhalation (answer #5).

ANSWER TO QUESTION 4 (COOPERATION WITH PULMONARY FUNCTION TESTING)

The correct answer is #2 (9-year-old girl with braces on her teeth). Braces do not interfere in any way with performance of pulmonary function testing. The other answers point out the need of a cooperative patient able to understand instructions and to give a forceful expiratory effort. Children younger than age 6 years (answer #1) are rarely able to perform the forced expiratory maneuver needed for spirometry. Inability to understand directions (answer #3), to take a maximal breath in due to chest pain (answer #4), or give a forceful effort due to sedation (answer #5) would preclude reliable test results.

ANSWER TO QUESTION 5 (DIAGNOSTIC TESTS FOR ASTHMA)

The correct answer is #5. Reversible airway narrowing (causing reversible airflow obstruction on pulmonary function testing) is a characteristic feature of asthma.

Multiple positive allergy skin tests (answer #1), an elevated eosinophil count in the peripheral blood (answer #2), and an increased immunoglobulin E (IgE) blood level (answer #3) all point to the presence of allergic disease (atopy). They do not, however, point specifically to asthma. A patient without asthma who has nasal, ocular, or skin allergies may have positive skin test reactions, peripheral blood eosinophilia, and increased blood IgE levels. And a patient with nonallergic asthma may have all negative allergy skin tests and normal blood eosinophil count and IgE level. Hyperinflation on chest x-ray (answer #4) is most suggestive of emphysema; it may also be encountered during a severe asthma attack.

ANSWER TO QUESTION 6 (ASSESSING FOR ASTHMA WHEN AN INITIAL PULMONARY FUNCTION TEST IS NORMAL)

The correct answer is # 3. Peak flow values that are normal before the workshift, then fall during and after exposure to wheat allergen, would suggest possible occupational asthma. In effect, peak flow monitoring allows measurement of lung function at times other than when the patient is at the doctor's office and particularly when the patient is actively experiencing symptoms. The chest CT scan (answer #1) is generally unremarkable in asthma. One would expect normal oxygen saturation at rest and with exercise (answer #2) if testing is performed when the patient feels well and has normal lung function. Demonstration of skin test allergy to wheat (answer #4) might suggest a susceptibility to developing asthma in a baker, but it would not document the presence (or absence) of asthma. Likewise, a strong family history of asthma and allergies (answer #5) may predispose to the development of asthma, but it does not help establish a diagnosis in our particular patient.

ANSWER TO QUESTION 7 (ASPECTS OF THE METHACHOLINE BRONCHO-PROVOCATIVE CHALLENGE)

The correct answer is #5. Almost all persons with asthma (approximately 95%) will develop airflow obstruction in response to methacholine. A negative methacholine challenge weighs strongly against a diagnosis of asthma. The test is usually performed only in persons with normal or near-normal lung function at the start of testing. The presence of significant airflow obstruction on initial pulmonary function testing (answer #1) would pose serious risk for precipitating a severe asthmatic attack during the testing. Methacholine testing is routinely performed in the outpatient setting; overnight hospitalization (answer #2) is not necessary. Airflow obstruction (due to bronchial muscle constriction) characteristically develops in response to inhalation of methacholine in persons with asthma; but the same response can also be found in other respiratory diseases, such as chronic obstructive pulmonary disease and cystic fibrosis. Some people with hay fever and even a small percentage of normal people will also react to high concentrations of methacholine (answer #3). Testing can safely be employed in children who are old enough to perform repeated spirometries (answer #4); methacholine is nontoxic.

ANSWER TO QUESTION 8 (CRITERIA FOR JUDGING THE STAGE OF ASTHMA SEVERITY)

The correct answer is #4. There is no stair climbing question included in the guidelines for assessing asthma severity! The four steps of asthma severity (mild intermittent asthma, mild persistent asthma, moderate persistent asthma, and severe persistent asthma) are based on the following: (1) frequency of daytime asthmatic symptoms (answer #1); (2) frequency of nighttime awakenings due to asthma (answer #2); (3) frequency and severity of asthmatic exacerbations (answer #3); and severity of airway narrowing as judged by peak expiratory flow or FEV_1 measured on spirometry (answer #5).

ANSWER TO QUESTION 9 (USING THE FOUR STAGES OR STEPS OF ASTHMA SEVERITY)

The correct answer is #3. Intense allergen exposure can worsen asthma severity; removal of allergens from a patient's environment can alleviate the severity of asthma. As a result, for some patients the intensity of asthma treatment may appropriately vary in different seasons. It is not known to what extent there is a genetic basis for asthma severity (answer #1); exposure to asthma triggers and inciters of asthmatic inflammation in the environment is known to play a major role. Patients with criteria for asthma severity that apply to more than one asthma step should be assigned to the most severe step to which *any* criterion applies (answer #2). The current system for staging asthma severity is best applied to patients who are using only quick-acting bronchodilators for relief of symptoms. Nonetheless, the use of inhaled steroids may be appropriate to patients with mild persistent asthma, moderate persistent asthma, or severe persistent asthma (answer #4). It is assumed that *every* patient can be assigned to one of the four categories of asthma severity (answer #5).

ANSWER TO QUESTION 10 (STAGING THE SEVERITY OF ASTHMA: CASE EXAMPLE 1)

The correct answer is #1 (mild intermittent asthma). This child with asthma has suffered an episode of exercise-induced bronchoconstriction. Though her symptoms were quite severe, they resolved quickly; and on further inquiry she generally has few daytime or nighttime symptoms of asthma. She uses her albuterol inhaler for relief of symptoms no more than twice weekly; she wakes from her sleep with asthmatic symptoms no more than two times each month. Her lung function is normal.

ANSWER TO QUESTION 11 (STAGING THE SEVERITY OF ASTHMA: CASE EXAMPLE 2)

The correct answer is #4 (severe persistent asthma). This child has severe disease, with symptoms nearly every night and frequent interference with his routine functioning (such as going to school or playing outdoors). As a consequence, it is likely that his mother has her sleep routinely disturbed and often has to miss work because of her son's illness. His wheezes heard on examination point to significant airway narrowing even when he is sitting quietly.

ANSWER TO QUESTION 12 (STAGING THE SEVERITY OF ASTHMA: CASE EXAMPLE 3)

The correct answer is #2 (mild persistent asthma). Although her chest is clear and her lung function is normal, the frequency of her daytime and nighttime symptoms indicates persistent disease. She has daytime symptoms more than twice weekly (but less than once daily, a finding that would put her in the moderate persistent asthma category), and she has nocturnal awakenings more than twice monthly (but not more often than once weekly, a frequency that would again put her in the next highest asthma step of severity). If we had not inquired about the frequency of her asthma symptoms—both daytime and nighttime—we might have been fooled into thinking that this healthy-appearing young woman had only mild intermittent asthma.

3

MEDICATIONS USED TO TREAT ASTHMA

C H A P T E R   O U T L I N E

I. Pharmacologic therapy: A brief historical perspective

II. Modern asthma medications—the bronchodilators
   a. Beta-adrenergic bronchodilators
      i. Short-acting beta-adrenergic bronchodilators
      ii. Long-acting beta-adrenergic bronchodilators
      iii. Are beta-agonist bronchodilators harmful?
   b. Other bronchodilators
      i. Theophylline
      ii. Oral-beta agonists
      iii. Anticholinergic bronchodilators

III. Modern asthma medications—the anti-inflammatory drugs
   a. Inhaled corticosteroids
   b. Mast cell stabilizers
   c. Leukotriene blockers
      i. Aspirin-sensitive asthma

"Am I taking the right medicines for my asthma?" "Which of these medicines am I supposed to be taking every day?" "I don't think that my child (or parent) is using her inhaler properly; can you show us how to do it correctly?" These and many similar questions come up daily in the care of patients with asthma. "Is it safe for me to be taking these medications every day? I don't want to get addicted to them." "My doctor told me to take steroids, but I don't want to grow big muscles." "I keep gaining weight. Do you think it could be from one of my asthma medicines?"

Medications are central to the treatment of asthma. With them we can prevent bronchoconstriction and reverse it when it occurs; we can reduce the underlying "twitchiness" of the airways that characterizes asthma; and we can protect our patients from asthmatic attacks. We have heard many patients with asthma say that their asthma medications "gave them back their lives." Instead of being chronically ill and watching life from the sidelines, they became able to lead fully active, participatory lives. At the same time, frequent or daily use of medications carries with it its own set of concerns and negative associations, including cost, side effects, sense of dependency, and worry regarding potential long-term harmful effects.

No wonder there exists a considerable gap between the doctor's prescription of asthma medications and the patient's faithful adherence to the prescribed treatment program. Many barriers get in the way, among them difficulty obtaining the medications, misunderstanding the directions, mistrust of the recommendations, and misuse of the medication devices. Perhaps it is not surprising that studies investigating long-term compliance with asthma medications have found abysmal rates of adherence. One recent retrospective study of pharmacy utilization in a health maintenance organization in Michigan found that only approximately half of the adult patients filled their prescriptions for inhaled corticosteroids regularly; and for every 25% increase in the proportion of time spent without inhaled corticosteroids, the number of hospitalizations for asthmatic attacks doubled.

Enter the asthma educator! Armed with an understanding of the various medications—their intended effects, proper use, and potential side effects—you are in an excellent position to advise patients about their use. You can clarify misconceptions, address points of concern, and help to make sense of what can be a bewildering array of instructions. In Chap. 8, "Inhalers and Inhalational Aids in Asthma Treatment," we will examine the details of proper inhaler use. In this chapter we emphasize the actions, potential side effects, and recommended role of the various medications used to treat asthma. In the next chapter we will discuss the topic of which medications are appropriate for which patients and introduce one additional treatment, anti-IgE monoclonal antibody.

As we begin our discussion of the medicines used to treat asthma, we wish to acknowledge that medical therapy is only one component of a comprehensive approach to asthma management. Good asthma control also involves avoidance of asthma triggers, monitoring lung function over time, preparation for dealing with asthma attacks, and patient-provider communication. In some cases it also includes allergen immunotherapy (allergy shots), which we will consider further in Chap. 4, "Treating Asthma in the Ambulatory Setting." The Expert Panel of the National Asthma Education and Prevention Program identifies four key components of effective asthma care:

Component 1: Measures of Assessment and Monitoring

Component 2: Control of Factors Contributing to Asthma Severity

Component 3: Pharmacologic Therapy

Component 4: Education for a Partnership in Asthma Care

PHARMACOLOGIC THERAPY: A BRIEF HISTORICAL PERSPECTIVE

Ask your patients about some of the medicines that they were given for their asthma years ago, and you will hear a rich medical history of asthma pharmacology over the last few decades. Some of your very old patients may even remember smoking stramonium cigarettes. The leaves of the *Datura stramonium* or Jimsonweed plant (also called loco weed!) were dried and rolled up into a cigarette. The cigarette smoke contained an atropine-line medicine that acted as a bronchodilator ... and it also contained a lot of irritating smoke particles that didn't help the lungs at all!

Others will remember receiving their bronchodilator medication via a bulb nebulizer device (Fig. 3-1). It wasn't until 1956 that the first metered-dose inhalers were introduced by 3M. Before then, medication was put into a glass container and made into a mist for inhalation by squeezing the attached rubber bulb. Or perhaps your patient remembers receiving inhaled bronchodilator in the emergency room using a small ventilator (a green, plastic box the size of a toaster) driven by compressed air, called an Intermittent Positive Pressure Breathing device, fondly known as an IPPB machine. (Perhaps you yourself remember some of these devices; you don't have to admit it to anyone!)

Theophylline has been available for treating asthma since the 1940s. Popular oral medications to treat asthma in the 1960s and 1970s were tablets containing the

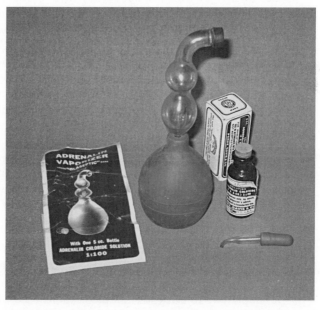

FIGURE 3-1 *An old-fashioned bulb nebulizer and medicine it was used to deliver. Reproduced with permission from www.inhalatorium.com.*

combination of theophylline and ephedrine. As you would predict, side effects included an anxious, jittery sensation, so some of the combination tablets incorporated a small amount of sedating antihistamine or barbiturate! Brand names (that can still bring a glimmer to your older patients' eyes) included Marax and Tedral.

Slow-release theophylline tablets and capsules had a major impact on asthma care through the 1970s and 1980s. Their long duration of action made possible twice- and even once-daily dosing of bronchodilator medication. Theophylline became the routine *next step* when short-acting inhaled bronchodilators provided insufficient relief of symptoms. Innumerable slow-release preparations became available, with brand names like Theo-dur, Slophylline, Slo-BID, Unidur, Uniphyl, Theo-24, and others.

Individuals vary greatly in how fast they metabolize theophylline. As a result, it is difficult to predict precisely the correct dose of theophylline for any given individual. The medical prescriber makes an estimate based on weight, then after a few days needs to check the resulting blood level and adjust the dose accordingly. Too much theophylline (too high a blood level) can cause myriad side effects, including heart racing, nausea, vomiting, diarrhea, and insomnia. Toxic blood levels, the result of accidental or deliberate overdoses, can lead to seizures, cardiac arrhythmias, and death. So, monitoring blood levels of theophylline—and adjusting the dose of theophylline accordingly—became part of the routine care of many people with asthma. Not surprisingly, some patients came to think of asthma as a theophylline-deficient condition, like iron-deficient anemia. If their blood level of theophylline became low, it might cause them to have worse asthma and so they needed to take more medicine to restore their level to *normal*!

In the early 1970s came introduction of the first inhaled corticosteroids that were active locally (in the airways) and not systemically. Beclomethasone was the first such inhaled steroid, marketed as Vanceril and Beclovent. The use of inhaled steroids to treat bronchial inflammation in asthma revolutionized modern asthma care, but the start was somewhat rocky. Beclomethasone was introduced as a medicine to be taken four times daily—not an easy assignment for daily administration of a medicine without any immediate symptomatic benefit—and each inhalation had only approximately 50 micrograms of medication, a relatively small amount. As the use of high-dose inhaled steroids to treat refractory asthma became popular in the 1980s, patients were asked to take as many as four, six, or even eight puffs four times daily. It is remarkable how quickly what seemed like "state-of-the-art" at the time becomes primitive and somewhat ridiculous in retrospect!

MODERN ASTHMA MEDICATIONS—THE BRONCHODILATORS

One simple way to categorize all medications used to treat asthma is into two groups: the bronchodilators and the anti-inflammatory medicines. We will use this model here as we discuss types of asthma medicines and individual examples of each category. In a sense, one goal of all of these medicines is to open wider the bronchial air passageways and to make them less predisposed to narrow again. But if we conceive of the cause of airway narrowing in asthma as partly due to constriction of the bronchial smooth muscles and partly due to swelling and inflammation of the bronchial walls, then it makes sense to separate medicines into two boxes: those that primarily act to relax the bronchial muscles (bronchodilators) and those that primarily work to reduce inflammation and mucus hypersecretion (anti-inflammatory medicines).

In fact, when it is time to talk to patients about their asthma medicines, it is recommended that we use a different model. We will talk about *controller* medicines (those taken every day to control asthma symptoms and prevent attacks) and *reliever* medicines (those taken only as needed for prompt relief of symptoms). We will see that some controller medicines are bronchodilators, others are anti-inflammatory medicines. Reliever medicines are the quick-acting bronchodilators.

Perhaps all that your patients will need to know about their medicines is which ones to take daily but leave at home in the medicine cabinet, and which ones to take only as needed but carry with them at all times. Or perhaps they will want to know more information such as, *What does this medicine do for me? How quickly will I know that it's working? What side effects can it cause?*, and so on. They will look to you as a trustworthy source of reliable information about their medicines. Our advice is that if you are uncertain about any of the information, don't guess. Misinformation is sometimes worse than no information at all. In addition to this book, there are many sources of accurate information at your disposal, including pharmacology texts, the *Physicians' Desk Reference* (PDR), online resources, and programs downloadable onto your personal digital assistant (PDA) device.

KEY POINT   Misinformation is sometimes worse than no information at all. If you are uncertain about the answer to a medication (or other) question, don't guess; look it up.

Beta-adrenergic bronchodilators

By way of review, the human autonomic nervous system—the part of the nervous system that regulates the involuntary functioning of organs throughout the body—is organized in a yin-yang balance between the sympathetic and parasympathetic nerves. Sympathetic nerve endings release (and sympathetic nerve receptors respond to) adrenaline-like chemicals; hence the name, *adrenergic* nerves and receptors. Parasympathetic nerve endings release acetylcholine; hence the name, *cholinergic*, to refer to that system of nerves, neurotransmitters, and receptor molecules.

On the surface of bronchial muscles are many adrenergic and cholinergic receptor molecules. Stimulate the adrenergic receptors with adrenaline (also called epinephrine), and the bronchial muscles relax, causing the bronchi to dilate. Stimulate the cholinergic receptors with acetylcholine (or its analog, methacholine, as used in bronchoprovocative challenge tests for asthma), and the bronchial muscles contract, causing the bronchi to narrow. It is clear that if you wanted to design a bronchodilator medicine, you might begin with either a stimulant (also called an agonist) of the adrenergic receptors or a blocker (also called an antagonist) of the acetylcholine-type stimulants of the cholinergic receptors. You would create adrenergic bronchodilators or anti-cholinergic bronchodilators—and you'd be on the right track. Remember, too, that people with asthma are uniquely sensitive to beta-adrenergic blocking drugs (beta blockers), like propranolol (Inderal). Block the normal amount of stimulation of adrenergic receptors on bronchial smooth muscles, and people with asthma develop bronchoconstriction.

SHORT-ACTING BETA-ADRENERGIC BRONCHODILATORS

Adrenaline (epinephrine) was first isolated from animal adrenal glands, purified, and made available for the treatment of asthma at the beginning of the twentieth century. For decades it was the mainstay of treatment of acute asthmatic attacks, given as a subcutaneous injection. It is also widely available as a metered-dose inhaler formulation, with brand names such as Primatene Mist and Bronkaid. It is the only inhaled bronchodilator sold over-the-counter in the United States. Because it is rapidly metabolized by enzymes in the stomach, epinephrine is not available as an orally administered tablet.

Epinephrine acts as a bronchodilator, but it can also elevate your blood pressure. When given by injection, it not only causes the bronchial muscles to relax, it also causes the muscles that surround our blood vessels to constrict. It turns out that some of the adrenergic receptors on blood vessels, when stimulated, cause vasoconstriction. To distinguish this effect from the dilating effect on muscles, the constricting-type receptors are referred to as *alpha-adrenergic* receptors and the dilating-type receptors as *beta-adrenergic* receptors. Epinephrine is both a beta- and an alpha-adrenergic stimulant. We take advantage of the latter effect in anaphylactic shock. We give epinephrine to raise the blood pressure quickly. Our patients with peanut allergy may carry a prefilled syringe containing epinephrine, called an "Epi-Pen" or "Twinject," to treat allergic swelling or shock with a powerful vasoconstrictor medicine. However, if our primary goal is bronchodilation, as in asthma, this effect of epinephrine on the alpha receptors of blood vessels becomes an undesirable side effect.

KEY POINT   Epinephrine is a bronchodilator with alpha- and beta-adrenergic effects. It raises blood pressure when given systemically.

Epinephrine inhalers begin to act within a minute or two. Their effect lasts approximately 3–4 hours. Their side effects, including elevated blood pressure and heart racing, make them less desirable than inhaled bronchodilators available only by prescription. Still, in a pinch, they can bring relief of acute asthma symptoms.

On the other hand, used to excess, they can be dangerous—and even potentially lethal if their transient benefit delays access to other needed medications.

Around 1950 researchers introduced the first purely beta-adrenergic bronchodilator medication, one that did not also stimulate the alpha-adrenergic receptors on blood vessels. It was called isoproterenol (Isuprel). It was made available in the first pressurized, metered-dose inhalers in the mid-1950s (the Isuprel Mistometer) and as a liquid for aerosolization by IPPB machine or, later, by continuous-flow, hand-held nebulizers. Rarely, in life-threatening asthmatic attacks, it was given as an intravenous infusion.

Although isoproterenol did not raise blood pressure, it continued to have one major adverse effect: tachycardia. Not only are there beta receptors on the bronchial muscles that lead to bronchodilation, there are also beta receptors on heart tissue that promote increased heart rate and more forceful heart contraction. Isoproterenol treatments improved the breathing in patients with asthma but often left them with an uncomfortable sensation of heart pounding and racing. And intravenous isoproterenol could occasionally precipitate myocardial injury, even in young people with normal coronary arteries.

KEY POINT   Isoproterenol is a nonselective beta-adrenergic bronchodilator; it stimulates bronchi and cardiac tissue with equal potency. It does not raise blood pressure, but it speeds heart rate.

The next advance in bronchodilator therapy came in the mid-1960s, when scientists were able to distinguish two distinct types of beta receptors: one found primarily on the heart (and blood vessels), called beta-1 receptors; the other found primarily on bronchial smooth muscle, called beta-2 receptors. Soon thereafter came the development of albuterol, a beta-2 selective adrenergic bronchodilator. Rapidly, the selective beta-2 agonists came to replace isoproterenol and dominate the inhaled bronchodilator market. Although not perfectly specific for the beta-2 receptors on bronchial tubes—and therefore not completely free of cardiac stimulatory effects—the beta-2 selective bronchodilators are a great improvement. At standard doses, they offer comparable bronchodilation with far less (if any) tachycardia compared to isoproterenol (Table 3-1).

TABLE 3-1

EVOLUTION OF BETA-2 SPECIFIC BRONCHODILATORS

	Alpha (Blood Vessels)	Beta-1 (Heart)	Beta-2 (Bronchi)
Epinephrine	+++	+++	+++
Isoproterenol	–	+++	+++
Albuterol	–	+	+++

THE INHALED BETA-2 ADRENERGIC AGONISTS AND THEIR ROUTES OF ADMINISTRATION

Generic Name	Brand Names	Metered-Dose Inhaler	Liquid for Nebulization
Albuterol	ProAir, Proventil, Ventolin	Yes	Yes
Pirbuterol	Maxair	Yes	No
Metaproterenol	Alupent	Yes	Yes
Levalbuterol	Xopenex	Yes	Yes

Inhaled beta-2 selective adrenergic bronchodilators (commonly referred to as "beta agonists" for short) are powerful bronchodilators, quick in onset (within 3–5 minutes), lasting 4–6 hours, with relatively few side effects (some jitteriness and muscle tremor may occur). Currently available beta-2 selective agonists and their routes of administration are listed in Table 3-2. Although albuterol has come to dominate the market, in our opinion there is relatively little distinction between the different agents. There are some differences between delivery devices (traditional metered-dose inhaler vs. CFC propellant-free metered-dose inhaler vs. breath-actuated inhaler), which will be discussed further in Chap. 8, "Inhalers and Inhalational Aids in Asthma Treatment."

KEY POINT Inhaled beta-2 selective adrenergic agonists (the current beta-agonist bronchodilators) are potent bronchodilators with little cardiac stimulatory effects. Examples include albuterol (Ventolin, Proventil, ProAir), pirbuterol (Maxair), metaproterenol (Alupent) and levalbuterol (Xopenex).

One reason why selective beta-2 agonist bronchodilators via metered-dose inhaler (MDI) have so few side effects is the small amount of medication that is needed to achieve bronchodilation. For instance, each actuation of an albuterol MDI delivers 90 mcg of albuterol. A standard dose is two puffs or 180 mcg, approximately one fifth of 1 mg. Because the inhaled route of administration deposits medication directly on airway surfaces, far smaller amounts of medication can be administered than would be needed to achieve the same effect via oral administration of albuterol (in tablet or liquid form). Thus, despite the frustrations of trying to master proper use of MDIs, the inhaled route of administration is quicker, produces greater bronchodilation, and entails fewer unpleasant side effects than oral administration.

The newest inhaled beta-agonist bronchodilator is called levalbuterol (Xopenex). It turns out that albuterol (and all of the beta-agonist bronchodilators) are a chemical mixture of molecules, all of which have the same chemical structure but half of which has one spatial arrangement, whereas the other half has a different spatial arrangement. The molecules differ like our left and right hands; they are mirror images of one another (called enantiomers) (Fig. 3-2). This difference in spatial orientation affects their function. All of the bronchodilator activity of albuterol is contained within its dextrorotatory molecules (enantiomers that bend polarized light to the right); the levorotatory molecules (enantiomers that bend polarized light to the left) do not act as bronchodilators and perhaps have undesirable effects on the beta receptors.

One pharmaceutical company has developed the technology to isolate and purify only the dextrorotatory (R-albuterol) molecules, called levalbuterol. Until recently, levalbuterol was only available as a liquid for nebulization; a metered-dose inhaler formulation has recently been released. Its special niche is that at doses that cause bronchodilation identical to albuterol (levalbuterol solution 0.63 mg compared to albuterol solution 2.5 mg), it is said to have slightly less cardiac stimulatory effects—although this difference is debated. And at doses that cause similar side effects (levalbuterol 1.25 mg compared to albuterol 2.5 mg), it may have slightly greater bronchodilator effect. Its major disadvantage is its increased cost compared to generic albuterol solution. We tend to restrict our use of levalbuterol to the elderly or those with known cardiac disease, in whom its possibly lesser cardiac stimulation becomes potentially important. Some

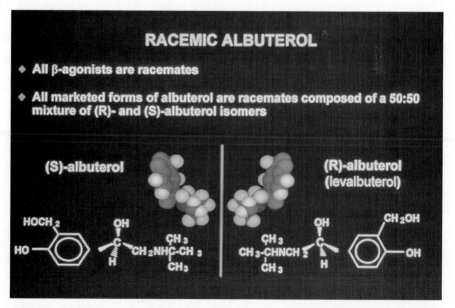

FIGURE 3-2 *Albuterol is a 50:50 mixture of molecules sharing the same chemical structure but with mirror-image spatial orientations. Levalbuterol (Xopenex) is a single-isomer preparation containing only the R-isomer. From: slide set, Sepracor.*

pediatricians find that children become less agitated with nebulized levalbuterol than they do with conventional albuterol solution.

LONG-ACTING BETA-ADRENERGIC BRONCHODILATORS

A major revolution in asthma care followed the introduction in the mid-1990s of inhaled beta-agonist bronchodilators with prolonged duration of action. The first of these was salmeterol (Serevent); a similar long-acting beta-agonist bronchodilator is formoterol (Foradil). Both are available only as dry-powder inhalers (as discussed in Chap. 8, "Inhalers and Inhalational Aids in Asthma Treatment"). Salmeterol is marketed in the multidose Diskus device; formoterol is sold with each dose contained in a gelatin capsule, individually loaded into an Aerolizer device for inhalation. When initially introduced, salmeterol was sold in a conventional metered-dose inhaler, but the Serevent MDI was subsequently withdrawn from the market (as part of a worldwide trend to decrease the use of medications containing ozone-harmful chlorofluorocarbons [CFCs]).

The long-acting beta-agonist bronchodilators stay attached to the beta receptor molecules on bronchial muscles for a prolonged period. Their duration of action is 12 or more hours. Consequently, they are recommended for twice-daily dosing, and more frequent use is discouraged. Salmeterol begins to work only 30–45 minutes after inhalation, whereas formoterol has a quick onset of action (within 5 minutes). Both are highly selective for the beta-2 receptors on bronchial muscle; they cause relatively little cardiac stimulation. Like the short-acting beta agonists, they can occasionally cause tremor, muscle cramps, and headache.

Use of the long-acting beta-agonist bronchodilators does not preclude intermittent use of short-acting beta agonists (such as albuterol) for quick relief of symptoms. The latter continue to exert their bronchodilator effect even in the presence of salmeterol or formoterol.

The impact of the long-acting inhaled beta agonists on current asthma care has been enormous. The reason: they have proved to be hugely effective in controlling asthma in patients who continued to be plagued by frequent symptoms despite use of inhaled corticosteroids and repeated doses of short-acting bronchodilators. They have none of the drawbacks of the alternative long-acting bronchodilator, slow-release theophylline. Unlike for theophylline, administration of the long-acting inhaled beta agonists does not entail frequent side effects, variable dosing, checking drug blood levels, concern about drug-drug interactions, and risk of dangerous overdoses because of a narrow therapeutic-to-toxic drug ratio. Their use in combination with an inhaled steroid helps to avoid the need for *high-dose* inhaled steroids, with the latter's potential long-term risk of serious side effects. And their long duration of action following an evening dose proves very effective in reducing nighttime awakenings due to asthma.

KEY POINT Salmeterol (Serevent) and formoterol (Foradil) are long-acting inhaled beta-agonist bronchodilators with durations of action of at least 12 hours. They have proved to be highly effective in reducing nighttime awakenings and controlling difficult asthma.

ARE BETA-AGONIST BRONCHODILATORS HARMFUL?

Our enthusiasm for the long-acting inhaled beta agonists comes in part from the many patients who have told us that their lives were changed by these medicines. They went from poorly controlled to well-controlled asthma with use of a well-tolerated medication taken only morning and night. What do we make, then, of the recent newspaper headlines that salmeterol has been identified by a drug safety researcher for the Food and Drug Administration (FDA) as one of five potentially lethal medications still approved for sale in this country. This assertion came in the wake of Merck's decision to withdraw its anti-inflammatory drug, rofecoxib (Vioxx), from the market because of evidence that its long-term use led to an increased incidence of heart attacks and strokes.

This expression of concern about the safety of salmeterol was prompted by the outcome of a study conducted by the manufacturer of salmeterol, GlaxoSmithKline. Stimulated by concerns over potential harmful effects of excess use of beta-agonist bronchodilators, GlaxoSmithKline conducted a large-scale, randomized trial to assess the safety of salmeterol. The study, called the Salmeterol Multicenter Asthma Research Trial (SMART), was begun in 1996, two years after salmeterol was approved by the FDA for sale in the United States. Patients were randomly assigned to receive salmeterol or placebo for 28 weeks, in addition to their usual asthma care, whatever it might be. After 26,000 patients had been enrolled (of the 60,000 initially planned for this study), the experiment was stopped. More of the patients who were assigned to receive salmeterol had suffered respiratory deaths or respiratory failure requiring intubation and mechanical ventilation than patients assigned to receive placebo. Although the number of deaths and near-deaths was very small in both groups, significantly more occurred in the salmeterol-treated group.

These findings led to a "black-box warning" that now appears on the package inserts of salmeterol and Advair (which contains salmeterol in combination with an inhaled steroid) and, just recently, formoterol as well:

> **WARNING**: Data from a large placebo-controlled US study that compared the safety of salmeterol (SEREVENT® inhalation aerosol) or placebo added to usual asthma therapy showed a small but significant increase in asthma-related deaths in patients receiving salmeterol (13 deaths out of 13,176 patients treated for 28 weeks) versus those on placebo (3 of 13,179) (see WARNINGS and CLINICAL TRIALS: Asthma: *Salmeterol Multicenter Asthma Research Trial*).

The reason for this outcome is unknown. One potential explanation has to do with the use of the bronchodilator, salmeterol, in the absence of any anti-inflammatory agent. Only a minority of subjects in this study were using an anti-inflammatory steroid inhaler. It is possible that by taking a bronchodilator only, these asthmatic subjects felt better, had improved lung function, and consequently allowed themselves to be exposed to allergens and irritants that progressively worsened the inflammation of their bronchi. As the inflammation worsened, so did swelling, mucus plugging, and hyperresponsiveness or twitchiness of their airways. Perhaps the long-acting bronchodilator allowed subjects to deceive themselves into thinking that their asthma was under control while the inflammatory aspects of their disease worsened to the point of no return.

In support of this interpretation is the observation shown in Table 3-3: the difference in asthma deaths between the two groups (salmeterol vs. placebo) was most striking in those not receiving anti-inflammatory steroids. These numbers are too small to be considered definitive proof of this interpretation, however; and other explanations are also possible. For instance, it is possible that some of us, because of variation in our genetic make up, have variant forms of our beta-receptor molecules that make us respond negatively to stimulation with beta agonists (preliminary experimental evidence is available to lend support to this explanation). Or perhaps some patients derive benefit from the long-acting inhaled beta agonists,

TABLE 3-3

SALMETEROL MULTICENTER ASTHMA RESEARCH TRIAL (SMART): NUMBER OF ASTHMA-RELATED DEATHS BY SUB-GROUP ANALYSIS

	Salmeterol-Treated Group (N = 13,176)	Placebo-Treated Group (N = 13,179)
Using Inhaled Steroids at Baseline	4	3
Not Using Inhaled Steroids at Baseline	9	0

but during an asthma attack they suddenly find that their quick-acting beta agonist (such as albuterol) no longer works. Somehow in these individuals the long-acting beta agonist blocks the activity of the shorter-acting drug (some anecdotal evidence supports this interpretation). In the end, at this point we are left with the observations made in the SMART study and only speculation as the why they occurred.

Our own response to this information has been to continue to prescribe salmeterol and formoterol in combination with anti-inflammatory drugs for patients with more than just mild asthma. We reassure our patients that when used together with inhaled steroids, the long-acting inhaled beta agonists appear to be safe and highly effective. We remind our patients that the deaths and near-deaths observed with salmeterol use in the SMART study were due to severe asthma attacks (not cardiac deaths or some other unexpected medication side effect). And we suggest that the best protection against severe, life-threatening asthmatic attacks is not to discontinue long-acting inhaled beta agonists but to maintain good asthma control, monitor for exacerbations, and communicate with your health care providers when your asthma begins to worsen.

KEY POINT The Salmeterol Multicenter Asthma Research Trial (SMART) found a small but significant increase in asthma deaths and near-deaths among salmeterol-treated patients compared to the placebo group. The explanation for these findings is uncertain. We continue to prescribe salmeterol and formoterol, but only in combination with anti-inflammatory medications (inhaled steroids).

Other bronchodilators

Inhaled beta-adrenergic agonists have come to dominate the bronchodilator treatment of asthma because they are effective, safe, and mostly free of side effects. In most instances these benefits have outweighed their primary disadvantage: the difficulty that so many people have in coordinating the use of inhaler devices. Teaching and reinforcing proper inhaler use—again and again—is an important function of asthma educators. We will address this subject in detail in Chap. 8, including the very special circumstance of administering inhaled medications to very young children (see also Chap. 5, "Special Considerations in Childhood Asthma").

THEOPHYLLINE

Other bronchodilator medications are available to treat asthma, but their serious drawbacks have led us in our practices to use them very infrequently (Table 3-4). We have already considered some of the disadvantages of theophylline, which for decades played a central role in asthma care. These include: (1) frequent unpleasant side effects; (2) a narrow gap separating blood levels that are therapeutic from those that are toxic (i.e., a narrow therapeutic window); (3) unpredictable dosing requirements necessitating measurement of blood levels to determine the proper dose for any given individual; (4) risk of dangerous

TABLE 3-4

OTHER BRONCHODILATORS

Category	Generic Name	Brand Name	Formulations
Oral Beta-Agonists	Albuterol	Proventil, Ventolin	Tablets, syrup
	Metaproterenol	Alupent	Tablets, syrup
	Terbutaline	Brethine	Tablets
Anticholinergics	Ipratropium	Atrovent	Metered-dose inhaler; liquid for nebulization
	Ipratropium combined with albuterol	Combivent; Duo-neb	Metered-dose inhaler; liquid for nebulization
	Tiotropium	Spiriva	Dry-powder inhaler
Methylxanthines	Theophylline	Uniphyl, Theo-24, others	Tablets, oral solution, intravenous

complications at toxic blood levels (such as seizures and cardiac arrhythmias); (5) major drug interactions that affect blood levels (e.g., theophylline blood levels rise when someone takes erythromycin or ciprofloxacin); and (6) limited potency as a bronchodilator.

A rapid-release formulation is available, in which theophylline is dissolved in alcohol for rapid absorption from the stomach (Elixophylline). Slow-release preparations, now including generic formulations, make theophylline a long-acting bronchodilator, with once- or twice-daily dosing possible. Theophylline and its derivative, aminophylline, can also be administered as a continuous intravenous infusion during severe asthmatic attacks (see Chap. 9, "Managing Asthmatic Attacks").

Some of our older patients continue to take—and do well on—sustained-release theophylline. We explore with them possibly discontinuing theophylline if they are doing well and if they are willing to consider alternative therapies. Rarely do we newly begin our patients on theophylline nowadays.

Theophylline is chemically related to caffeine, which explains some of its more common side effects, like insomnia and a jittery, racy feeling. On the flip side, it is true that caffeine is a weak bronchodilator. In a jam, three cups of coffee will open bronchoconstricted airways somewhat—but don't expect to sleep that night. Curiously, it is still not entirely known by what biochemical pathway theophylline exerts its effects in asthma. One of its actions is to block the enzyme, phosphodiesterase. When there is less phosphodiesterase activity, levels of cyclic-adenosine monophosphate (cyclic-AMP) increase within the cell, the amount of calcium available for muscle contraction decreases, and muscle cells relax. Current research is pursuing the development of novel phosphodiesterase inhibitors that will be more specific for airway smooth muscle, with fewer undesired effects outside of the lungs.

KEY POINT   Caffeine and theophylline are chemically related. Three cups of coffee contain enough caffeine to open constricted airways somewhat—but at the cost of a sleepless night!

ORAL-BETA AGONISTS

Not all beta agonists are like epinephrine and isoproterenol, metabolized in the stomach and thereby rendered inactive when taken in tablet form. Some, like albuterol (Ventolin, Proventil), terbutaline (Brethine), or metaproterenol (Alupent), are available as tablets or syrups for oral administration. Direct comparison of the bronchodilating effects of oral versus inhaled beta agonists gives interesting results. For instance, if one compares the effect of 2 puffs of metaproterenol (1.3 mg) from a metered-dose inhaler with that of a metaproterenol tablet (20 mg), the inhaled route of delivery gives more rapid onset and achieves greater improvement in lung function. It's quicker and stronger, and it produces fewer side effects (less heart racing and jumpy feeling). By administering the medication directly to the bronchial tubes, one can use a smaller dose and cause fewer side effects beyond the bronchi themselves. As a consequence, we very rarely if ever use the orally administered beta agonists as quick-acting, quick-relief bronchodilators, even in very young children.

KEY POINT   Compared to the inhaled route of administration, orally administered beta agonists (as tablets or syrup) take longer to begin working, are less effective, and have more side effects.

Slow-release tablets containing albuterol are available for sustained bronchodilator activity (approximately 8 hours); a brand name preparation is VoSpire ER. Their role has largely been supplanted by the long-acting inhaled beta agonists, which are more potent bronchodilators with a longer duration of action. Although these patented sustained-release formulations are designed to make the albuterol available for absorption at a slow and steady rate, occasionally imperfections will lead to sudden release of a large amount of medication, with unpleasant stimulatory side effects.

ANTICHOLINERGIC BRONCHODILATORS

As noted earlier, another mechanism by which one might cause bronchi to dilate is by blocking the nervous system input that stimulates them to contract.

Cholinergic nerves release acetylcholine at their nerve endings along bronchial muscles (and mucous glands); acetylcholine acts as a bronchoconstrictor (and stimulant for mucus production). Anticholinergic drugs are bronchodilators; they block acetylcholine from reaching its receptor on the airway smooth muscle (as well as on mucous glands).

The oldest known anticholinergic drug is atropine. Atropine acts (weakly) as a bronchodilator in asthma, but it also has many undesirable side effects. One of the concerns about anticholinergic drugs like atropine is that they tend to dry up (i.e., reduce the water content of) airway secretions, potentially making them thicker, stickier, and harder to raise. You may know that many over-the-counter cold remedies have warning labels that advise people with asthma not to use them unless they first check with their physician. The reason is that the older, first-generation antihistamines contained in these cold remedies have atropine-like side effects. Although they are not effective bronchodilators, they pose a slight risk of drying airway secretions, causing mucus plugging and more difficult breathing in someone with asthma and lots of mucus production.

A derivative of atropine is ipratropium (Atrovent). Ipratropium represents a chemical modification of atropine such that this newer anticholinergic drug continues to exert a bronchodilator effect without drying airway secretions or causing confusion (an undesirable central nervous system effect of atropine). Ipratropium is available only via inhalation, as a metered-dose inhaler and solution for nebulization. It too has disadvantages compared to beta agonist bronchodilators for treating asthma: slower to begin working (15–20 minutes after inhalation) and less effective in opening airways. As a result, the FDA approved ipratropium for use in chronic obstructive pulmonary disease (COPD) but not in asthma.

Despite this recommendation, in urgent care settings you will commonly see ipratropium used in combination with albuterol for quick relief of asthmatic attacks. For *severe asthmatic attacks*, the combination of ipratropium and albuterol via nebulization (sold in combination as a nebulizer solution with the brand name Duoneb) achieves slightly greater bronchodilation than albuterol alone. However, for routine use in the ambulatory setting, we do not prescribe ipratropium or Combivent, the combination of ipratropium and albuterol in metered-dose inhaler formulation, for our patients with asthma. We do not find an advantage over a beta agonist like albuterol alone, and prescribing an additional inhaler just leads to greater expense and confusion about their different roles.

Here's a fine point: a patient taking a monoamine oxidase (MAO) inhibitor drug such as phenelzine (Nardil) or tranylcypromine (Parnate), used to treat depression, or the anti-Parkinsonian medication, selegiline (Eldepryl), should avoid beta agonists. These MAO inhibitors accentuate the stimulatory effects of the beta agonists, including cardiac effects. One might consider using ipratropium rather than an inhaled beta agonist as your bronchodilator of choice in someone for whom no alternative to a MAO inhibitor were available. Similarly, in someone forced to avoid any and all cardiac stimulation because of tachyarrhythmias, ipratropium offers an alternative to a beta agonist because of its negligible effect on heart rate or rhythm.

The newest anticholinergic bronchodilator is a remarkable drug. It is an ultra long-acting bronchodilator, with a duration of action of 24 hours! The medication is called tiotropium (Spiriva); it is supplied in individual capsules (like the long-acting beta-agonist bronchodilator, formoterol) and administered via a dry-powder inhaler, called a Handihaler. Other than sometimes causing a dry mouth, it is virtually free of side effects. But in asthma it is not as strong a bronchodilator as the long-acting inhaled beta agonists. Like ipratropium, it has been approved for use in COPD, not asthma. Just as with ipratropium, we tend to use tiotropium in patients with asthma only in those unusual circumstances when for some reason a long-acting inhaled beta agonist is contraindicated.

KEY POINT The anticholinergic bronchodilators, ipratropium (Atrovent) and tiotropium (Spiriva), are not as effective in the treatment of asthma as the inhaled beta agonists are. The FDA has approved their use in COPD, not asthma.

MODERN ASTHMA MEDICATIONS—THE ANTI-INFLAMMATORY DRUGS

As you know well by now, asthma is a chronic inflammatory disease of the airways. In some way this inflammation—involving mast cells, lymphocytes, and eosinophils—confers upon the airways their tendency for bronchial muscle constriction (bronchospasm) or at least it heightens or accentuates that tendency. Armed with that understanding, it would seem incredibly obvious now that to treat asthma only with bronchodilators would be like treating gastrointestinal bleeding only with transfusions or severe pneumonia only with oxygen. It treats one of the manifestations of the disease, but not the underlying problem. If the manifestations of asthma are mild and infrequent, such an approach is acceptable. If they are more intense or more frequent, it is clearly not—because bronchodilators do not treat swelling of the walls of the bronchial tubes, they do not reduce mucus hypersecretion, and they do not reduce the twitchiness of the airways that represents the underlying vulnerability of asthma.

When the only option for reducing asthmatic inflammation of the airways was use of oral corticosteroids, such as prednisone, there was understandable reluctance to administer this anti-inflammatory therapy on a regular basis. Prolonged oral steroid use (for months and years) is a disaster. The list of common and serious side effects is lengthy: weight gain and redistribution of fat ("moon facies," "buffalo hump," and excess fat in the supraclavicular areas), mood swings, tendencies to elevated blood pressure and blood sugar, cataracts, glaucoma, thinning of the skin and easy bruisability, loss of scalp hair and increased facial hair, muscle weakness (steroid myopathy), fluid retention, osteoporosis, and avascular necrosis of the long bones—to name a few! The likelihood of developing these adverse reactions depends on the dose and duration of treatment. In general, there is a cumulative dose effect, and few if any people taking 10 mg/day or more of prednisone for a year or more escape without some of these sequelae.

Inhaled corticosteroids

You can imagine, then, the impact of a drug that for the first time exerted anti-inflammatory effects on asthmatic airways without causing any of the harmful effects associated with orally administered steroids. Here was a drug—an inhaled corticosteroid preparation—that could be safely taken for years. By administering the medication directly onto the surface of airways (by inhalation), it can be given in microgram rather than milligram quantities (a 1000-fold less). Yes, some of the medication is swallowed and absorbed into the bloodstream from the gastrointestinal tract, but most of that absorbed medicine is metabolized as it passes through the liver, leaving little to be carried to other parts of the body. Since only a small amount of medicine is absorbed into the bloodstream from the surfaces of the bronchial tubes (bypassing the liver), the amount of medicine delivered systemically is minute.

KEY POINT   Only a minute amount of medication is absorbed into the bloodstream and delivered systemically when corticosteroids are administered by inhalation.

There is a footnote that needs to be added here: when given in *high doses* for several months or more, inhaled steroids can have a small but detectable effect on other organs besides the lungs. At these high doses, some systemic absorption does occur. We will return to this point subsequently. It is mentioned here as a "footnote" because our emphasis is that at low and moderate doses of inhaled steroids, long-term adverse effects have not been observed—even 30-plus years after they were first introduced. Inhaled steroids improve lung function, reduce asthmatic symptoms, decrease the risk of asthmatic attacks, and save lives (fewer asthmatic deaths were observed among those regularly using inhaled steroids than among those who were not). They improve the quality of life of persons with asthma. Our job as asthma educators is to communicate these benefits and attempt to help patients understand the distinction between the effects of inhaled and oral steroids.

   In fact, as we start teaching about steroids, we often need to begin by distinguishing the anti-inflammatory steroids from the muscle-building (anabolic) steroids that are used illicitly by some bodybuilders and competitive athletes. When the newspapers and other news media are full of stories about professional athletes taking steroids, it is easy to see how patients might get confused when you suggest that they should begin taking steroids, whatever the route of administration. The anabolic steroids are derivatives of testosterone; they do not reduce inflammation. The anti-inflammatory steroids are derived from cortisol (made by the adrenal glands); hence the name, corticosteroids. They do not make your muscles grow bigger. Corticosteroids are used to treat numerous different inflammatory diseases, from arthritis to glomerulonephritis to tendonitis. Many patients will already be familiar with topical steroid skin creams sold over-the-counter for the treatment of poison ivy and other inflammatory reactions of the skin (e.g., Cortaid cream). They do not consider these superficially applied steroid preparations dangerous, and neither should they view the inhaled steroids in that way.

KEY POINT   We need to clarify for our patients the distinction between the anti-inflammatory steroids used to treat asthma (and many other inflammatory conditions) and the muscle-building (anabolic) steroids used illicitly by some bodybuilders and competitive athletes.

Inhaled steroids can have some side effects, but they tend to be minor. Well-known is the risk of the fungal infection of the mouth, candidiasis. Steroids promote the growth of candida species, especially when antibiotics (that kill off the normal bacteria living in the mouth) are administered simultaneously. The risk of oral candidiasis (also called thrush) can be greatly reduced by rinsing one's mouth with water after each dose of the inhaled steroid. Many people who are prescribed their steroid medication for use morning and night simply leave the device in the bathroom and use it before tooth brushing. Hollow chambers called spacers can be attached to the metered-dose inhalers used to deliver some of the steroid preparations. From the spray released by the metered-dose inhaler, spacers collect some of the steroid medicine that would otherwise settle in the mouth. In this way they decrease the risk of developing thrush. (We will speak more about the use of spacers in Chap. 8.)

Thrush most commonly develops on the roof of the mouth (the hard and soft palate) and/or the tongue. It typically manifests as whitish papules or plaque with surrounding erythema. Symptoms may include a sore throat or simply a dry mouth. Highly effective treatment is available with anti-fungal mouthwash (nystatin [Mycostatin]), oral troches dissolved in the mouth (nystatin or clotrimazole [Mycelex]), or oral anti-fungal tablets (fluconazole [Diflucan]).

Another relatively common side effect from inhaled steroids is a hoarse or altered voice (dysphonia). As it makes its way down onto the bronchial tubes, the medication passes through the larynx and some of the medication deposits directly onto the vocal cords, causing a reversible deformity of the cords (a characteristic bowing when the cords are brought together for phonation). This change in voice quality tends to come and go over the course of the day or vary from day to day. It is not preventable by rinsing one's mouth after medication use (because the water or other mouthwash does not reach the vocal cords). Sometimes adding a spacer can help, but the problem may persist; and adding a spacer is not an option when the steroid preparation is delivered by dry-powder inhaler. The best that we can offer our patients is the option of stopping their inhaled steroids for a few days, allowing their vocal quality to return to normal, and then resuming the inhaled steroid. For some people the dysphonia may recur, an unavoidable annoyance that accompanies this highly effective asthma therapy.

Finally, occasional patients will find that they are unable to use their steroid inhaler because it causes them to cough immediately, resulting in loss of most of the medication intended for the airways because of this uncontrollable rapid exhalation. This side effect is rare with the currently available inhaled steroid preparations and can be easily overcome by switching to another steroid, pre-medication with an inhaled bronchodilator, or—for patients with highly twitchy airways—getting their asthma under better control first with a brief oral steroid course.

KEY POINT   Common side effects of the inhaled steroids include oral candidiasis (thrush) and hoarse voice or altered voice quality. Other potential long-term side effects relate only to the use of high-dose inhaled steroids.

So far we have focused on communicating the safety of inhaled steroids and the relatively few and minor side effects that one may encounter. What about the benefits?

Using bronchial biopsies and bronchial lavage samples, it has been possible to document that the inhaled steroids achieve their desired effect: they reduce the allergic-type inflammation of the bronchi that characterizes all asthma. After a few weeks of therapy, one finds fewer allergy cells (mast cell, eosinophils, and type-2 helper lymphocytes) in these samples, and the appearance of the bronchial tissue looks more like normal. Many other indicators of asthmatic bronchial inflammation tell the same story: fewer eosinophils in expectorated (induced) sputum; less nitric oxide in exhaled breath; and lower concentrations of various chemical mediators, such as histamine and leukotrienes. Like steroids used to treat inflammation elsewhere in the body, inhaled steroids are highly effective in treating this type of allergic inflammation when it occurs in the airways.

Admittedly, patients don't complain of inflammation in their bronchial tubes. What they experience is cough, shortness of breath, tightness in the chest, and wheezing, including nighttime awakenings with some or all of these symptoms. By reducing airway inflammation, the inhaled steroids reduce these symptoms. Patients feel better (generally within a week or two). They experience fewer symptoms, they sleep better, and they need their quick-acting bronchodilator less often. They feel as though their asthma were going away. If you ask them about the quality of their life (with validated, asthma-specific survey questionnaires), they report that it improves significantly with regular use of inhaled steroids.

The other very important benefit of inhaled steroids is that bronchial hyper-responsiveness lessens. The airways become less twitchy, less sensitive to developing bronchoconstriction in response to exposure to the various asthmatic triggers, such as exercise, allergen exposure, or second-hand smoke exposure. It's not that one becomes immune to them, but with regular use of inhaled steroids one finds that the bronchoconstriction that occurs is less, and it occurs only after a larger or stronger triggering stimulus. Partly, this decreased airway sensitivity translates into fewer day-to-day symptoms, and partly it means less vulnerability to asthmatic attacks. Many studies have shown that regular use of inhaled steroids results in fewer emergency room visits and fewer hospitalizations for asthma. In one retrospective review of asthma medication use among nearly 17,000 asthmatic patients enrolled in a health maintenance organization in New England, the number of hospitalizations for severe asthmatic attacks among those prescribed (and filling their prescriptions for) inhaled steroids was half that among those not using inhaled steroids.

Each year in the United States as many as 5000 people die of asthma. In most instances, they die of severe asthmatic attacks. The risk of death due to asthma is significantly reduced by the regular use of inhaled steroids. One large-scale retrospective analysis of all asthmatic deaths in the province of Saskatchewan, Canada, between 1975 and 1991 found that the risk of death due to asthma decreased in proportion to the number of inhaled steroid prescriptions filled within the preceding year. Even low-dose inhaled steroids, taken regularly, protected against fatal asthma (Fig. 3-3).

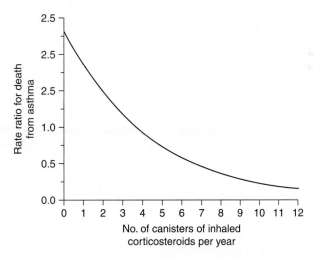

FIGURE 3-3   *The risk of death from asthma is significantly reduced (below a relative risk of 1) among persons using inhaled steroids on a regular basis, even in low doses. Reproduced with permission from Suissa S, et al. Low-dose inhaled corticosteroids and the prevention of death from asthma. N Engl J Med 2000; 343:332–6. Copyright 2000 Massachusetts Medical Society. All rights reserved.*

KEY POINT   Inhaled steroids have numerous beneficial effects, including fewer symptoms, improved quality of life, less hyperresponsiveness of the airways, and fewer asthmatic attacks, including the severe attacks that can result in emergency department visits, hospitalizations, and even death.

The currently available steroid preparations are listed in Table 3-5, along with the number of micrograms delivered from the device with each puff or inhalation and the number of doses provided in each purchased inhaler. (A smaller number of doses is provided in some inhalers distributed free of charge as samples). We anticipate that soon one other inhaled steroid may receive approval for sale in the United States: ciclesonide (Alvesco). Also, the fluticasone-salmeterol combination (Advair) has recently been released in a metered-dose inhaler formulation (Advair-HFA).

TABLE 3-5

INHALED CORTICOSTEROIDS

Generic Name	Brand Name	Delivery System	Individual Dose	Doses per container
Beclomethasone	Qvar	Metered-dose inhaler	40 mcg/puff 80 mcg/puff	100
Budesonide	Pulmicort	Dry-powder inhaler	200 mcg/inhal'n	200
		Liquid for nebulization	250 mcg/vial 500 mcg/vial	
Flunisolide	Aerobid, Aerobid-M	Metered-dose inhaler	250 mcg/puff	100
Fluticasone	Flovent	Metered-dose inhaler	44 mcg/puff 110 mcg/puff 220 mcg/puff	120
Fluticasone combined with salmeterol	Advair	Dry-powder inhaler	100 mcg/inhal'n 250 mcg/inhal'n 500 mcg/inhal'n	60
Mometasone	Asmanex	Dry-powder inhaler	220 mcg/inhal'n	30, 60, or 120
Triamcinolone	Azmacort	Metered-dose inhaler	100 mcg/puff	240

What might make a health care provider choose one inhaled steroid medication over another? Cost may be one factor. The convenience or ease of use of the delivery device may be another (to be considered further in Chap. 8). In terms of medication strength and side effects, there are relatively few differences. Microgram for microgram, fluticasone (Flovent, Advair) and mometasone (Asmanex) appear to be more potent inhaled steroids than the other currently available preparations (approximately twice as potent at any given dose). Budesonide (Pulmicort Turbuhaler) and mometasone (Asmanex) have approval for once-daily dosing. Budesonide (Pulmicort) has the most favorable rating for use in pregnancy (category B). Budesonide (Pulmicort Respules) is the only steroid available as a liquid to be administered as an aerosol via nebulizer. Fluticasone is the only inhaled steroid available combined with a long-acting beta-agonist bronchodilator (salmeterol) in a single device, the Advair Diskus.

When they were first introduced, the inhaled steroids were prescribed to be taken four times daily (q.i.d.). Subsequent studies and clinical experience showed that when the same total daily dose was delivered twice daily (b.i.d.), the same benefits were obtained—with greatly improved patient adherence to the treatment plan. More recently, budesonide (Pulmicort) and mometasone (Asmanex) have been approved by the FDA for administration on a once-daily schedule. In our opinion, it is likely that once-daily dosing will likewise prove effective in mild asthma with any of the other inhaled steroids given in adequate doses.

There was a time when the best treatment for patients who continued to have troubling asthmatic symptoms despite taking an inhaled steroid was more inhaled steroids. Thinking that the inflammation of the airways had not been adequately suppressed, we asked our patients to take more puffs of their steroid inhaler: six puffs twice daily, eight puffs twice daily, and even more. When steroid preparations became available with more micrograms delivered with each inhalation, it became easier to administer high doses of inhaled corticosteroids, by which we mean here more than 1,000 mcg/day (in adults). More than four puffs/day of the fluticasone (Flovent) 220 metered-dose inhaler, more than five puffs/day of the budesonide (Pulmicort) Turbuhaler, and more than two inhalations/day from the Advair Diskus (500/50) put you into this category. (Children are more susceptible to the effects of corticosteroids; high doses are defined by a lower mcg/day value, as discussed in Chap. 5, "Special Considerations in Childhood Asthma.")

Fortunately, for patients with all but the most severe asthma, we now have better strategies for bringing their asthma under control than simply escalating their dose of inhaled steroids. Specifically, by adding a long-acting inhaled beta agonist to the low- or medium-dose inhaled steroid, better asthma control is achieved than with high doses of inhaled steroids. Similarly, by adding a leukotriene blocker (to be discussed below) without increasing the dose of inhaled steroids, one can often achieve better lung function and fewer symptoms than by raising the dose of inhaled steroids. It turns out that the dose-response curve for inhaled steroids is relatively flat. As one increases the dose above conventional levels, there is comparatively little added improvement in asthma.

On the other hand, as doses of inhaled steroids rise, so does the likelihood that enough medication will be absorbed into the bloodstream and delivered throughout the body to cause systemic side effects. Perhaps you have seen patients given high-dose inhaled steroids who inquire about their new "black-and-blue" skin marks (ecchymoses). If you measure adrenal function, you can find subtle evidence for an effect of high-dose inhaled steroids on adrenal cortisol production. Over a period of many months to years, we worry about ocular side effects, specifically increased intraocular pressures, open-angle glaucoma, and cataracts. And particularly in women and older individuals of either gender, we are concerned about altered calcium metabolism and loss of bone mass (as relates to the development of osteoporosis). Not on this list (despite the concerns of some of our patients) is liver or kidney disease; neither organ is significantly affected by long-term steroid use.

KEY POINT   At high doses (more than 1000 mcg/day in adults, less in children), inhaled steroids pose some risk of long-term adverse effects, including ecchymoses, elevated intraocular pressure, open-angle glaucoma, cataracts, and accelerated bone loss. Fortunately, alternative therapeutic strategies are often available.

What should you advise your patient who is receiving high doses of inhaled steroids? Certainly, we do not recommend that you suggest that they stop their inhaled steroid; its use may indeed be necessary, and the long-term side effects of high-dose inhaled steroids are certainly *far less* than daily oral steroids, which the patient might otherwise need. You might inquire whether their physician has explored alternative therapeutic approaches, and you should help those at risk for osteoporosis (including women of any age) to take preventive measures, such as adequate intake of calcium and vitamin D and periodic radiographic measurement of their bone density (bone densitometry).

Mast cell stabilizers

Remember that when an allergic patient encounters an allergen (such as during a visit with her sister and the sister's pet cat), the allergen binds to immunoglobulin E (IgE) molecules on the surface of mast cells, triggering an explosive release of inflammatory chemicals from the mast cells. When the patient has asthma, these chemicals cause bronchial muscle constriction and heightened airway inflammation. Were it possible, it would be desirable to administer a medicine that prevents the mast cell from releasing all these chemicals, despite the occurrence of allergen-IgE interaction. In fact, this is the mechanism by which cromolyn (Intal) and nedocromil (Tilade), "mast cell stabilizers," are thought to work.

As you might predict, mast cell stabilizers are only effective preventively. Once an asthmatic reaction has taken place, they bring no acute relief. Unfortunately, for cromolyn and nedocromil to be effective maintenance therapies, they needs to be taken four times daily, a major drawback for any medication administered for more than just a few days. For a time, cromolyn was the mainstay of asthma therapy in children, primarily because of its remarkable safety profile. It is virtually free of adverse effects, short-term or long-term. However, it is also of only modest efficacy in controlling asthma symptoms. Because it is not as effective as the inhaled steroids and not as convenient as the leukotriene blockers (which we will consider momentarily), its role as routine maintenance therapy for asthma has dwindled.

Early on, cromolyn was made available as a dry-powder inhaler. One medication-filled capsule at a time was placed in a plastic delivery device, called a Spinhaler. The force of a breath in caused a small propeller to spin, aerosolizing the powder for inhalation. Unlike modern dry-powder inhalers, the cromolyn Spinhaler produced a rather coarse and unpleasant powder. Patients were advised to stop its use during asthmatic attacks, because the irritant effects of the coarse powder could trigger more bronchoconstriction. Subsequently, cromolyn became available as a liquid for nebulization (20 mg per glass vial) and as a traditional metered-dose inhaler (to be taken two puffs four times a day).

It turns out that cromolyn has another potential role in asthma care. A single dose of cromolyn administered approximately 20 minutes prior to exercise provides significant protection against exercise-induced bronchoconstriction. It has the advantage over beta-agonist bronchodilators, which can also be used preventively prior to exercise, of not causing any unpleasant side effects (such as jitteriness or heart racing). It has the disadvantages of being less effective than inhaled beta agonists and of providing no benefit should exercise-induced bronchoconstriction occur. Unlike albuterol, for instance, cromolyn would provide no acute relief from exercise-induced cough, chest tightness, or wheeze. In some instances, patients benefit from combining both cromolyn and an inhaled beta-agonist bronchodilator prior to exercise, when neither one alone seems to provide adequate protection.

Cromolyn is also sometimes used as a preventive medication prior to an anticipated allergen exposure, such as the trip to visit the in-laws and their pet cats. Although the safest choice would be total avoidance, the mast cell stabilizing properties of cromolyn may help to blunt the allergic asthmatic response. Have the patient start taking two inhalations from the metered-dose inhaler four times daily beginning on the day of the visit and continuing until after he or she is safely home again!

KEY POINT   Cromolyn has fallen from favor as maintenance therapy for asthma because of its limited effectiveness and need for four-times-daily dosing. It can be used (alone or in addition to a beta-agonist bronchodilator) prior to exercise for prevention of exercise-induced bronchoconstriction; and its preventive use can help minimize asthmatic symptoms during a known and unavoidable allergenic exposure.

Nedocromil (Tilade) is similar to cromolyn in its actions and efficacy. It too is recommended for administration four times daily, a major drawback. Some patients experience an unpleasant taste from this medication.

Leukotriene blockers

In 1996 the first of a new class of antiasthmatic medications, called leukotriene modifiers or leukotriene blockers, was introduced for sale in the United States: zafirlukast (Accolate). Soon thereafter followed zileuton (Zyflo) and montelukast (Singulair). At that time these medications represented the first entirely new approach to asthma treatment developed in over 30 years. They also represent a triumph of studies in airway biology and physiology resulting ultimately in new drugs that improve patient care—"from bench to bedside," as is said.

In the 1960s it was known that substances other than histamine were important in causing bronchoconstriction in asthma. Antihistamines proved effective in controlling certain allergic reactions (e.g., allergic rhinitis), but they did not work to treat asthma. It was evident that other chemicals were being released from mast cells and eosinophils, provoking airway inflammation and smooth muscle contraction. Early on, one of these chemicals was identified as "slow-reacting substance of anaphylaxis." The contraction of bronchial muscles that it caused was greater and sustained longer than that induced by histamine. Intensive research, including much contributed by physicians now practicing at Partners Asthma Center, identified the specific components of slow-reacting substance of anaphylaxis: the leukotrienes C_4, D_4, and E_4, together called the cysteinyl leukotrienes.

So, simply, leukotrienes are like histamine; they are chemical mediators of inflammation produced by mast cells and eosinophils. They cause bronchial muscle contraction, stimulate mucus production from bronchial mucous glands, and attract more eosinophils to travel out of the bloodstream and into the bronchi. They are approximately 1000-fold more potent than histamine in provoking bronchoconstriction. Wouldn't it be good if we had antileukotrienes to inhibit the effects of leukotrienes in the same way that antihistamines block the effects of histamine?

Zafirlukast (Accolate) and montelukast (Singulair) do just that. They block the cysteinyl leukotrienes from interacting with their receptor molecules. They are officially cysteinyl leukotriene receptor antagonists, which by agreement are all designated as –lukasts. They can also be appropriately called leukotriene blockers.

We think it worthwhile considering very briefly the biochemistry of leukotriene production, in part because it will help you to understand (and explain to patients) the differences among leukotriene modifying drugs and in part because it helps to clarify the condition, aspirin-sensitive asthma.

ASPIRIN-SENSITIVE ASTHMA

You have met patients with asthma who have been told by their doctors never to take aspirin. Why is that? It is because some patients with asthma—probably only 3–5% of all adults with asthma—will develop a severe asthmatic attack beginning 30–180 minutes after ingesting aspirin or any of the nonsteroidal anti-inflammatory drugs (NSAIDs), like ibuprofen (Advil, Motrin) and naproxen (Aleve, Naprosyn). Some doctors believe that because it is unpredictable when someone with asthma will become aspirin-intolerant, it is best to advise all patients with asthma to avoid aspirin and NSAIDs. Others (like us) feel that it is probably inappropriate to tell all patients with asthma to avoid these drugs when 95% or more will be able to take them without any harmful effect on their asthma.

KEY POINT   Three to five percent of adult asthmatic patients have aspirin sensitivity. They develop a severe asthmatic attack shortly after ingesting aspirin or any of the nonsteroidal anti-inflammatory drugs (NSAIDs).

Some patients with asthma and aspirin sensitivity also have nasal polyps. These three features (asthma, aspirin sensitivity, and nasal polyps) tend to run together; as many as 25% of patients with asthma and nasal polyps are aspirin sensitive. Dr. Samter and colleague described these associations in 1968, referring to them as "triad asthma." Others have since referred to asthma, aspirin sensitivity, and nasal polyps as Samter's triad or Samter's syndrome. We would certainly encourage patients with asthma and nasal polyps to be cautious about use of aspirin or NSAIDs if they have not taken either medication in several years.

An anecdote about one of our patients may help to keep this syndrome of asthma and aspirin sensitivity in mind. One of our patients with asthma and aspirin sensitivity underwent dental extraction. Her dentist recommended Motrin for post-procedure pain control. She mentioned that she was *allergic to aspirin*, but he thought that the Motrin would be fine. She took her prescription for Motrin to her pharmacist to be filled. She asked if he thought it would be OK for her to take the Motrin, given her allergy to aspirin, and he saw no reason for her not to take it. She went home, took two tablets of Motrin, and within a few hours was in the local hospital's intensive care unit with a life-threatening asthmatic exacerbation!

Now what does aspirin-sensitive asthma have to do with leukotrienes? Here's where a look at the biochemical pathways involved with leukotriene formation is informative. When mast cells and eosinophils are stimulated or activated, enzymes cause the fatty acid called arachidonic acid to be released from cell membranes. Arachidonic acid is the source of important chemicals involved in inflammatory processes. As shown in Fig. 3-4, when metabolized by the *5-lipoxygenase* enzyme, arachidonic acid is transformed via a series of chemical reactions to the cysteinyl leukotrienes, LTC_4, LTD_4, and LTE_4. This same arachidonic acid, when metabolized by the enzyme, *cyclooxygenase*, produces other families of chemicals, called the thromboxanes and prostaglandins.

Of note, in persons with asthma and aspirin sensitivity, an imbalance of these metabolic pathways leads to excess production of the leukotrienes. Aspirin-sensitive asthmatics are leukotriene overproducers. And if they ingest aspirin or any of the NSAIDs, they pour out lots more of the leukotrienes than

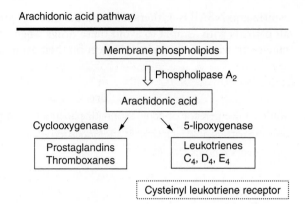

FIGURE 3-4 *The lipoxygenase enzyme metabolizes arachidonic acid toward the formation of the leukotrienes. The cyclooxygenase enzyme leads down another pathway, toward the formation of thromboxanes and prostaglandins. Aspirin and nonsteroidal anti-inflammatory drugs (NSAIDs) inhibit the action of cyclooxygenase, and in a small percentage of asthmatic patients can trigger severe asthmatic attacks.*

usual, in a burst of excess metabolism down this pathway. The reason is apparent when one remembers that aspirin and NSAIDs act by inhibiting the cyclooxygenase enzyme. In aspirin-sensitive asthma, if you block the metabolism of arachidonic acid down the cyclooxygenase pathway, you get excess leukotriene manufacture and a severe asthmatic attack.

KEY POINT   People with aspirin-sensitive asthma overproduce leukotrienes at baseline and make even greater amounts of leukotrienes after ingestion of aspirin or nonsteroidal anti-inflammatory drugs.

Persons with aspirin-sensitive asthma are not *allergic* to aspirin in the traditional sense of allergy. Their immune systems do not make an allergic reaction to aspirin (and ibuprofen, naproxen, sulindac, etc) in the way that they might to penicillin or sulfa drugs. Rather, they overproduce leukotrienes in response to cyclooxygenase inhibitors, also called COX inhibitors. Of interest, the selective cyclooxygenase 2 inhibitor, celecoxib (Celebrex), called a COX-2 inhibitor, generally does not provoke asthmatic attacks in persons with aspirin-sensitive asthma. Also, acetaminophen (Tylenol) is a very weak cyclooxygenase inhibitor and is generally safe for use in aspirin-sensitive asthma.

As asthma educators we need to help patients with asthma and aspirin sensitivity to be careful medication "bottle readers." Aspirin and NSAIDs are widely available over-the-counter in numerous cold remedies, pain relievers, and anti-inflammatory preparations. Without thinking, a patient with aspirin-sensitive asthma might take Alka-Seltzer for indigestion, unaware that at least some of the formulations contain aspirin. For these patients strict avoidance of aspirin and NSAIDs can be life-saving, and it requires considerable vigilance. Some patients may find a medical alert bracelet ("Asthma with Sensitivity to Aspirin and NSAIDs") useful.

The leukotriene-modifying drug, zileuton (Zyflo), was introduced in 1997, withdrawn from sale in the United States in 2003, and reintroduced onto the market by another pharmaceutical manufacturer in 2005. It works not by blocking the action of the leukotrienes at their receptor (like montelukast [Singulair] and zafirlukast [Accolate]), but by inhibiting the formation of the leukotrienes from arachidonic acid. It acts to inhibit the action of the 5-lipoxygenase enzyme (Table 3-6).

Zileuton (Zyflo) is an oral medication, and the tablet needs to be taken four times daily—a major drawback that in the past contributed to low "market share." A slow-release preparation for twice-daily administration is "in the works." Another negative is that zileuton has a small incidence (3–5%) of mild liver toxicity, such that blood studies to monitor liver function tests are recommended during the first few months of its use. Still, for some patients it has proved to be a highly effective medication, including some who do not benefit from the leukotriene receptor antagonists.

KEY POINT Montelukast (Singulair) and zafirlukast (Accolate) are leukotriene receptor antagonists; zileuton (Zyflo) is a lipoxygenase enzyme inhibitor. They are oral medications that block the action or formation of leukotrienes.

Leukotriene-modifying drugs cause some bronchodilation within hours of ingesting the first dose, and they exert some anti-inflammatory effects (for instance, fewer eosinophils found in blood and in expectorated sputum). Thus,

TABLE 3-6

LEUKOTRIENE MODIFIERS

Mechanism	Generic Name	Brand Name	Route of administration	Dosage strengths
Leukotriene-receptor antagonists	Montelukast	Singulair	Tablet, chewtab, sprinkles	4, 5, and 10 mg
	Zafirlukast	Accolate	Tablet	10 and 20 mg
Lipoxygenase inhibitor	Zileuton	Zyflo	Tablet	600 mg

they are not easily classified as "bronchodilators" or "anti-inflammatory drugs"; they seem to be some of both. They can be used alone as the only controller medication or in combination with inhaled steroids, providing additive benefit. And how effective are they, especially in comparison with inhaled steroids, for relief of symptoms, improvement in lung function, and prevention of asthmatic attacks?

The answer to this question appears to depend in large measure on how much of the leukotrienes a particular patient with asthma makes? Evidence from research studies suggests that some patients respond very well to leukotriene-modifying drugs whereas others respond not at all, depending at least in part on the extent of their leukotriene production. Leukotriene overproducers, including (but not restricted to) patients with aspirin-sensitive asthma, are most likely to do well with these drugs. Unfortunately, as of yet we have no way to predict which patients make lots of leukotrienes (with the exception of the subgroup with aspirin-sensitive asthma). We are left with the need to employ a *therapeutic trial*. Patients who benefit will do so within the first few weeks of use. If there is no improvement after 2–4 weeks, the medication can be discontinued.

In general—overall—inhaled steroids at low and moderate doses are more potent than leukotriene-modifying drugs in suppressing inflammation, improving lung function, and reducing the risk of asthmatic attacks. We often find ourselves prescribing leukotriene-modifying drugs for the following groups: those patients who are *steroid-phobic* and refuse use of any form of corticosteroids, including inhaled steroids; those who insist on medication in tablet form; those troubled by repeated bouts of oral candidiasis or hoarse voice due to their inhaled steroids; persons requiring high doses of inhaled steroids or oral steroids to control their asthma, where we are seeking ways to reduce the dose of steroids; and persons with aspirin-sensitive asthma. Montelukast (Singulair) has also been approved for the treatment of seasonal and perennial allergic rhinitis, conditions commonly associated with asthma in atopic individuals. The use of leukotriene-modifying drugs in children, including children as young as 6 months of age, will be discussed in Chap. 5, "Special Considerations in Childhood Asthma."

The efficacy of montelukast (Singulair) was proven in clinical trials where the time of administration of this once-daily medication (or placebo) was specified to be in the evening. The thinking, it appears, was that the drug would exert a maximal effect on nocturnal airway inflammation when given in this way. Often, montelukast continues to be prescribed as a medication for use in the evening or at bedtime. It is likely that once-daily administration in the morning would be equally effective, and most important is having the patient fit regular medication use into his or her schedule—in the morning, afternoon, or evening—in a way that maximizes adherence to daily usage.

Side effects are almost nonexistent with the following curious exception. Very, very rarely, a patient begun on one of the leukotriene receptor antagonists develops a serious systemic illness, called Churg-Strauss syndrome, within the first few months of beginning its use. Churg-Strauss syndrome is a vasculitis that can cause pneumonia-like pulmonary infiltrates, cardiomyopathy, renal injury, neuropathy, and skin rash. It occurs in persons with preexisting asthma, and it is characterized by eosinophils and granulomas in blood vessel walls throughout the body. There continues to be debate as to the relationship between leukotriene blockers and Churg-Strauss syndrome: do the medications cause the vasculitis, or does withdrawal of prednisone around the time that the leukotriene blockers were introduced unmask what has been a long-standing predisposition to this vasculitis? The incidence of this complication is thought to be one case per 64 million patient-years of treatment, comparable to the risk of an anaphylactic reaction to penicillin. Because it is so exceedingly rare, this association between leukotriene blockers and Churg-Strauss syndrome has not caused us to alter our prescribing pattern for montelukast (Singulair) or zafirlukast (Accolate), nor do we routinely discuss this complication with our patients when prescribing these drugs.

KEY POINT   A very rare complication associated with use of the leukotriene blockers is Churg-Strauss syndrome, an eosinophilic vasculitis with the potential for multisystem involvement (lungs, heart, kidneys, nerves, and skin).

We have not yet discussed the newest medication introduced for treatment of asthma, a medication designed to remove most of the allergy protein, immunoglobulin E (IgE), from the blood. This remarkable new immune-modulating molecule, called omalizumab (Xolair), has recently become available to treat allergic asthma that responds incompletely to traditional asthma medications. We will discuss it in detail in the following chapter, after we have a chance to address our approach to the patient with difficult-to-control asthma.

Self-Assessment Questions

QUESTION 1

The Expert Panel of the National Asthma Education and Prevention Program has identified four key components of effective asthma care. Which of the following is not one of these four key components?

1. Measures of assessment and monitoring.
2. Control of factors contributing to asthma severity.
3. Pharmacologic therapy.
4. Education for a partnership in asthma care.
5. Advocacy for asthma-safe housing and workplace environments.

QUESTION 2

In the 1970s and 1980s, slow-release theophylline preparations were commonly prescribed to asthmatic patients as the next step in therapy after inhaled beta-agonist bronchodilators. Some of the common side effects and other difficulties associated with theophylline include all of the following except:

1. Weight gain and mood swings.
2. Nausea.
3. Jittery, racy sensation.
4. Need to measure blood levels to find the proper dose.
5. Risk of seizures and cardiac arrhythmias from overdoses.

QUESTION 3

The current model for categorizing and teaching about asthma medications used in the ambulatory setting is which of the following?

1. Alpha-agonists and beta-agonists.
2. Bronchodilators and corticosteroids.
3. Bronchodilators and anti-inflammatories.
4. Controllers and quick-relievers.
5. Inhaled medications and orally-administered medications.

QUESTION 4

Medications that stimulate beta-adrenergic receptors on airway smooth muscle cause bronchodilation. An example of a medication that causes bronchoconstriction in asthmatics via this same pathway is:

1. Quinidine
2. Aspirin

3. Propranolol (Inderal)

4. Lisinopril (Zestril, Prinivil)

5. Magnesium

QUESTION 5

Unlike epinephrine (adrenaline) or isoproterenol (Isuprel), albuterol is a beta-2 selective adrenergic agonist. This implies that:

1. Albuterol is designed to cause less cardiac (beta-1) stimulation than the older bronchodilators.

2. Albuterol is preferred for intravenous administration.

3. Epinephrine is effective for treatment of anaphylaxis but not for asthma.

4. Albuterol can be expected to raise blood pressure to a similar degree as the older bronchodilators.

5. Albuterol is the preferred bronchodilator for ambulatory asthma management; epinephrine or isoproterenol is preferred for treatment of acute asthmatic attacks.

QUESTION 6

Levalbuterol (Xopenex) differs from albuterol in that it:

1. Causes no cardiac stimulation.

2. Contains only one of the two mirror-image molecules that make up albuterol.

3. Takes less time to administer because the dose is lower.

4. Can be made and sold at a lower cost.

5. Is indicated only for persons under age 14 or over age 60.

QUESTION 7

A 35-year-old woman comes to you concerned about a recent prescription that her doctor has written for combination fluticasone-salmeterol (Advair). She read in the package insert a warning about the potential harmful effects of salmeterol, including death. Her doctor made no mention of this possibility to her when he prescribed the medication. She asks whether you think that she should take it. You explain that:

1. Salmeterol is safe to use, but it will block the effect of other beta-agonist bronchodilators, such as albuterol.

2. Salmeterol and formoterol are dangerous; she should ask her physician for a prescription for fluticasone alone (Flovent).

3. The principal danger of salmeterol relates to cardiac arrhythmias that, because of its long duration of action, can be prolonged; she is safe to use Advair if she has no history of cardiac disease.

4. Advair is safe to use except prior to exercise.

5. Salmeterol should not be used in the absence of an anti-inflammatory medication such as an inhaled corticosteroid like fluticasone.

QUESTION 8

The mother of a 4-year-old boy with asthma worries that her son gets very little of the inhaled albuterol that she administers to him via a spacer and attached face mask. She wonders whether you would recommend that her doctor prescribe albuterol formulated as a syrup instead. She is sure that her son would swallow the liquid without difficulty. You suggest to her that there are disadvantages to the orally-administered liquid, including all of the following except:

1. More unpleasant side effects (jitteriness, heart pounding).

2. Slower onset of action (takes longer to begin to work).

3. Less powerful bronchodilation.

4. Greater potential for dependency.

5. Larger dose is needed to achieve the same bronchodilator effect.

QUESTION 9

Your 60-year-old patient is concerned about long-term effects of prednisone. Which of the following is not considered a potential adverse effect of long-term oral corticosteroids?

1. Kidney failure

2. Osteoporosis

3. Proximal muscle weakness (myopathy)

4. Cataracts

5. Glaucoma

QUESTION 10

A 21-year-old patient with newly-diagnosed asthma has been prescribed an inhaled steroid to be taken twice daily. She wonders whether it will cause her to build large muscles. You reassure her that steroids that cause athletes to enhance muscle growth are entirely different. At the same time, there are many advantages to taking inhaled steroids in asthma. You mention to her that the anti-inflammatory steroids can be expected to have all of the following effects in asthma except:

1. Improve lung function

2. Reduce risk of asthmatic attacks

3. Reduce the risk of progression to emphysema

4. Decrease airway hyperresponsiveness to exercise

5. Improve asthmatic symptoms and quality of life

QUESTION 11

The patient described in Question 10 has additional concerns about inhaled steroids. She has a friend who developed a yeast infection in her mouth (thrush) from use of an inhaled steroid. She asks if you have seen any other side effects from inhaled steroids. You mention as a possibility, even at low doses:

1. Glaucoma
2. Hoarse voice
3. Adrenal insufficiency
4. Glucose intolerance
5. Tolerance (need for increasing doses with chronic use)

QUESTION 12

Cromolyn [Intal] is thought to act by stabilizing mast cells. It prevents the release of inflammatory chemicals even when the triggering stimulus of IgE antibodies on the cell surface encounter allergens to which the antibodies have been formed. Cromolyn is best used:

1. Twice daily by nebulizer
2. Twice daily by metered-dose inhaler
3. Prior to exercise to block exercise-induced bronchoconstriction
4. After exercise to relieve exercise-induced bronchoconstriction
5. By patients with aspirin-sensitive asthma

QUESTION 13

A 13-year-old girl has been prescribed montelukast (Singulair) by her pediatrician, who explained to her that the medication is a leukotriene blocker. She comes to you to ask, "What's a leukotriene?" You explain that leukotrienes are chemicals released by inflammatory cells as part of allergic reactions in the body, including in the bronchial tubes. Effects caused by the leukotrienes include all of the following except:

1. Bronchoconstriction.
2. Stimulation of production of IgE antibodies to common inhaled allergens.
3. Secretion of extra mucus by bronchial mucous glands.
4. Attraction of more inflammatory cells (eosinophils) to the bronchial tubes.
5. Contraction of bronchial muscles at 1/1000th the concentration of histamine.

QUESTION 14

A young man with asthma and aspirin sensitivity comes to the emergency room following a fall from a ladder. He has suffered a contusion to his chest wall without rib fracture. You recommend for pain relief:

1. Low-dose aspirin only (no more than 650 mg/day)
2. Ibuprofen (Motrin)
3. Naproxen (Aleve)
4. Codeine
5. A single injection of keterolac (Toradol)

Answers to Self-Assessment Questions

ANSWER TO QUESTION 1 (GOALS OF ASTHMA MANAGEMENT FROM THE NATIONAL ASTHMA EDUCATION AND PREVENTION PROGRAM)

The correct answer is #5. Advocacy for asthma-safe housing and workplace environments, though a worthy goal, was *not* identified by the National Asthma Education and Prevention Program as one of its four key components of asthma care. They emphasized: (1) Making measurements of lung function to assess and monitor the severity of obstruction in patients with asthma (answer #1); (2) Control of factors contributing to asthma severity (answer #2), such as avoidance of allergens and irritants that make asthma worse; (3) Pharmacologic therapy (answer #3), the medications that we use to treat asthma; and (4) Education for a partnership in asthma care (answer #4), the concept of asthma comanagement involving medical provider and well-informed patient in a collaborative relationship. An asthma educator can contribute to achieving all of these goals and is absolutely crucial to the last one.

ANSWER TO QUESTION 2 (THEOPHYLLINE)

The correct answer is #1 (weight gain and mood swings). Systemic corticosteroids, not theophylline, can cause weight gain and mood swings. Theophylline side effects commonly include nausea (answer #2) and a jittery, racy sensation (answer #3). Because of the seriousness of overdosage and the differences in rates of metabolism of theophylline among different people, it is necessary in any given individual to adjust the dose according to measured theophylline blood level (answer #4). At very high (toxic) blood levels of theophylline, seizures and serious cardiac arrhythmias can develop (answer #5).

ANSWER TO QUESTION 3 (MODEL FOR CATEGORIZING—AND TEACHING ABOUT—ASTHMA MEDICATIONS)

The correct answer is #4 (controllers and quick-relievers). Controller medications are to be taken regularly to prevent or control asthma symptoms; quick-relievers are to be used intermittently for quick relief of asthma symptoms when they occur. Alpha-agonists and beta-agonists (answer #1) refer to medications that stimulate the alpha-adrenergic receptors (on blood vessels) or the beta-adrenergic receptors (on bronchi, blood vessels, and the heart). Bronchodilators and corticosteroids (answer #2) are two major categories of medications to treat asthma, but this model would omit several other types of medicines (e.g., mast cell stabilizers and leukotriene blockers). Bronchodilators and anti-inflammatories (answer #3) is the old model for discussing asthma medications. It refers to how medications work rather than how they are to be taken. One problem with this model is that leukotriene blockers, such as montelukast (Singulair) and zafirlukast (Accolate), appear to act as *both* bronchodilator and anti-inflammatory. Inhaled versus orally-administered tablets and syrups (answer #5) as a model to teach about asthma medications would fail to bring any new or useful information to patients, and would exclude the novel medication, omalizumab (Xolair), given by injection.

ANSWER TO QUESTION 4 (BETA-ADRENERGIC ANTAGONIST OR BLOCKER)

The correct answer is #3 (propranolol [Inderal]). Propranolol is a beta-adrenergic antagonist or blocker (beta-blocker). It acts at the same receptors as beta-adrenergic agonists such as albuterol. Stimulate the beta-adrenergic receptor on airway smooth muscle, and you get bronchodilation. Block the beta-adrenergic receptor on airway smooth muscle and you get—in asthmatics—bronchoconstriction. Quinidine (answer #1), aspirin (answer #2), lisinopril (Zestril, Prinivil) (answer #4), and magnesium (answer #5) do not operate via beta-adrenergic receptors. Incidentally, anyone (whether or not they have asthma) can develop a cough as a side effect of angiotensin converting enzyme inhibitors (ACE inhibitors) such as lisinopril. There are no special effects from ACE inhibitors in people with asthma.

ANSWER TO QUESTION 5 (MEANING OF "BETA-2 SELECTIVE ADRENERGIC AGONIST")

The correct answer is #1 (less cardiac [beta-1] stimulation than older bronchodilators). Older bronchodilators, such as isoproterenol (Isuprel), caused heart racing by stimulating beta-1 receptors on the heart as well as bronchodilation by stimulating beta-2 receptors on bronchial tubes. Newer bronchodilators such as albuterol and pirbuterol (Maxair) cause less tachycardia because they more selectively stimulate the beta-2 receptors on the bronchi. Albuterol is not available for intravenous administration in this country (answer #2). Epinephrine (answer #3) is an effective bronchodilator as well as treatment for anaphylaxis. Its nonselective beta-adrenergic stimulatory effect causes bronchodilation; its alpha-adrenergic agonist effect raises blood pressure and reduces swelling by causing blood vessels to constrict. Despite popular misconception, albuterol and other beta-2 selective adrenergic agonists do *not* cause elevation of blood pressure (answer #4). Even patients who become jittery with their use do not generally have rises in blood pressure from albuterol. Feeling jittery or having heart pounding is different than hypertension. Inhaled albuterol is preferred over epinephrine or isoproterenol in both the ambulatory management of asthma and the treatment of acute asthmatic attacks (answer #5) because it has fewer side effects.

ANSWER TO QUESTION 6 (LEVALBUTEROL [XOPENEX])

The correct answer is #2 (contains only one of two mirror-image molecules that make up albuterol). Levalbuterol is a single-isomer form of albuterol. Its advantage over albuterol depends on whether—as some say—the eliminated isomer has harmful effects, or whether—as others say—it is simply inert. Levalbuterol is meant to cause *less* cardiac stimulation (at doses causing equal bronchodilation) compared to albuterol, but not *no* cardiac stimulation (answer #1). The time needed to complete a nebulizer treatment (answer #3) depends on the volume of liquid placed into the nebulizer cup. Levalbuterol does not differ from albuterol in this regard. Levalbuterol is more expensive to make (and to buy) than albuterol (answer #4). Levalbuterol is often used in young children (in the hope of causing less agitation than albuterol) and in the elderly (in the desire to cause less cardiac stimulation), but levalbuterol has no special indications for these age groups (answer #5). According to the Food and Drug Administration (FDA), it is indicated for use in anyone 12 years of age or older.

ANSWER TO QUESTION 7 (SAFETY CONCERNS ABOUT LONG-ACTING INHALED BETA-AGONIST BRONCHODILATORS)

The correct answer is #5 (salmeterol should not be used in the absence of anti-inflammatory medications such as an inhaled corticosteroid like fluticasone). It is felt that effective bronchodilation without an anti-inflammatory medication can *mask* worsening airway inflammation and predispose to severe, potentially life-threatening asthmatic attacks. The long-acting inhaled beta-agonist bronchodilators do not prevent the shorter-acting bronchodilators such as albuterol from working (answer #1). The long-acting beta-agonist bronchodilators salmeterol and formoterol have benefits that exceed their risks (according to recent FDA review), are highly effective for many patients with asthma, and do not need to be considered dangerous (answer #2). The concern about long-acting beta-agonist bronchodilators that arose from the Salmeterol Multicenter Asthma Research Trial (SMART) was risk of respiratory failure and death due to severe asthmatic exacerbations, not cardiac arrhythmias (answer #3). Advair is not dangerous to use prior to exercise (answer #4).

ANSWER TO QUESTION 8 (ORAL VS. INHALED MEDICATION ADMINISTRATION IN A YOUNG CHILD)

The correct answer is #4 (greater potential for dependency). Neither oral nor inhaled administration of bronchodilators leads to a dependency on the medication. The disadvantages of taking a quick-acting bronchodilator, such as albuterol, as a tablet or liquid over inhaling the medication are the following: more unpleasant side effects, such as jitteriness and heart pounding (answer #1); slower onset of bronchodilator action (answer #2); and less powerful bronchodilation (answer #3).

It is also true that a larger dose of oral medication is needed to achieve the same bronchodilator effects as when the medication is inhaled (answer #5).

ANSWER TO QUESTION 9 (LONG-TERM SIDE EFFECTS OF ORAL CORTICO-STEROIDS)

The correct answer is #1; kidney failure is *not* a side effect of long-term oral steroid use. On the other hand, systemic steroids over time can indeed cause osteoporosis (answer #1); proximal muscle weakness (particularly in the thighs and shoulders), called "steroid-induced myopathy" (answer #3); cataracts (answer #4); and elevated intraocular pressure and open-angle glaucoma (answer #5).

ANSWER TO QUESTION 10 (BENEFICIAL EFFECTS OF INHALED STEROIDS IN ASTHMA)

The correct answer is #3. As you know, asthma does not develop into emphysema. Some people with asthma can develop an irreversible airway narrowing over time, which is different from emphysema; it is not known whether long-term use of inhaled corticosteroids can prevent this irreversible bronchial obstruction from occurring. Inhaled steroids can improve lung function (increase FEV_1) (answer #1), reduce the risk of asthmatic attacks (answer #2); decrease airway hyperresponsiveness to any triggering stimulus, including exercise (answer #4); and improve asthmatic symptoms and quality of life (answer #5).

ANSWER TO QUESTION 11 (SIDE EFFECTS FROM INHALED STEROIDS, EVEN AT LOW DOSES)

The correct answer is #2 (hoarse voice). The inhaled steroids can deposit on the vocal cords, leading to intermittent hoarse voice or change in the quality of one's voice. Glaucoma (answer #1) has been associated with long-term use of *high-dose* steroids only (more than 1500 mcg of beclomethasone per day or the equivalent for more than 3 months). Oral but not inhaled steroids are associated with adrenal insufficiency after several weeks of use (answer #3). Oral but not inhaled steroids can cause glucose intolerance and diabetes in susceptible individuals (answer #4). Neither oral nor inhaled steroids lead to medication tolerance and the need for gradually increasing doses over time (answer #5).

ANSWER TO QUESTION 12 (MAST CELL STABILIZER, CROMOLYN [INTAL])

The correct answer is #3. Taken as a single dose 20–30 minutes prior to exercise, cromolyn (Intal) partially blocks exercise-induced bronchoconstriction. As a daily controller medication, cromolyn is to be taken four times daily and is not recommended for twice-daily use by nebulizer (answer #1) or metered-dose inhaler (answer #2). Cromolyn acts entirely as a preventive medication; it does not act to reverse bronchoconstriction once it has occurred (answer #4). Leukotriene modifiers, not a mast cell stabilizer like cromolyn, are recommended for aspirin-sensitive asthma because the latter is associated with abnormally high amounts of leukotriene production (answer #5).

ANSWER TO QUESTION 13 (LEUKOTRIENES AND THEIR ACTIONS)

The correct answer is #2. Interleukins produced by lymphocytes, not leukotrienes, stimulate B-lymphocytes to produce IgE antibodies. It is true that leukotrienes stimulate bronchoconstriction (answer #1), secretion of extra mucus from bronchial mucous glands (answer #3), and attraction of eosinophils into the airways (answer #4). Leukotrienes are 1000-fold more potent than histamine in causing bronchoconstriction (answer #5).

ANSWER TO QUESTION 14 (CHOOSING AN ANALGESIC FOR A PATIENT WITH ASPIRIN-SENSITIVE ASTHMA)

The correct answer is #4 (codeine). Persons who have asthma and aspirin-sensitivity can develop an asthmatic attack following even small doses of aspirin (answer #1). Remember that aspirin sensitivity in asthma refers to a sensitivity to any medication that inhibits the cyclooxygenase enzyme, including all of the nonsteroidal anti-inflammatory drugs (NSAIDs). NSAIDs include ibuprofen (Motrin) (answer 2), naproxen (Aleve) (answer 3), and keterolac (Toradol) (answer 5).

CHAPTER

4

TREATING ASTHMA IN THE AMBULATORY SETTING

CHAPTER OUTLINE

I. Step-care approach to asthma therapy
   a. Mild intermittent asthma
      i. Exercise-induced bronchoconstriction
   b. Mild persistent asthma
   c. Moderate persistent asthma
   d. Severe persistent asthma
      i. Specialist referral
      ii. Approach to difficult-to-control asthma
      iii. Allergen immunotherapy
   e. Stepping down asthma therapy
II. New biologics: monoclonal anti-IgE antibody
III. Complementary and Alternative Therapies for Asthma
IV. Case examples

STEP-CARE APPROACH TO ASTHMA THERAPY

The current model for thinking about—and teaching about—the medications used to treat asthma divides the available drugs into two categories: *controllers* and *relievers*. The distinction is based on the purpose of the medications and how they are to be taken (rather than on their mechanism of action as an anti-inflammatory or bronchodilator). Controllers are used to control and prevent asthma symptoms; relievers are meant to provide quick relief from asthmatic symptoms. Controllers are to be taken every day on a preventive basis, regardless of the presence or absence of symptoms; relievers are to be used only when one is having asthma symptoms, to alleviate them. Leave the controllers at home in the medicine cabinet (except, of course, when you are away from home overnight); carry your quick-reliever with you at all times in your pocket or handbag.

Controller medications may be anti-inflammatory drugs (such as inhaled steroids or cromolyn), long-acting bronchodilators (such as long-acting inhaled beta-agonists, slow-release oral beta agonists, and theophylline), and leukotriene-modifying drugs. The quick-relievers are the inhaled beta-agonists with a quick onset of action and relatively short duration of action, like albuterol. (Formoterol [Foradil] is a curious hybrid in this regard: it has a quick onset of action but also a long duration of action. In this country we use it only as a controller medication.)

"Which are the right medications for me?" asks your patient. "That depends," you might reasonably answer, "on how severe your asthma is." Some patients with asthma have infrequent symptoms, normal lung function, and rare asthmatic attacks. They certainly will need a medication regimen for their asthma that is less intense than those who have frequent symptoms, impaired lung function, and repeated asthmatic attacks. We try to match the intensity of treatment to the severity of asthma. Using the four-stage system for categorizing asthma severity outlined in Chap. 2, national and international treatment guidelines recommend a four-step treatment approach. The treatment recommendations, summarized below, offer the best prediction of what medications will be needed to achieve good control in a patient with asthma of that particular level of severity.

Let's review one more time what is considered *good control* of asthma:

- Prevention of persistent and troublesome symptoms (e.g., coughing or breathlessness in the night, in the early morning, or after exertion);
- Maintenance of normal or near-normal lung function;
- Maintenance of normal activity levels (including exercise and other physical activity);
- Prevention of recurrent exacerbations of asthma, thereby minimizing the need for emergency department visits or hospitalizations.

If our initial treatment program fails to meet these goals, it may be necessary to *step up* the intensity of treatment. If good control is achieved for a period of weeks to months, it may be possible to *step down* the treatment. As part of a comprehensive treatment program, all patients can benefit from an effort at reducing their exposures to the inciters and triggers of their asthma, whether that means quitting cigarette smoking, finding another home for the pet cat (or the classroom pet bunny), or ridding the apartment of cockroaches. Likewise, most patients will benefit from a review of their use of their inhaled medications—are they inhaling them in a way that effectively delivers the medication to their airways or is their technique such that little medicine actually passes beyond the uvula?

Mild intermittent asthma (Step 1)

Patients with mild intermittent asthma can be treated simply with use of a quick-acting bronchodilator on an as-needed basis (Table 4-1). They have normal

T A B L E   4 - 1

SUMMARY OF STEP-CARE APPROACH

Stepwise Approach for Managing Asthma in Adults and Children Older Than 5 Years of Age: Treatment

Classify Severity: Clinical Features Before Treatment or Adequate Control			Medications Required To Maintain Long-Term Control
	Symptoms/Day Symptoms/Night	PEF or FEV$_1$ PEF Variability	Daily Medications

Step 4
Severe Persistent
	Continual
	Frequent
		≤ 60%
		> 30%
			■ Preferred treatment:
			  – High-dose inhaled corticosteroids
			    AND
			  – Long-acting inhaled beta$_2$-agonists
			    AND, if needed,
			  – Corticosteroid tablets or syrup long term (2 mg/kg/day, generally do not exceed 60 mg per day). (Make repeat attempts to reduce systemic corticosteroids and maintain control with high-dose inhaled corticosteroids.)

Step 3
Moderate Persistent
	Daily
	> 1 night/week
		> 60% – < 80%
		> 30%
			■ Preferred treatment:
			  – Low-to-medium dose inhaled corticosteroids and long-acting inhaled beta$_2$-agonists.
			■ Alternative treatment (listed alphabetically):
			  – Increase inhaled corticosteroids within medium-dose range
			    OR
			  – Low-to-medium dose inhaled corticosteroids and either leukotriene modifier or theophylline.
			
			If needed (particularly in patients with recurring severe exacerbations):
			■ Preferred treatment:
			  – Increase inhaled corticosteroids within medium-dose range and add long-acting inhaled beta$_2$-agonists.
			■ Alternative treatment (listed alphabetically):
			  – Increase inhaled corticosteroids within medium-dose range and add either leukotriene modifier or theophylline.

Step 2 Mild Persistent	> 2/week but < 1x/day > 2 nights/month	≥ 80% 20–30%	■ Preferred treatment: – Low-dose inhaled corticosteroids. ■ Alternative treatment (listed alphabetically): cromolyn, leukotriene modifier, nedocromil, OR sustained-release theophylline to serum concentration of 5–15 mcg/mL.
Step 1 Mild Intermittent	≤ 2 days/week ≤ 2 nights/month	≥ 80% < 20%	■ No daily medication needed. ■ Severe exacerbations may occur, separated by long periods of normal lung function and no symptoms. A course of systemic corticosteroids is recommended.

Quick Relief All Patients	■ Short-acting bronchodilator: 2–4 puffs **short-acting inhaled beta$_2$-agonists** as needed for symptoms. ■ Intensity of treatment will depend on severity of exacerbation; up to 3 treatments at 20-minute intervals or a single nebulizer treatment as needed. Course of systemic corticosteroids may be needed. ■ Use of short-acting beta$_2$-agonists >2 times a week in intermittent asthma (daily, or increasing use in persistent asthma) may indicate the need to initiate (increase) long-term-control therapy.

Step down
Review treatment every 1 to 6 months; a gradual stepwise reduction in treatment may be possible.

Step up
If control is not maintained, consider step up. First, review patient medication technique, adherence, and environmental control.

Goals of Therapy: Asthma Control

■ Minimal or no chronic symptoms day or night
■ Minimal or no exacerbations
■ No limitations on activities; no school/work missed
■ Maintain (near) normal pulmonary function
■ Minimal use of short-acting inhaled beta$_2$-agonist
■ Minimal or no adverse effects from medications

Note
■ The stepwise approach is meant to assist, not replace, the clinical decisionmaking required to meet individual patient needs.
■ Classify severity: assign patient to most severe step in which any feature occurs (PEF is % of personal best; FEV$_1$ is % predicted).
■ Gain control as quickly as possible (consider a short course of systemic corticosteroids); then step down to the least medication necessary to maintain control.
■ Minimize use of short-acting inhaled beta$_2$-agonists. Overreliance on short-acting inhaled beta$_2$-agonists (e.g., use of approximately one canister a month even if not using it every day) indicates inadequate control of asthma and the need to initiate or intensify long-term-control therapy.
■ Provide education on self-management and controlling environmental factors that make asthma worse (e.g., allergens and irritants).
■ Refer to an asthma specialist if there are difficulties controlling asthma or if step 4 care is required. Referral may be considered if step 3 care is required.

From: National Asthma Education and Prevention Program Expert Panel Report: Guidelines for the Diagnosis and Management of Asthma—Update on Selected Topics 2002 (www.nhlbi.nih.gov/guidelines/asthma/index.htm).

lung function, rare or no asthmatic attacks, and infrequently experience symptoms of their asthma. It is assumed that they will need their quick-acting bronchodilator for relief of symptoms no more than twice per week (or two nights per month). An albuterol inhaler, with 200 sprays in a full canister, should last all year. Although they too have chronic allergic-type inflammation of their bronchi, this inflammation is sufficiently mild that it does not require treatment.

Perhaps you know a person with mild intermittent asthma. She may have a story like the following. As a child she had troublesome asthma. She made many visits to her pediatrician for cough and wheezing and recalls several trips to an allergist, where allergy tests showed her sensitive to "just about everything." In early adolescence her asthma became less severe, and when she left home for college it seemed to disappear. Now at age 28, she very rarely experiences asthmatic symptoms. She knows that she still has asthma: if she ever comes in close contact with a cat, she develops wheezing and a tight chest, along with tearing and nasal congestion. And occasionally with chest colds she finds herself using her albuterol inhaler because of cough and shortness of breath. She enjoys mountain biking, but when the weather gets cold, she finds that she needs to take her albuterol inhaler during strenuous bike trips because the exertion predictably brings on chest symptoms. Her sleep is not disturbed by symptoms of asthma, and she has never had a severe asthmatic attack requiring emergency care.

We would remind her—and anyone with asthma—that she can use her quick-acting bronchodilator not only to relieve the symptoms of exercise-induced bronchoconstriction but also to prevent them. Approximately 10–15 minutes before exercise, take two puffs of albuterol or other quick-acting bronchodilator. She will then find that the exertion that would otherwise have caused her to cough or feel chest constriction now does not do so. Shoveling snow from her driveway no longer provokes cough and wheezing; a jog with friends can be accomplished without needing to stop to use her inhaler. If the medication is helpful but makes her uncomfortable because of side effects (jitteriness and heart racing), she can try one puff instead of the usual two.

KEY POINT   Use of a quick-acting bronchodilator 10–15 minutes prior to exertion is an effective strategy for prevention of symptoms associated with exercise-induced bronchoconstriction.

We are often asked about the patient with exercise-induced bronchoconstriction who works out 5–6 days per week and consequently uses his or her quick-acting bronchodilator *preventively* 5–6 times/week. Does this frequency of bronchodilator use put the patient in the category of mild persistent asthma?

Our answer is "no." If this patient continues to feel well, free of asthmatic symptoms, and uses his or her bronchodilator not for relief but for prevention of symptoms, this is still mild intermittent asthma. On the other hand, if—despite preventive use of albuterol—this patient experiences asthmatic symptoms for which he/she needs albuterol for relief or *rescue* several times per week, whether the symptoms are being provoked by exercise or other triggers, this patient would be considered to have mild persistent asthma. The intent here is prevention of frequent asthmatic symptoms. If preventive use of albuterol achieves that goal, continue that strategy. If not, begin use of a regular controller medication as the preferred strategy.

EXERCISE-INDUCED BRONCHOCONSTRICTION

Exercise-induced bronchoconstriction is a nearly universal experience among persons with asthma. For some it is also the most troubling aspect of their asthma. They find that asthmatic symptoms provoked by physical exertion limit their regular exercise, their recreational sports, or their competitive athletics. What should one consider in the patient who reports that despite use of a quick-acting bronchodilator prior to exercise, asthma continues to interfere with his or her physical activities?

Here is a 7-point checklist of things to consider:

1. Is the quick-acting bronchodilator being used properly? Always a good place to start is to review the patient's inhalational technique. (We will discuss in detail the proper use of metered-dose inhalers in Chap. 8, "Inhalers and Inhalational Aids in Asthma Treatment.") Is the inhaler empty? Has it expired?

2. Consider air temperature. Many people find that they can jog without difficulty in the summer, but come winter and a drop in air temperature (and humidity), the same level of exertion now provokes asthmatic symptoms. As we discussed in Chap. 1, the colder and drier the inspired air and the higher the level of ventilation during exercise (i.e., the heavier one's breathing), the more potent the stimulus to bronchoconstriction. It may be possible to find a venue (e.g., indoor gym) where exercise can continue without cold air exposure. For others, simple advice may suffice: cover your mouth and nose with a scarf (or cold weather mask) when walking outside.

3. Warm up and cool down periods before and after exercise are helpful. The same good advice for preparing your muscles for exercise seems to help to condition the airways as well.

4. Other medications taken prior to exercise can be useful in blocking exercise-induced bronchoconstriction. Cromolyn (two puffs) taken 20–30 minutes before exercise exerts additive protection when used in combination with a beta-agonist bronchodilator. Montelukast (Singulair) has also been shown to block exercise-induced bronchoconstriction, although this is not a Food

and Drug Administration (FDA)-approved indication for the drug. The long-acting beta-agonist bronchodilators are appealing in that their protective effect lasts essentially all day. A dose of salmeterol (Serevent) or formoterol (Foradil) administered at 9:00 in the morning can help block exercise-induced bronchoconstriction during gym class at 2:00 in the afternoon. However, a curious observation about the long-acting inhaled beta-agonists is that with daily use, this protective effect quickly (within 1 week) wears off.

5. The extent to which exercise provokes bronchoconstriction is influenced greatly by the underlying state of twitchiness of the airways. Airways that are very sensitive will react with more bronchoconstriction than airways that are only minimally hyperresponsive—whether to exercise or to any other asthmatic trigger. If one can reduce bronchial hyperresponsiveness, the same exercise stimulus may no longer provoke troubling airway narrowing. *Regular* use of an inhaled steroid or a leukotriene blocker can achieve this goal.

6. Is it possible that something other than asthma is limiting exercise? Shortness of breath that goes away in 2–3 minutes after resting is probably due to deconditioning, not exercise-induced bronchoconstriction (which typically takes 30–60 minutes to resolve, in the absence of bronchodilator use). Sometimes a functional abnormality of the upper airway (vocal cord dysfunction syndrome) gets in the way of exercising; it manifests as cough and loud wheezing—sometimes inspiratory, sometimes expiratory—emanating from the throat area rather than the chest. Cardiac issues may limit exercise in older persons and may cause symptoms (cough, chest tightness, and shortness of breath) that overlap with those of asthma. When assessing refractory exercise-induced bronchoconstriction, we need at least to consider alternative diagnoses.

KEY POINT Symptoms of exercise-induced bronchoconstriction tend to last for 30–60 minutes in the absence of bronchodilator treatment; breathlessness from being "out-of-shape" lasts only a minute or two.

7. Exercise-induced bronchoconstriction can readily be assessed in the pulmonary function laboratory. Exercise on a treadmill, and we can measure the degree to which exercise provokes airway narrowing by measuring spirometry before and after the exercise. If bronchoconstriction develops, repeat the experiment after premedication with albuterol or other treatments. If necessary, this sort of formal testing is available to recreate the conditions of exercise and to assess the role of various preventive strategies.

Mild persistent asthma (Step 2)

Patients with symptoms of asthma more than twice a week or nocturnal awakenings due to asthma more than twice per month should begin regular controller therapy for their asthma. That is the recommendation of experts written in national and international guidelines for asthma management. The preferred controller medication is an inhaled steroid in low doses.

KEY POINT   The preferred treatment for patients with mild persistent asthma is use of an inhaled steroid once or twice daily; once- or twice-daily administration of a leukotriene blocker is a potential alternative.

This is not a trivial decision: when to switch from reacting to asthmatic symptoms with a rescue bronchodilator to preventing asthmatic symptoms with a daily controller medication. Asking a young, otherwise healthy person to take a medication every day for the foreseeable future is a major intervention, especially if the medication that you recommend is a "steroid," with all the associated misgivings that people hold regarding steroids. *Will the medication have side effects? What about long-term effects? Will I become dependent on the medication; or will it lose its effectiveness if I take it every day? What happens if I skip a dose? If I want to stop its use, do I have to taper off gradually? What if I want to become pregnant?* You may be called upon to address these and many other questions about regular medication use for asthma.

In addition, patients with mild persistent asthma will still need to carry with them their quick-acting inhaled beta-agonist bronchodilator for rapid relief of symptoms, should they occur. Now your patient has two different medications to manage, doubling the possibility for confusion and error. We have all encountered patients who are using their rescue bronchodilator routinely twice daily and taking their preventive inhaled steroid as needed for relief of symptoms!

We need to remind ourselves that the pay off for regular use of a controller medication is worth it, even when persistent asthma is mild. Our patients will feel better. They will have fewer symptoms of asthma; they will need their quick-acting bronchodilator less often; they will be able to have good nights' sleep uninterrupted by asthmatic symptoms; and they will have some degree of protection from asthmatic attacks. Some have argued that long-term inhaled steroid use will also help protect from "airway remodeling" and potential loss of lung function over the years. Although this last benefit may be true, we believe it to be unproven and at present only a theoretical advantage to anti-inflammatory therapy.

Potential choices for initiating therapy with low-dose inhaled steroids include the following: beclomethasone (QVAR 40), two puffs twice daily; triamcinolone (Azmacort), two puffs twice daily; flunisolide (Aerobid/Aerobid M) one puff twice daily; fluticasone (Flovent 44), two puffs twice daily; budesonide

(Pulmicort Turbuhaler), one to two inhalations once daily; and mometasone (Asmanex), one inhalation once daily. We encourage use of a spacer device with flunisolide and fluticasone (QVAR has ultrafine particle delivery; Azmacort has a built-in spacer, and the Pulmicort Turbuhaler and Asmanex Twisthaler are dry-powder devices.)

An alternative strategy for mild persistent asthma is daily treatment with a leukotriene blocker. The appeal of this approach is use of a tablet rather than an inhaler, once-daily dosing (for montelukast [Singulair]), and virtual freedom from side effects. The disadvantage is that overall—in the majority of patients— it does not prove as effective as an inhaled steroid in relieving symptoms, preventing attacks, or improving overall quality of life.

As for the medication-related questions posed above, here are the answers that we would provide:

Will the medication (an inhaled steroid) have side effects? There is a small chance of dry mouth, hoarse voice, or a yeast infection of the mouth and throat, called candidiasis or thrush. To prevent these side effects, it is best to rinse your mouth with water after each use of your steroid inhaler. The yeast infection is easily treated with a medicated mouthwash or other prescription medication.

What about long-term effects? Inhaled steroids have been used to treat asthma for more than 30 years now. No long term harmful effects have emerged when they are used at the doses prescribed for mild persistent asthma.

Will I become dependent on the medication? No, the medication does not create a dependency on itself (like, for example, sleeping pills or narcotic pain relievers). If your asthma were to get better on its own, you could stop the medication immediately without any difficulty.

Will it lose its effectiveness if I take it every day? No, the medication will not lose its effectiveness at all; nor will you need to take more and more of it over time because of long-term use. If the medicine stops helping you, it will be because your asthma has changed, not because you have been taking the medication for a long time.

What happens if I skip a dose? There is no problem if you miss an occasional dose. You can simply resume use with the next scheduled dose. And note that when your doctor recommends that you use your medication twice daily, you do not have to adhere precisely to an every-12-hour schedule. Take the medicine sometime in the morning and again sometime in the evening, even if the interval between doses is more like 8 and 16 hours or even 6 and 18 hours. The main goal is to match medication use with your lifestyle so that you can remember to take two doses each day.

If I want to stop its use, do I have to taper off gradually? No, unlike oral steroids taken for a long time, there is no need to "wean off" inhaled steroids. If you no longer need them, you can simply stop them, without risk of experiencing the side effects of adrenal insufficiency.

What if I want to become pregnant? There is no evidence that any of the inhaled steroids causes problems during pregnancy; and good asthma control is the key to successful outcomes in pregnancy—for both mother and child. Still, the safety of inhaled steroids during pregnancy is not proven. Of the available inhaled steroids, the two that are considered to have the greatest safety for use during pregnancy are beclomethasone and budesonide. Budesonide (Pulmicort Turbuhaler) has the most favorable rating from the FDA for use in pregnancy (Category B), and many physicians ask their asthamatic patients to switch to this preparation if they are pregnant or are attempting to become so.

KEY POINT   Inhaled steroids do not lose their effectiveness over time, do not create a medication dependency, and do not have any known long-term harmful effects (in the doses prescribed for mild persistent asthma).

Recently, the recommendations from national and international guidelines regarding the treatment of mild persistent asthma have been called into question. A study published in the *New England Journal of Medicine* in the Spring of 2005 tested these recommendations in a group of approximately 200 patients carefully chosen for having mild persistent disease. In this study, called the Improving Asthma Control or IMPACT trial, patients were divided into three groups. For 1 year, the first group received the inhaled steroid, budesonide (Pulmicort 200 mcg twice daily), the second group received the leukotriene blocker, zafirlukast (Accolade 20 mg twice daily), and the third group received placebo. All patients were given a symptom-based asthma action plan to follow, with recommendations for use of inhaled or oral steroids during exacerbations of their asthma.

The IMPACT study found no differences between the three groups in frequency or severity of exacerbations, asthma quality-of-life symptom scores, or lung function measurements. The budesonide-treated group had slightly more symptom-free days (26/year) compared to the other two groups, and fewer signs of airway inflammation (based on measurements of sputum eosinophil concentration and exhaled nitric oxide levels). These findings will challenge the current recommendations for management of mild persistent asthma. They raise the possibility that in patients whose disease is truly mild, episodic treatment based on asthma symptoms may be acceptable in many patients. With this model, controller medications can be used for a period of a few weeks, until the increased symptoms abate, rather than taken daily all year-round. The authors of this research report (from the NIH-funded Asthma Clinical Research Network) suggest further study involving larger numbers of patients. In the meantime, physicians will likely negotiate with their patients about the lowest doses of preventive medication needed to keep them feeling well, sleeping well, using their rescue beta agonists infrequently, and maintaining normal or near-normal lung function. In some patients with mild persistent asthma, this dose may be zero.

Moderate persistent asthma (Step 3)

Patients with moderate persistent asthma will need more intensive therapy than recommended for mild persistent asthma. So, too, patients with mild persistent asthma who do not achieve good asthma control despite low-dose inhaled steroids will need to have their treatment program stepped up. You've ensured proper inhaler technique and regular medication compliance. You've helped the patient to reduce exposure to asthma triggers at home and at work or school, but still he or she is symptomatic. What's the next step in the step-care approach to asthma management?

There are three options at this point. The first is to increase the dose of the inhaled steroid. For example, switch from beclomethasone (QVAR) 40 to QVAR 80 mcg/puff, or increase from fluticasone (Flovent) 44 to Flovent 110 mcg/puff. Still the patient need only take two inhalations twice daily. The second is to continue the low-dose inhaled steroid and add one of the long-acting inhaled beta agonists, either salmeterol (Serevent) or formoterol (Foradil). The combination of fluticasone and salmeterol in a single dry-powder inhaler, the Advair Diskus, makes this particularly easy. Moderate persistent asthma can often be brought under good control with a regimen as simple as one puff twice daily of Advair 100/50 or 250/50. The third option is to begin a leukotriene-modifying drug in addition to the inhaled steroid in low doses. This regimen can be as easy as one pill once or twice daily and one or two puffs of a steroid inhaler twice daily. All patients continue to use a quick-acting bronchodilator as needed for "rescue therapy."

All three of these options are effective, relatively easy to comply with, and safe. Still, there are differences among them that have been demonstrated by carefully conducted clinical experiments. From these studies has emerged the consistent finding that the combination of a low-dose inhaled steroid with a long-acting inhaled beta agonist provides the best asthma control, and this approach succeeds in maintaining minimal long-term exposure to inhaled steroids. The combination of any of the inhaled steroids with either of the two long-acting inhaled beta agonists achieves this effect. The appeal of putting the combination in a single device—the Advair Diskus—is its convenience. With just one inhalation morning and night, even stubborn asthma can become well controlled. The device is easy to use; side effects are infrequent. For patients who at one time required complicated and potentially toxic regimens—for example, oral theophylline and six puffs of their beclomethasone (Vanceril) inhaler (delivering only 50 mcg/puff) twice daily—this modern therapy has had a life-altering effect. Safe, convenient, easy to use, and highly effective: asthma therapy has made huge strides forward in the last decade.

KEY POINT The preferred treatment for moderate persistent asthma is combination inhaled steroid (in low to medium doses) and a long-acting inhaled beta-agonist bronchodilator. The Advair Diskus provides this combination in a formulation that is easy to use, convenient, and highly effective. We anticipate the release of other devices combining an inhaled steroid with a long-acting inhaled beta agonist in the near future.

Severe persistent asthma (Step 4)

When asthma is severe, we tend to throw at it everything in our disposal, with the purpose of avoiding regular use of the oral corticosteroids, such as prednisone, prednisolone (Prelone), or methylprednisolone (Medrol). This often means "triple controller therapy": an inhaled steroid at high doses, a long-acting inhaled beta agonist, and a leukotriene-modifying drug. The recommended treatment of first choice is a high-dose inhaled steroid plus a long-acting inhaled beta agonist, such as is made available in the Advair 500/50 device (containing in each inhalation 500 mcg of fluticasone and 50 mcg of salmeterol). Alternatively, salmeterol (Serevent) or formoterol (Foradil) can be added to a separate steroid inhaler, such as beclomethasone (QVAR) 80 four puffs twice daily, flunisolide (Aerobid) four puffs twice daily, budesonide (Pulmicort Turbuhaler) four puffs twice daily, or fluticasone (Flovent) 220 two puffs twice daily.

As noted earlier in this chapter, when given in high doses for a long period of time (months to years), inhaled steroids can have some adverse consequences, including increased risk of cataracts, elevated intraocular pressure and glaucoma, and bone thinning. Still, the risk if far less than the myriad harmful effects that inevitably accrue from regular use of oral steroids. And our treatment plan includes the hope that once the patient's asthma is well controlled, we will be able to step down the dose of inhaled steroids.

SPECIALIST REFERRAL

Perhaps this would be also a good time for this patient to consider specialist consultation, especially if control of asthma symptoms has not been fully satisfactory. In general, referral is made to either an allergist or pulmonologist. Besides his or her special expertise in treating asthma, the specialist offers time and focus: an entire visit devoted strictly to helping manage the patient's asthma.

Patients appropriate for specialist referral include the following:

- Needing oral steroids on a regular basis;
- Frequent emergency room visits or hospitalizations for asthma;
- Uncertainty about the diagnosis of asthma;
- Intolerant of conventional medications because of adverse side effects; and
- Complicating comorbidities.

KEY POINT Patients with severe persistent asthma who do not achieve satisfactory control of their asthma despite recommended therapy should be referred for specialist consultation. This includes all asthmatic patients needing regular *oral steroids* to treat their asthma.

Asthma complicated by severe hay fever or food allergy might prompt referral specifically to an allergist. Asthma in a long-term cigarette smoker or a diagnostic puzzle requiring sophisticated pulmonary testing might appropriately lead to referral to a pulmonologist. Often local referral patterns are based more on historical affiliations than subtleties of the medical question being asked. In our opinion, the best referral is to the best asthma doctor, regardless of specialty.

APPROACH TO DIFFICULT-TO-CONTROL ASTHMA

At our Partners Asthma Center, we encourage a systematic approach to difficult asthma, using the following four steps:

1. *Assess for continued exposure to inciters of asthmatic inflammation.*

    In those with an allergic tendency, continued allergic exposures lead to more severe asthma, and reduction in environmental exposures results in better asthma control. Although these assertions seem intuitively obvious, only recently have scientific data from controlled clinical trials provided convincing scientific evidence in support of them. In particular, researchers found that a comprehensive program to reduce allergic exposures in the homes of children living in the inner city significantly improved their asthma control. Severe persistent asthma may be refractory to appropriate therapy because of continued pet exposure in the pet-allergic patient, cockroach infestation of the home of a cockroach-allergic patient, on-going cigarette smoking, or daily exposure to diesel exhaust fumes in a first-floor apartment outside a bus depot. Methods to reduce allergic and irritant exposures in the home are discussed in detail in Chap. 7, "Identifying Allergic Sensitivities and Promoting Allergen Avoidance."

2. *Check for aggravating medical conditions.*

    Some medical conditions make it difficult to get good control of asthma. Chronic rhinosinusitis worsens asthmatic symptoms. Gastroesophageal reflux can cause cough and chest tightness and may provoke worsened bronchoconstriction. Illicit drug use, especially inhaled cocaine, can provoke severe asthmatic attacks. Allergic bronchopulmonary aspergillosis is a rare complication of asthma, in which airway infection with the fungus, aspergillus, causes an intense inflammatory reaction in the lungs and bronchi. Depression and/or alcoholism make compliance with medical treatment plans difficult. These are some of the confounding medical conditions that may need attention before asthma can become well controlled.

3. *Ensure adherence with the prescribed medical regimen.*

    Medication noncompliance is a common finding in poorly controlled asthma. Inhaled medications are not always easy to coordinate; medication schedules can be excessively complicated; and asthma may be only one of a number of medical problems that the patient is trying to address all at the same time. Barriers to full adherence with the proposed treatment plan may also include the following: failure to understand the instructions; misgivings about the safety of the medications taken on a daily basis; cultural differences relating to health care beliefs; not enough money to obtain medication on a regular basis; and psychosocial handicaps, including alcoholism, depression, and social isolation. Overcoming these barriers often requires a team approach, involving multiple medical and social service resources.

4. *Confirm that asthma is the correct diagnosis.*

It is appropriate for the specialist to step back and ask, "Is this really asthma that we are dealing with?" Perhaps the medications aren't working well and airflow obstruction remains severe because the patient has chronic obstructive pulmonary disease (COPD), not asthma. Or because antibiotics are needed to treat chronic airway infection (bronchiectasis), rather than anti-inflammatory drugs to treat asthma. Or perhaps the cough and wheezing are due to congestive heart failure, multiple pulmonary emboli, or focal endobronchial narrowing due to an aspirated foreign body or bronchogenic carcinoma. These are a few of the examples of patients whom we have personally seen with a misdiagnosis of asthma, failing to improve on what should have been appropriate therapy for asthma.

ALLERGEN IMMUNOTHERAPY

Another consideration for the patient whose asthma is not responding to conventional medical therapy might be referral to an allergist for allergen immunotherapy (also called allergy desensitization injections or "allergy shots"). The rationale for this approach is the following. If one can identify an allergen to which a patient with asthma is sensitive and to which he or she is being exposed (e.g., house dust mite), one might be able to overcome that sensitivity by repeated injections of gradually increasing amounts of that allergen. If dust mite allergy were an important force driving the activity of the patient's asthma, and if by repeated injections of dust mite allergen the patient could be made no longer sensitive to that allergen, the overall allergic inflammation of the bronchial tubes (i.e., asthma) might lessen.

Despite more than 90 years of incorporation into clinical practice, the role of allergen immunotherapy in the treatment of asthma remains controversial. Ask many allergists, and they will tell you of the unquestionable successes that they have achieved with this technique. Ask other asthma specialists, and they may express skepticism as to its benefits and even concerns about its safety. The debate is reflected in the words of experts. One authority offers this viewpoint: "*Immunotherapy is the only treatment available today that has the potential to suppress the basic mechanism and to reduce the underlying cause of allergic asthma. Many studies have unequivocally shown that properly administered immunotherapy reduces both asthma symptoms and the need for concomitant medications*" (Dr. Philip Fireman). Another expert expresses the opposite viewpoint: "*There can be few indications for the use of allergen immunotherapy in the routine management of asthma in view of its low efficacy, the risk of adverse effects, the relatively high cost of treatment, and the availability of safer and more effective drug therapy*" (Dr. Peter Barnes).

KEY POINT   Even today, controversy surrounds the role of allergen immunotherapy ("allergy shots") in the treatment of asthma.

The premise on which allergen desensitization is founded seems sound. In patients with anaphylactic reactions to stinging insects (e.g., bee sting anaphylaxis), allergen desensitization is of proven benefit and can be life-saving. With repeated injections of very small amounts of the appropriate allergen, the life-threatening reactions to bee stings subside. In immunologic terms, patients can be made to synthesize immunoglobulin G (IgG) in reaction to the injected antigen, rather than immunoglobulin E (IgE). IgG antibodies do not trigger allergic reactions; they act to block the allergic response. By choosing the right doses and frequency of administration of the allergen, the allergist in essence can switch the patient's immune response from primarily IgE- to primarily IgG-mediated.

Sounds good, but does it work in asthma? Therein lies the debate, even when discussing the results of published research experiments. One carefully controlled clinical trial was conducted by medical researchers at Johns Hopkins School of Medicine. They enrolled approximately 120 children between the ages of 5 and 12 years, all of whom had asthma and allergic sensitivities. For slightly more than $2^1/_2$ years, half the children received allergen immunotherapy, the other half received placebo injections. The patients and their primary doctors were kept blinded as to which group the patients were assigned. According to a written protocol, the doctors tried to reduce the children's asthma medications as much as possible, without causing any worsening of their symptoms.

In the end, there were no significant differences between the two groups. Both groups were able to have their medications reduced somewhat. Thirty-one percent of the children who received allergen immunotherapy experienced what was considered partial or complete remission of their asthma; but similar results were found in the placebo group. If there was a benefit from the allergy shots, it seemed to be confined mostly to the subgroups of children younger than $8^1/_2$ years and having mild asthma. As you might predict, interpretation of these results falls into two camps. Some find that the results indicate a lack of benefit from allergen immunotherapy when it is added to good medical care; others point to the benefit observed in some children and to flaws in the design of the study that prevented even greater utility from being seen.

It is not entirely surprising that so much confusion surrounds the role of allergen immunotherapy in treating asthma. Many different variables will influence the outcomes.

Is the patient definitely allergic to the allergen(s) being chosen for the immunotherapy treatments? Are these allergic sensitivities crucial to the allergic-type inflammation of the airways? (It will probably do no good to undergo desensitization to dust mite allergen if one continues to smoke cigarettes and have exposure to cat allergen and mold.) Is there a standardized version of that allergen available for use in allergen immunotherapy, or does the allergen preparation vary from one physician's practice and another's? Are the doses and frequency of administration properly chosen? And is the patient compliant with the regimen, including in many instances weekly medical visits for the first 3–6 months of treatment?

Nor is this treatment without its risks. Sometimes injection of the allergen provokes allergic reactions, including asthmatic attacks, throat swelling, and low blood pressure (anaphylaxis). Very rarely, fatal reactions occur, with those who have the most severe asthma being at greatest risk. Therein lies a major dilemma regarding the role of allergen immunotherapy. In those patients with the most severe disease, in whom an alternative to treatment with systemic steroids is being sought, allergen immunotherapy poses the greatest risk for dangerous allergic reactions—and is probably best avoided.

KEY POINT The greatest risk for serious adverse reactions from allergen immunotherapy, including death, is among those with severe asthma.

Stepping down asthma therapy

The step-care approach to asthma therapy allows one to choose an initial medication or set of medications based on disease severity. If there is incomplete improvement, the treatment regimen can be stepped up to the next highest level, until good control of asthma symptoms is achieved. When the patient is feeling well and lung function has been optimized, one can then continue that intensity of treatment—but for how long? Forever? Or is it sometimes possible to cut back on some of the medications, to step down the intensity of treatment?

For some patients, there is a clear-cut seasonal variability to their asthma. For instance, they can predict improvement every spring and summer, with worsening as soon as central heating comes on and life moves indoors for late fall and winter. Others report predictable worsening with grass and tree pollen season (e.g., May through September in New England), then improvement with the first frost. It is entirely appropriate to step up treatment at the beginning of allergy season (e.g., begin an inhaled steroid) and then step down treatment when out of allergy season (e.g., stop the inhaled steroid).

Another patient reports moving into a new home free of dust and mold exposures; or perhaps she has found a new home for the pet cat. She is feeling well, and perhaps has missed some doses of medication without noting any change in symptoms. Is it possible that the intensity of her asthma has lessened and that some of her anti-asthmatic medications are no longer necessary? The answer is, sadly, no more definite than "yes, maybe." We have no good test to predict whether cutting back or stopping this patient's inhaled steroid, for example, will lead to worse asthma control or not. Is it possible that we will be putting the patient at greater risk for an asthma attack by reducing preventive medications?

It would be good if we could monitor the degree of airway inflammation to determine whether it remains adequately suppressed with less medication. As we reduce the dose of inhaled steroids for example, from fluticasone (Flovent) 220 mcg/puff, four puffs per day to 110 mcg/puff, four puffs per day does the allergic inflammation of the bronchial tubes worsen, heightening bronchial hyperresponsiveness and making the patient more susceptible to asthma exacerbations?

As of yet, we have no simple and reliable measure to answer this question. Perhaps some day we will measure the concentration of an important biomarker (e.g., nitric oxide) in the exhaled breath or the percentage of eosinophils in a sample of induced sputum. For the time being it is a matter of trial and error. If the patient is doing well and therapy is stepped down, we need to monitor closely for deterioration (and the need to resume the previous level of treatment).

We tend to follow the following three rules in stepping down asthma therapy. First, our priority is to reduce the most toxic medications first. Consequently, we work hardest to have patients who require daily or alternate-day oral steroids withdraw from their systemic steroids; and we try to cut back from high-dose steroids to low or medium doses, which are safer in the long run. Second, when reducing medications, besides asking patients to watch for increased symptoms or increased frequency of need for their rescue bronchodilator, we ask them to monitor their lung function with measurements of peak flow at home. Gradually falling peak flow values can be a good warning sign that the lower dose of medication is insufficient for good asthma control.

KEY POINT   When stepping down asthma therapy, we target first those medications with the greatest risk of serious harmful side effects.

Third, patients on dual controller therapy with an inhaled steroid and long-acting inhaled beta-agonist bronchodilator may be able to reduce their dose of inhaled steroid, but they should not stop the steroid all together. For example, a patient with moderate persistent asthma may have achieved good control by adding salmeterol (Serevent) to his steroid inhaler (triamcinolone [Azmacort]). It would be tempting to reduce the dose of triamcinolone, and, if the patient is doing well, to stop it entirely. This approach turns out to be a bad idea. When tested in a controlled experiment where good asthma control was achieved with addition of a long-acting inhaled beta agonist, the number of subsequent treatment failures over a 4-month period was fourfold greater in those whose inhaled steroid was stopped compared to those whose steroid dose was maintained unchanged. Some minimal treatment of the allergic-type inflammation of the airways is necessary in moderate and severe persistent asthma, probably with no fewer than 200 mcg/day of most inhaled steroids or 88 mcg/day of fluticasone (Flovent).

KEY POINT   In patients with moderate or severe persistent asthma, it is a mistake to stop inhaled steroids while continuing a long-acting inhaled beta-agonist bronchodilator. The risk of an asthma flare is unacceptably high with this approach. Long-acting beta-agonist bronchodilators should only be used in combination with concurrent anti-inflammatory medication (inhaled steroids).

NEW BIOLOGICS: MONOCLONAL ANTI-IGE ANTIBODY

We have already spoken of the central importance of the allergy protein, immunoglobulin E (IgE), in allergic (atopic) asthma and in other atopic diseases. Allergens and the IgE antibodies that recognize them are like lock and key to initiation of the allergic process. When IgE molecules, bound at one end to their receptors on the surface of mast cells, encounter and bind at their other end to allergens, the allergic cascade is triggered. Inflammatory chemicals are made and released from mast cells; other inflammatory cells, especially eosinophils, are recruited into the airways; and the allergic response is launched. In the airways it manifests as asthma; in the eyes as allergic conjunctivitis; in the nose as allergic rhinitis; in the skin as allergic dermatitis or eczema; and in the bloodstream as anaphylaxis.

What if you could design a molecule that would bind to IgE and remove it from the blood? It would have to be a highly targeted molecule, an antibody that would recognize only IgE molecules. It would have to bind IgE in such a way that it did not act like an allergen and trigger off an allergic reaction. It would need to be created in mice, all of the antibody molecules exactly the same (monoclonal antibodies), but then modified with mostly human amino acids substituted for mouse amino acids so that the human immune system would not recognize it as a foreign protein. And the IgE—anti-IgE complexes that it formed with IgE would need to be sufficiently small so that they could be readily cleared from the system and not settle, as immune complexes sometimes do, in joints or the kidneys.

What sounds like an impossible task has been achieved by scientists working in the pharmaceutical industry. These scientists have created an anti-IgE monoclonal antibody called omalizumab (Xolair), marketed by Genentech and Novartis. As an aside, you will notice that the names of all monoclonal antibodies end in -mab, whether they are the monoclonal antibodies used for treatment of lymphomas (rituximab [Rituxin]), for antiplatelet effects (abciximab [Reopro]), or for rheumatoid arthritis (infliximab [Remicaide]). Omalizumab binds to IgE molecules at exactly the site where they would otherwise have bound to their receptors on the surface of mast cells (Fig. 4-1). The omalizumab- IgE complexes are relatively small and are readily cleared by the reticuloendothelial system (lymph nodes and spleen) (Fig. 4-2). This humanized monoclonal antibody is 95% human amino acid sequence and only 5% mouse amino acid sequence (Fig. 4-3). It is not recognized as a foreign protein by our immune system; we rarely make anti-omalizumab antibodies despite repeated injections of omalizumab.

Omalizumab (Xolair) cannot clear from our system the IgE molecules that are already tightly bound to the surface of mast cells. It can, however, remove the IgE molecules circulating in our blood, and it does so with 95% efficacy. And it removes all IgE molecules, regardless of the target to which they have been formed. So it reduces the level of circulating IgE to cat dander, IgE to mold, IgE to cockroach, IgE to dust mite, and the like.

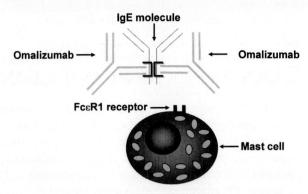

FIGURE 4-1 *Binding of the allergy protein, IgE, to its receptor (FcɛR₁) on the surface of a mast cell is prevented when omalizumab binds to IgE molecules at precisely the site where they would otherwise attach to this receptor molecule. From: slide set, Genentech/Novartis.*

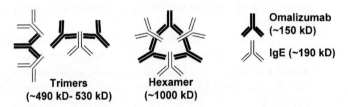

FIGURE 4-2 *Omalizumab and its target, IgE, form small molecular complexes (timers and hexamers) that are removed from the blood without settling in the kidneys or joints (as larger immune complexes sometimes do). kD = kilodaltons, a measure of the size of molecules. From: slide set, Genentech/Novartis.*

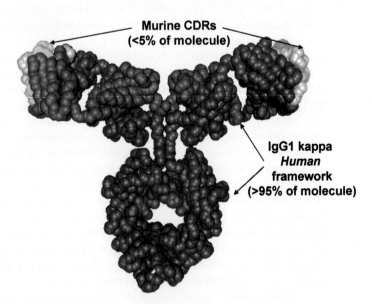

FIGURE 4-3 *The anti-IgE monoclonal antibody, omalizumab, is created by genetically manipulated mouse cells. This diagram showing the structure of omalizumab illustrates that most of the amino acids in the structure of this protein have been substituted with human amino acids, with <5% continuing as mouse amino acids. CDR = "complementarity-determining region," the part of the molecule that "recognizes" the specific attachment site on IgE molecules. From: slide set, Genentech/Novartis.*

KEY POINT Omalizumab (Xolair) clears circulating IgE molecules from the blood, regardless of the specific allergen to which they have been formed.

Omalizumab (Xolair) has been approved for use in moderate persistent and severe persistent asthma. It is indicated for patients who have documented allergy to at least one perennial allergen (year-round allergens include animal danders, dust mite, cockroach, and mold) and who have blood IgE levels in the range of 30 to 700 units. In most instances it is used to treat asthma that has failed to come under good control with conventional antiasthmatic therapies. If your patient is already taking an inhaled steroid, long-acting inhaled beta-agonist bronchodilator, and leukotriene blocker, what else do we have to offer? One answer is the anti-IgE antibody, omalizumab (Xolair). In our opinions, it should only be offered in concert with specialist (allergist or pulmonologist) consultation regarding asthma.

The medication is administered as a subcutaneous injection. Depending on the dose required, it is given every 2 weeks or every 4 weeks. The dose is determined by patient weight and blood IgE level. Once it is given, unfortunately we cannot monitor blood IgE levels. Most available assays will measure the sum of both free IgE and IgE bound to omalizumab, giving values that do not decrease from baseline. The injections are well tolerated, with very few local reactions (swelling or hives). Early concerns about a possible association between use of omalizumab and an increased incidence of neoplasia have not been born out by careful scrutiny of the data or by subsequent experience. There is a very small risk of anaphylactic reactions to omalizumab (occurring in 1 in 1000 patients), prompting us to observe our patients for two hours after they receive their omalizumab injections and to request them to carry with them an epinephrine autoinjector (EpiPen or Twinject) for a day afterwards.

And how well does omalizumab (Xolair) work? In our experience and review of published clinical trials, we would answer: very well for some people, but overall only modestly well. Overall, patients treated with omalizumab (Xolair) have a small increase in lung function, a small improvement in symptoms, and a small decrease in their need for rescue bronchodilator; and they achieve this while reducing their need for inhaled steroids. The most consistent outcome is that omalizumab-treated patients have fewer and shorter asthmatic exacerbations (despite reducing their inhaled steroid dose). Because of the enormous cost of the drug (tens of thousands of dollars each year, prescribed for chronic use, indefinitely), we have reserved its prescription for our most severe patients, especially those needing frequent or continuous oral corticosteroids. It is possible that even more dramatic beneficial effects can be obtained in a population of asthmatic patients less severely ill.

KEY POINT Omalizumab (Xolair) offers a new therapeutic option for patients with allergic asthma of moderate and severe intensity, one that does not involve corticosteroids and appears to be free of significant side effects. It comes at great financial cost.

With this new anti-IgE monoclonal antibody we can offer our patients with allergic asthma a novel medication, one that is not a steroid and appears to be free of significant side effects. Because of its route of administration, medication compliance can be assured. At the same time, we can also wonder why this "designer molecule" has not been more miraculously effective, essentially eliminating all allergic reactions. The answer may be that enough IgE molecules remain bound to mast cells to continue to trigger allergic responses. It is also possible that IgE molecules bound to omalizumab are still able to bind to mast cells, using other binding proteins along the mast cell surface (called their "low affinity receptors"). And perhaps there are other pathways via which allergic reactions can be triggered, even in the absence of IgE molecules (as occurs in genetically IgE-deficient mice).

COMPLEMENTARY AND ALTERNATIVE THERAPIES FOR ASTHMA

Even with the remarkable advances that have been made in asthma care over the last few decades—even with the introduction of drugs that are safe, easy to use, and highly effective—modern asthma therapy is not perfect. Coordinating inhaled medications can be frustrating. Sometimes patients experience unpleasant side effects from their medications, whether thrush, heart racing, or muscle cramps. And not everyone achieves full relief with his or her prescribed treatments. Emergency room visits and hospitalizations for asthma remain commonplace, and school and work absences are all too frequent. Given these shortcomings it is not surprising that many people explore nontraditional avenues to treat their asthma. They look about for something better.

Other patients are driven by different motivations. They wish to avoid putting *foreign chemicals* in their bodies and so explore dietary, herbal, or homeopathic remedies. They are attracted to the idea that these treatments seem safer and more *natural* to them. From drugstores we get drugs, with concerns about toxicity, dependency, and addiction. From health food stores, we seek health-promoting natural remedies. And this is just one example of culturally-derived health care beliefs. Other cultures believe just as strongly in the value of other folk remedies, whether keeping Chihuahuas to fend off asthma (Mexican) or swallowing live sardines to clear up phlegm (Indian).

As medical providers trained in Western medicine, we tend to view these nontraditional approaches with some skepticism. Hucksterism is as old as humanity. Wherever there is illness, there will be shysters willing to sell worthless "remedies" with fabulous claims about their miraculous curative powers. You may remember laetrile, the "cancer cure" that turned out to be nothing more than ground-up apricot pits. Glossy advertisements, dramatic patient testimonials, and endorsements by authorities with impressive degrees—these are some of the draws that can be used to sell unregulated products with no worth whatsoever.

And yet, is it possible that there is merit to some of these nontraditional treatments? Many modern drugs were first isolated from plants. Acupuncture may be based on primitive, prescientific concepts of energy flow through *meridians* in our body, but it clearly provides effective pain control in certain circumstances. The mind-body connection is incredibly complex; how the brain interacts with our immune system is understood only superficially. We should not close our minds to the possibility that stress-relaxation and biofeedback techniques may favorably influence the course of asthma. How do we achieve a healthy balance between skepticism and open-mindedness, accepting cultural biases different from our own while not encouraging useless and potentially dangerous quack remedies?

In our practices we are guided by three main principles. First, we ask for scientific evidence about effectiveness. Complementary and alternative therapies should be held to the same standards as any new medicine or procedure. It is possible to test whether chiropractic manipulation is more effective in asthma than sham manipulations (no, it is not). Randomized trials can test whether acupuncture for asthma produces better outcomes than random placement of acupuncture needles at irrelevant body sites (no, it does not). When patients ask about herbal treatments or special diets (e.g., diets rich in fish oil or eicosapentaenoic acid), we ask about published results in peer-reviewed journals. Scientific methodology is a powerful tool to determine the truth of advertising claims.

KEY POINT   One can ask of an alternative or complementary remedy, as we do of all of our traditional practices, for scientific evidence of efficacy and safety based on controlled clinical trials.

Second, we seek to ensure the safety of the nontraditional medication or practice. Because in the United States herbal treatments are not regulated by the FDA, their safety cannot be guaranteed. Recall the disastrous consequence (eosinophilic myositis) that some people suffered when using the "natural" sleep remedy, tryptophan. Remember that ephedra seemed like a harmless weight-control remedy until studies documented an associated risk of strokes and heart attacks. Acupuncture administered by skilled practitioners is safe, but cases of poor technique have resulted in pneumothoraces and asthma fatalities. To the extent that we can, we seek to steer our patients away from treatments that are potentially dangerous.

KEY POINT   Herbal remedies are not regulated by the FDA and cannot be presumed safe even though they are marketed as "natural."

Third, we encourage our patients not to abandon their traditional prescribed medications while pursuing nontraditional approaches. We tell them: "Make this nontraditional therapy complementary to your usual care, not an exclusive alternative. Find a homeopathic physician or massage therapist or energy-field practitioner who can accept your contact with mainstream medical practitioners and conventional medications. Your pursuit of good health should have room to encompass both approaches."

CASE EXAMPLES

Whether you are in a position to write prescriptions or simply to review someone's medication plan to help assess its appropriateness, you will likely have the opportunity to consider application of the asthma *Guidelines* to a particular patient. Is he or she being appropriately treated? Are there concerns that you and the patient have that should be brought to the treating asthma care provider? As you consider these case examples, a good place to start is by asking yourself into which step or category of asthma severity this patient fits. Then think about the treatment options recommended for someone of that severity. Another equally helpful approach is to ask whether the treatment regimen that the patient is receiving is (1) achieving good asthma control; (2) as free as possible of side effects; and (3) safe for long-term use. If not, might something better be available?

▶ ▶ ▶ **CASE 1**

A Frightened Sister
A 21-year-old secretary comes for reassurance after her sister's death from asthma.

While in high school, she developed symptoms of asthma triggered mainly by exercise. She was prescribed an albuterol inhaler to use prior to exercise and as needed for relief of symptoms. She has some seasonal rhinitis, no pets, and no unusual exposures at home or at work. She considers her asthma quite mild; her visit is prompted by the death of her sister, who had severe asthma for many years.

Her past medical history is unremarkable. She takes no medications other than albuterol by metered-dose inhaler.

Her physical examination is normal. Spirometry reveals normal lung function with a forced expiratory volume in 1 second (FEV_1) 114% of predicted.

Is her treatment appropriate?
We hope that your reaction to this question is: "I need more information." Before you can judge the appropriateness of her treatment, you need more information to categorize the severity of her asthma and to assess the adequacy of her asthma control. You will need to ask how often she experiences symptoms of her asthma in a typical week (4–5 times/week, she answers). How often does she need her albuterol inhaler to relieve cough, chest tightness, or wheezing?

She uses it preventively every time that she goes to the gym and 4–5 times/week for her chest symptoms. How often does she awaken from her sleep because of asthma symptoms? Two or three times a month, she responds. Can she tell you about her peak flow measured at home? No, she does not check her peak flow.

KEY POINT   You need sufficient details about asthma symptoms and frequency of rescue bronchodilator use to judge the severity of asthma and the adequacy of asthma control. You can't make an adequate assessment based solely on the patient's appearance at one moment in time.

With this information you have a much better sense about how her asthma is affecting her life. According to the asthma *Guidelines*, she has mild persistent asthma, and albuterol used as needed is providing inadequate control of her symptoms. Asthma therapy is available such that she does not need to experience symptoms as often as she does; she does not need to have this many disturbed nights' sleep. With regular use of a controller medication, it is predicted that she will soon begin to feel better. She will have fewer asthma symptoms; she will rarely need her albuterol inhaler except prior to exercise; and she will sleep the night through virtually every night. She will feel as though her asthma is "going away."

For these reasons it is recommended that she begin a daily controller therapy for her asthma. Asking an otherwise healthy 21-year-old woman to take a medicine every day for years to come is not an easy sell. But the reason for her to do it, you might suggest to her, is that it will improve the quality of her life. In addition, it will help to protect her against asthmatic attacks. Although her risk of severe attacks is small—and unrelated to her sister's recent death from asthma—it is not zero. Even people with mild asthma can experience serious asthmatic exacerbations, and the risk is reduced with regular use of controller medication.

There will be considerable need for asthma education if her physician prescribes an inhaled steroid as her controller medication. She will need to learn how to use the inhaler device, perhaps together with a spacer. She will need to be reminded to rinse her mouth after each use (with plain tap water is fine). She will want to know about *steroids*, about possible side effects (scratchy or hoarse voice, sore throat, and dry mouth), and about harmful consequences of long-term use (none when used at low to medium doses). She will need to distinguish between her controller medication and her quick-acting bronchodilator and know that she can still use her albuterol as before (prior to exercise and for rapid relief of asthmatic symptoms). What if I miss a dose? (No problem; simply resume the usual schedule with the next dose.) What if I want to become pregnant? (These medicines are generally safe, but she will want to discuss the choice of specific asthma medicines during pregnancy with her doctor.) How will I know when the inhaled steroid is empty? (She can calculate the number of puffs/day and the number of doses provided in one canister; then mark the day when it will become empty on the device.) In brief, she will need an asthma educator!

▶ ▶ ▶ **CASE 2**

Breathless in Boston
A 35-year-old lawyer seeks your help with management of her asthma.

She has had asthma since early childhood. She has multiple known allergic sensitivities, including dust mites, and she has made an effort to keep her apartment very clean, especially the bedroom. She develops typical symptoms of wheeze, cough, and shortness of breath with respiratory tract infections and allergic exposures (dust, animals, and mold), and she has required courses of oral corticosteroids as often as every 1–2 months to control her symptoms. She received allergen immunotherapy for several years, but stopped 2 years ago believing that the treatments were making her worse.

She has aspirin-sensitivity and nasal polyposis and 2 years ago underwent endoscopic nasal polypectomy. Her medical regimen includes inhaled triamcinolone (Azmacort) 4 puffs twice daily, oral slow-release theophylline twice daily, and albuterol by metered-dose inhaler.

Currently, she has some early morning cough with clear phlegm. She notes some shortness of breath when out in cold weather. She is using her albuterol inhaler 2–3 times/day and infrequently overnight.

Her physical exam is remarkable for small nasal polyps and a few scattered expiratory wheezes. She has mild airflow obstruction on pulmonary function testing, with a peak flow = 74% of predicted.

Is her treatment appropriate?
There can be little debate that this patient has severe persistent asthma and that it is poorly controlled. Despite moderate doses of the inhaled corticosteroid, triamcinolone (Azmacort), and a long-acting bronchodilator, slow-release theophylline, she has daily symptoms and frequent need for oral steroids. Hers is an example of "difficult-to-manage" asthma, and the reason may be her aspirin sensitivity (she has triad asthma: asthma, nasal polyps, and aspirin sensitivity). A disproportionate number of patients with aspirin-sensitive asthma have severe disease.

You spring into action. You ask her to show you how she uses her inhaled steroid, thinking it important that she use it correctly in order to derive maximal benefit. You inquire about her medication compliance, knowing that 4 puff twice daily can be somewhat time consuming. And you review with her environmental exposures in her home and at work. Is there carpeting in her bedroom? Has she obtained allergy-proof wraps for her mattress, box springs, and pillows (to be discussed further in Chap. 7, "Identifying Allergic Sensitivities and Promoting Allergen Avoidance")?

You also are aware that her medication regimen is somewhat outdated. The long-acting inhaled beta-agonist bronchodilators, salmeterol (Serevent) and formoterol (Foradil), have largely replaced theophylline because they are more effective, easier to use (for instance, no need to monitor drug blood levels), and safer. Inhaled steroid preparations more potent and with more mcg/puff than triamcinolone (Azmacort), are available—fluticasone (Flovent) 220 and mometasone (Asmanex). And you know that one device, the Advair Diskus, offers both the long-acting inhaled beta agonist, salmeterol, and the potent inhaled steroid, fluticasone, in one dry-powder inhaler. She may wish to discuss with her doctor whether she might try the Advair Diskus 500/50, taken 1 inhalation twice daily, in place of her theophylline and inhaled triamcinolone.

In addition, you may remember that patients with aspirin-sensitive asthma are distinguished by their tendency to have high levels of leukotriene production. Perhaps she might benefit from a trial of a leukotriene blocker. Her doctor may consider "triple controller" therapy with a high-dose inhaled steroid, long-acting bronchodilator, and leukotriene blocker. The primary goals will be to decrease her frequent need for oral steroids, improve her lung function, and decrease the frequency of her need for albuterol. Once her asthma comes under good control, it may then be possible to step down her therapy, especially to reduce her dose of inhaled steroids.

KEY POINT Patients with aspirin-sensitive asthma tend to be leukotriene overproducers.

As her asthma educator, you won't stop with medication review. You will also want to discuss her bone health with her. Given her need for multiple courses of oral steroids, she will need to pay attention to her bone mass and risk of osteoporosis. Does she have adequate calcium intake each day? Is she taking any vitamin D supplements? Has she ever had a bone density x-ray? If not, she may want to raise the subject with her physician.

And one last thing: be sure to be a good listener. This young woman has had a lot to deal with in terms of asthma morbidity and medication side effects. Her asthma has had a big impact on her life. She will surely find it helpful to share some of this burden with a sympathetic listener who understands about asthma and its impact. It may be that what she remembers most about your time together, even more than your helpful suggestions, are the kindness of your questions and the caring expressed by your listening to her responses.

KEY POINT Part of being a good asthma educator is being a good listener: engaged and caring, as well as well-informed.

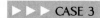 **CASE 3**

Having a Baby

A 28-year-old woman whom you have known for several years is eager to share with you her good news. "I'm pregnant," she gleefully announces.

You remember when you first met her. Following an emergency room visit for her asthma, she was referred to the medical office where you work. She felt as though she had no control over her asthma, that attacks would seem to come on unpredictably, interfering with her life. She used her quick-acting bronchodilator, metaproterenol (Alupent), once or twice every day. Every night when she went to bed, she would check to see that her inhaler was there on her nightstand or tucked under her pillow, so that when she woke with cough and wheezing she would have it ready to use. Several times a week her sleep was disturbed by symptoms of her asthma. She found it difficult to exercise on a regular basis because the exertion set off wheezing and chest tightness.

At the time, her doctor started her on a moderate dose of inhaled steroid together with a long-acting inhaled beta agonist, in the form of the Advair Diskus 250/50. The medication had a huge impact on her life. She found that she needed her metaproterenol (Alupent) inhaler far less often, perhaps once or twice per week, and that she could sleep the night through with very rare asthma symptoms (except when she suffered a chest cold). She now enjoys going to the gym and can walk on the treadmill without difficulty. She has not experienced a severe asthmatic attack in several years. Last year the dose of her inhaled steroid was reduced to 100 mcg/inhalation (Advair Diskus 100/50), without any change in the frequency of her symptoms or decline in her peak flow (which has been normal, at 400 L/min).

Is her treatment appropriate, and what advice can you share with her about her asthma and its treatment during pregnancy?

When she first sought medical care, her history indicated moderate persistent asthma. She was started on the preferred treatment for moderate persistent asthma: a long-acting inhaled beta-agonist bronchodilator and low-to-medium doses of an inhaled corticosteroid. She had an excellent response, with good control of her symptoms, freedom from serious asthmatic exacerbations, and maintenance of normal lung function. A successful effort was made to step down her therapy to a lower dose of inhaled steroids, minimizing her long-term exposure to even minute concentrations of systemically absorbed corticosteroids.

What can she expect about the course of her asthma during her pregnancy? How likely is it that pregnancy will be associated with worsening of her asthma control? In fact, it is difficult to predict. Sometimes asthma becomes more troublesome during pregnancy. Sometimes just the opposite occurs, and patients report that their asthma is the best that it has been in years. For others, pregnancy seems to have no impact on the course of their asthma. Very roughly, each pattern can be seen in about one third of pregnancies.

And does asthma pose a risk to the outcome of pregnancy? Yes, there is a slightly increased likelihood of preeclampsia, preterm birth, low birth-weight infants, and perinatal mortality due to maternal asthma. But the risk is greatest when asthma is out of control and can be minimized by good asthma control and prevention of severe asthmatic attacks. If ever there were a time to be attentive to your asthma symptoms, monitor your condition, be compulsive about taking your asthma medications, and stay in close communication with your healthcare providers, it is when you are breathing for two.

Pregnancy itself can make one feel short of breath. In part, the high sex hormone levels maintained during pregnancy can stimulate a sense of breathlessness; in part, during the third trimester the gravid uterus pushes up on the diaphragm, increasing the work of breathing. How can an asthmatic patient know whether asthma or the normal course of pregnancy is making her feel short of breath? Fortunately, it is not difficult: simply measure lung function, such as with a peak flow meter. It turns out that pregnancy does not cause a significant change in peak flow, even late in pregnancy. If the peak flow has declined significantly, asthma and not pregnancy is the cause.

KEY POINT   Peak expiratory flow does not change significantly during pregnancy. A decrease in peak flow is due to asthma (or some other respiratory problem), not pregnancy.

A major question in the mind of your patient will be: "Should I stop my asthma medications now that I am pregnant? I don't want to hurt my fetus; should I take only my prenatal vitamins? Is it safe to use my inhalers during my pregnancy?"

Much of what we know about asthma medications in pregnancy is derived from experiments in pregnant animals. Some information comes from cohort studies, in which a large group of pregnant women are followed through their pregnancies, and those with asthma are compared with others who are healthy. Some information is derived from registries of pregnant women taking specific medications. The outcomes in these asthmatic women are compared with the general population of healthy pregnant women. Very little information derives from randomized, controlled clinical experiments.

As you may know, the FDA uses a 4-category rating system (A-D) to describe the safety of medications for use in pregnancy (Table 4-2). Category A indicates that a medicine is safe in pregnancy based on controlled experiments conducted in humans. Category B suggests that a medicine is probably safe, based on its safety in animal experiments and the lack of human studies demonstrating harm. Category C points to potential harmful effects based on animal experiments using supra-therapeutic doses of medication, even in the absence of human data indicating harmful outcomes. Category D indicates that a medicine is known to have harmful effects on the developing fetus in humans. Most asthma medications are either category B or C. Oral steroids are thought to pose a slight increased risk of cleft lip and palate when administered in the first trimester.

In 2004 a Working Group of the National Asthma Education and Prevention Program prepared a document that reviews modern evidence regarding the use of asthma medications during pregnancy (and lactation). This report provides recommendations based on modern scientific data, where available, and on the best opinion of experts, where clinical experience and judgment are needed. It is available on line at: www.nhlbi.nih.gov/health/prof/lung/asthma/astpreg.htm.

In brief summary, the Working Group indicated that inhaled beta-agonists appear to be safe in pregnancy, and that albuterol is preferred because we have the

TABLE 4-2

FOOD AND DRUG ADMINISTRATION'S RATING SYSTEM FOR SAFETY OF MEDICATIONS TAKEN DURING PREGNANCY

Category A:	Proven safe based on human studies of pregnant women.
Category B:	Probably safe based on the lack of harmful effects at very large doses in pregnant animals and the absence of any known harmful effects in pregnant women.
Category C:	Possibly safe based on some harmful outcomes observed only at very large doses in pregnant animals and the absence of any known harmful effects in pregnant women.
Category D:	Unsafe based on known harmful effects for the developing human fetus.

From: National Asthma Education and Prevention Program Expert Panel Report: Guidelines for the Diagnosis and Management of Asthma—Update on Selected Topics 2002 (www.nhlbi.nih.gov/guidelines/asthma/index.htm).

KEY POINT   A recently released NIH document, the Working Group Report on "Managing Asthma during Pregnancy: Recommendations for Pharmacologic Treatment," provides state-of-the-art recommendations about managing asthma during pregnancy.

longest clinical experience with it. The inhaled steroids given in low-to-medium doses are also thought to be safe; the best evidence of safety is for budesonide (Pulmicort) (which has a Category B rating). Budesonide is preferred if inhaled steroids need to be given in high doses. There is relatively little experience with the long-acting inhaled beta agonists. However, because their pharmacology and toxicology are similar to the short-acting inhaled beta agonists, it is felt that they are likely safe. The leukotriene blockers and omalizumab (Xolair) are both rated Category B in pregnancy, despite their relative newness.

In sum, based on current recommendations, we would recommend that our pregnant patient (described above) continue her current treatment regimen (daily low-dose inhaled fluticasone plus inhaled salmeterol, and inhaled albuterol used as needed). We would assure her of their safety in pregnancy based on our present state of knowledge, and emphasize to her that good asthma control is the key to the successful outcome of her pregnancy. (Other physicians might favor switching her from Advair to budesonide [Pulmicort] with close monitoring for any worsening of her asthma.) We would also encourage close communication between her obstetrician and the practitioner primarily treating her asthma. Finally, we would heartily congratulate her on her pregnancy. The prospects for a successful pregnancy, a labor and delivery without respiratory complications, and a healthy baby are exceedingly good.

Self-Assessment Questions

QUESTION 1

Medications chosen to treat asthma will vary according to the severity of disease. In all patients with asthma, it is also appropriate for the asthma educator to do all of the following except:

1. Help develop and review an asthma action plan.
2. Review the proper use of inhaled medications.
3. Discuss allergen and irritant avoidance measures.
4. Encourage allergen immunotherapy.
5. Recommend vaccination against influenza.

QUESTION 2

The expressions, "step-up" and "step-down" therapy, refer to adjusting the intensity of medical treatment in an individual patient. Stepping-down therapy often focuses on attempting to limit the dose of:

1. Long-acting beta-agonist bronchodilators (e.g., salmeterol [Serevent]).
2. Quick-acting beta-agonist bronchodilators (e.g., albuterol).
3. Theophylline.
4. Corticosteroids, inhaled or orally administered.
5. Leukotriene blockers (e.g., montelukast [Singulair]).

QUESTION 3

Patients with mild intermittent asthma do not need to take a daily controller medication. They should be reminded about their quick-acting inhaled bronchodilator:

1. Never use two doses fewer than 4 hours apart.
2. Its use prior to exercise and cold air exposure can prevent asthmatic symptoms.
3. Over-the-counter inhaled bronchodilators are available at lower cost.
4. Wash and air-dry your medication canister and its plastic holder daily.
5. Always order two inhalers at a time so that you will have a back-up inhaler available in case you lose or misplace one.

QUESTION 4

Exercise-induced asthma is:

1. A separate form of asthma, with its own biology and pathophysiology.
2. Best referred to an asthma specialist for treatment.
3. Made worse equally by hot, humid weather and cold, dry weather.

4. Tends to resolve around the age of puberty.

5. Can be blocked by pretreatment with beta-agonists or cromolyn.

QUESTION 5

A 22-year-old woman has been advised to begin daily controller therapy for her mild persistent asthma. Her doctor has prescribed one of the following medications. You are most enthused about which of these recommendations?

1. Slow-release theophylline 200 mg p.o. b.i.d.

2. Budesonide (Pulmicort Turbuhaler) 2 inhalations q.D.

3. Salmeterol (Serevent Diskus) 1 inhalation b.i.d.

4. Tiotropium (Spiriva) 1 inhalation q.D.

5. Fluticasone-salmeterol combination (Advair 250/50) 1 inhalation b.i.d.

QUESTIONS 6

The patient described in Question 5 has many reservations about taking an inhaled steroid. You attempt to dispel some of her concerns. All of the following reassurances about inhaled steroids for asthma are true except:

1. They do not cause muscle building and aggressive behavior.

2. They can be stopped suddenly without fear of withdrawal.

3. They do not cause a chemical dependence.

4. They are not absorbed into the bloodstream.

5. They do not lose their effectiveness if taken every day.

QUESTION 7

Despite regular use of his inhaled steroid medication, beclomethasone (QVAR 40, 2 puffs twice daily), a 30-year-old electrician continues troubled by asthmatic symptoms. He has cough and chest tightness each day and finds that he needs his quick-acting bronchodilator, pirbuterol (Maxair Autohaler) 3–4 times per day. He is frustrated by his illness and wonders out loud whether he should just "throw out all of his inhalers and start over." You suggest that there are other medications that might help him. All of the following might prove beneficial, except:

1. Increase his beclomethasone dose (QVAR 80, 2 puffs twice daily).

2. Switch to a different inhaled steroid, such as fluticasone (Flovent 220, 2 puffs twice daily).

3. Add a mast cell stabilizer, cromolyn (Intal 2 puffs four times daily).

4. Add a long-acting inhaled beta-agonist bronchodilator, such as formoterol (Foradil Aerolizer 1 capsule inhaled twice daily).

5. Add a leukotriene modifier, such as zafirlukast (Accolate 20 mg one tablet p.o. twice daily).

QUESTION 8

Allergen immunotherapy (allergy shots) for asthma:

1. Blunts allergic asthmatic reactions by creating alternative (immunoglobulin G) antibodies, called "blocking antibodies," directed at the offending allergen.
2. Should be recommended for cat-allergic patients as an alternative to giving up their pet cat.
3. Should be reserved for patients with severe asthma and persistent expiratory airflow obstruction.
4. Is most effective for asthma triggered by food allergies.
5. Typically provides relief of symptoms within the first few weeks of treatment.

QUESTION 9

Treatment of asthma with an anti-IgE monoclonal antibody:

1. Is an exciting research tool not yet approved by the Food and Drug Administration (FDA).
2. Is indicated only for allergic asthma.
3. Can be taken once weekly as a tablet or liquid.
4. Is most effective against IgE antibodies formed to seasonal allergens (e.g., plant pollens and mold spores).
5. Is convenient because it can be self-administered at home.

QUESTION 10

A 45-year-old woman is referred for asthma education because her asthma has been so difficult to control. Despite multiple oral and inhaled medications and repeated courses of oral corticosteroids for her asthma, she has required frequent hospitalizations for asthmatic exacerbations. Because of her frequent need for prednisone, she has gained 30 pounds and has developed non-insulin-dependent diabetes mellitus. As you consider why her asthma has been so unusually severe, you plan to address with her all of the following topics except:

1. Proper technique(s) for use of her inhaled medications.
2. Avoidance of allergens and irritants in her home environment.
3. Potential complicating conditions, such as sinusitis or gastroesophageal reflux.
4. Review of medications that may aggravate her asthma.
5. Racial differences that may contribute to severe asthma.

QUESTION 11

A 51-year-old business executive has been seeing an acupuncturist for her asthma. She hasn't felt comfortable discussing this subject with her doctor and asks your opinion about its value in asthma. You refrain from sharing your own biases about complementary and alternative therapies for asthma and offer the following advice:

1. Evidence suggests that chiropractic manipulations give better outcomes than acupuncture in asthma.
2. Try to overcome your reluctance and discuss acupuncture with your doctor.
3. Avoid acupuncture because it is associated with the spread of AIDS and hepatitis B via contaminated needles.
4. Acupressure techniques are preferred in asthma over acupuncture with needles.
5. If acupuncture works for you, you will be able to discontinue your inhalers and avoid their potential long-term side effects.

QUESTION 12

A 21-year-old woman with asthma seeks your advice about becoming pregnant. She has mild persistent asthma treated with an inhaled steroid taken once daily. She uses her quick-relief bronchodilator as needed, on average approximately 3–4 times per week. In response to her questions, you tell her correctly that:

1. With good control of her asthma, the risk of complications to her pregnancy is no greater than for a woman without asthma.
2. She should delay her pregnancy until her asthma is better controlled.
3. All of the inhaled steroids are contraindicated in pregnancy.
4. She can anticipate that, in general, asthma tends to flare at the time of labor and delivery.
5. The severity of her asthma is likely to worsen slightly throughout the course of her pregnancy.

Answers to Self-Assessment Questions

ANSWER TO QUESTION 1 (MANAGEMENT STRATEGIES FOR ALL PATIENTS, REGARDLESS OF ASTHMA SEVERITY)

The correct answer is #4. Allergen immunotherapy is not appropriate for all patients with asthma, only a carefully selected subset of those with allergic asthma. On the other hand, all patients with asthma would benefit from discussion of an asthma action plan (answer #1); review of the proper use of inhaled medications (with or without spacers) (answer #2); allergen and irritant avoidance (answer #3); and vaccination against influenza (answer #5).

ANSWER TO QUESTION 2 (THE MAIN FOCUS OF "STEPPING-DOWN" ASTHMA THERAPY)

The correct answer is #4. Of the asthma therapies most likely to cause long-term adverse side effects, corticosteroids lead the way (especially oral or high-dose inhaled steroids). Our chief focus in stepping-down asthma care is minimizing side effects while maintaining good asthma control and preventing asthmatic exacerbations. Long-acting beta-agonist bronchodilators (answer #1), quick-acting beta-agonist bronchodilators (answer #2), theophylline (answer #3), and leukotriene blockers (answer #4) are not known to have long-term adverse side effects at routinely recommended doses. If you thought that it would be good to limit the dose of quick-acting beta-agonist bronchodilators because frequent use is usually an indicator of poor asthma control, or if you thought to limit the dose of theophylline because it is frequently associated with unpleasant side effects and can be dangerous at toxic blood levels, give yourself part credit!

ANSWER TO QUESTION 3 (USE OF QUICK-ACTING INHALED BRONCHODILA-TORS IN MILD INTERMITTENT ASTHMA)

The correct answer is #2. It is worthwhile reminding all asthmatic patients that they can sometimes *pre-treat* with their quick-acting bronchodilator to prevent anticipated bronchoconstriction, such as may occur with exercise or activities in very cold air. In an acute asthmatic attack patients may be encouraged to use their quick-acting bronchodilator more often than every 4 hours (answer #1). We do not encourage substitution of over-the-counter inhaled bronchodilators such as epinephrine (Primatene Mist) because of the greater cardiovascular side effects of epinephrine compared to prescription-only selective beta-2 adrenergic agonists (answer #3). It is not necessary to wash the canister and plastic holder of your metered-dose inhalers every day (answer #4). Although it may not sound like a bad idea, ordering two canisters at a time is in most instances wasteful—and will not be approved by most third-party payors (answer #5). Our hope is that in mild intermittent asthma, one canister of the quick-relief bronchodilator will last for nearly a full year (used no more than two times [4 puffs] per week).

ANSWER TO QUESTION 4 (EXERCISE-INDUCED ASTHMA)

The correct answer is #5. Beta-agonist bronchodilators, leukotriene modifiers, and the mast cell stabilizer, cromolyn, have all been shown to blunt the bronchoconstriction induced by exercise. Exercise-induced asthma is asthma for which exercise has been identified as a dominant trigger. Its biology and pathophysiology are indistinguishable from asthma in which other triggers play a more important role. It would be more precise to refer to exercise-induced bronchoconstriction, which is a part of all asthma (answer #1). Exercise-induced asthma can be treated by pediatricians, family physicians, and other generalists; it does not require specialist referral (answer #2). Although people with exercise-induced bronchoconstriction may find it uncomfortable to exercise in hot, humid weather, in fact warm, moist air breathed during exercise is far less of a trigger for bronchoconstriction than cold, dry air (answer #3). Exercise-induced bronchoconstriction does not tend to resolve around the age of puberty (ask any number of Olympic athletes with asthma!) (answer #4).

ANSWER TO QUESTION 5 (TREATMENT FOR MILD PERSISTENT ASTHMA)

The correct answer is #2. The preferred treatment for mild persistent asthma is an inhaled steroid prescribed at a low dose. A leukotriene blocker is an alternative option. Slow-release theophylline (answer #1), a long-acting inhaled beta-agonist bronchodilator (salmeterol) (answer #3), and a long-acting anticholinergic bronchodilator (tiotropium) (answer #4) would not provide the same protection as an anti-inflammatory controller medication. Tiotropium is FDA-approved for the treatment of COPD, but not for asthma. The fluticasone-salmeterol combination (Advair) would be effective and convenient, but probably represents *overkill* (answer #5). One medication rather than two would be sufficient; and the dose of inhaled steroids is probably too high. Advair might be a good choice if her low-dose inhaled steroid proved inadequate, and she needed to step-up her asthma therapy.

ANSWER TO QUESTION 6 (SAFETY OF LONG-TERM USE OF INHALED STEROIDS)

The correct answer is #4. A small portion of the dose of inhaled steroids is indeed absorbed into the bloodstream. The portion that is absorbed from the stomach is largely rendered inactive when it passes from the stomach through the liver on its way to the arterial circulation. The portion that is absorbed into the blood from the bronchial tubes bypasses the portal circulation through the liver and remains in its active form. It is true that inhaled corticosteroids do not cause muscle building and aggressive behavior (unlike the anabolic steroids used by some competitive athletes and weight lifters) (answer #1). They can be stopped suddenly—even after long-term use—without fear of adrenal insufficiency (answer #2). They do not cause a chemical dependence (answer #3); and they do not lose their effectiveness if taken every day (answer #5).

ANSWER TO QUESTION 7 (STEPPING-UP THERAPY FOR MODERATE PERSISTENT ASTHMA)

The correct answer is #3. There are no studies that demonstrate additive benefit from cromolyn combined with inhaled steroids; the 4-times-daily schedule for cromolyn is difficult to follow; and the other choices are all simpler and more effective. Options for stepping-up therapy in patients whose asthma is not well controlled on appropriate therapy for mild persistent asthma (low-dose inhaled steroids) include: increasing the dose of inhaled steroid (answers #1 and #2); adding a long-acting inhaled beta-agonist bronchodilator to a low-dose inhaled steroid (answer #4); and adding a leukotriene modifier to a low-dose inhaled steroid (answer #5).

ANSWER TO QUESTION 8 (ALLERGEN IMMUNOTHERAPY)

The correct answer is #1. One way in which allergen immunotherapy appears to blunt the allergic response is by inducing the formation of immunoglobulin G (IgG) antibodies against the antigen injected under the skin. Unlike IgE antibodies, when IgG antibodies bind to allergens, they do not set off an allergic response. Cat immunotherapy remains to be perfected and is not a satisfactory alternative to finding another home for the pet cat (answer #2). Patients with severe asthma and persistent expiratory airflow obstruction are at greatest risk for adverse reactions to allergen immunotherapy, including life-threatening and fatal allergic reactions (answer #4). Allergen immunotherapy is most effective for desensitization to inhaled allergens and stinging insects, not food allergies (answer #4). Benefit from traditional allergen immunotherapy may take many months to become manifest (answer #5).

ANSWER TO QUESTION 9 (ANTI-IGE MONOCLONAL ANTIBODY THERAPY)

The correct answer is #2. Treatment with the anti-IgE monoclonal antibody, omalizumab (Xolair), is indicated only for allergic asthma, in which IgE antibody is thought to play a major role in disease pathogenesis. It is an FDA-approved treatment for allergic asthma (answer #1). It involves subcutaneous injections administered every 2 or 4 weeks (depending on the dose required) (answer #3). This treatment modality leads to a decrease in blood levels of all IgE molecules, regardless of the allergens to which they were formed (answer #4). At present, administration requires special medication reconstitution and post-administration observation in a medical office (answer #5).

ANSWER TO QUESTION 10 (DIFFICULT-TO-CONTROL ASTHMA)

The correct answer is #5. The contribution of genetic differences based on race to difficult-to-control asthma is uncertain. Although severe asthma of this sort is more common in African-Americans and Hispanics than in Caucasians, the explanation may relate to socioeconomic differences among the population groups. Besides, racial differences cannot be modified with the help of asthma education! On the other hand, this patient will likely benefit from your review of her inhaler technique(s) (answer #1); discussion of allergen and irritant avoidance in her home (answer #2); exploration of sinusitis, gastroesophageal reflux, and other potential conditions that may be aggravating her asthma (answer #3); and certainty that none of her other medications (e.g., beta blockers) is making her asthma worse (answer #4).

ANSWER TO QUESTION 11 (COMPLEMENTARY AND ALTERNATIVE ASTHMA THERAPIES)

The correct answer is #2. If she follows your advice and asks our opinion about acupuncture, we will tell her that we are unaware of any evidence that it helps in asthma (and we do know of experiments indicating that it does not help). If she finds acupuncture beneficial, she should certainly continue with it, but also continue to use her asthma medications. She should use acupuncture as an adjunct to traditional therapy, not as a substitute. Chiropractic manipulations have not been shown to give better outcomes in asthma than acupuncture; direct comparisons have not been made (answer #1). A certified acupuncturist uses sterilized or disposable needles; the risk of spread of blood-borne viral infections is very low (answer #3). There is no published evidence favoring acupressure over acupuncture (or vice versa) in the treatment of asthma (answer #4). Patients who discontinue their controller medications in favor of acupuncture are at risk of asthmatic exacerbations and worse asthma control (answer #5).

ANSWER TO QUESTION 12 (ASTHMA AND PREGNANCY)

The correct answer is #1. You can offer her the reassurance that with good asthma control, her risk of complications during her pregnancy (to her or to the fetus) is no greater than for a woman without asthma. The frequency of her quick-relief inhaler use (3–4 times per week) is more than we would like to see (target = two or fewer times per week), but it is not so frequent that we would recommend delay in pursuing conception (answer #2). Budesonide (Pulmicort) is given Category B rating in pregnancy and is considered safe; other inhaled steroids may also prove to be safe during pregnancy, although adequate data are not available (answer #3). The course of asthma during pregnancy is somewhat unpredictable, but the time around labor and delivery is *not* usually associated with an asthma flare (answer #4). More women have their asthma remain unchanged or improve during pregnancy than have it worsen (answer #5).

CHAPTER

5

SPECIAL CONSIDERATIONS IN CHILDHOOD ASTHMA

C H A P T E R   O U T L I N E

I. Epidemiology of Asthma in Children
   a. Prevalence, mortality, and healthcare impact
   b. Effect on daily lives of children and parents/caregivers

II. Diagnosis of Childhood Asthma—A Case Example
   a. History and physical examination
   b. Diagnostic testing
   c. Diagnosis in children too young to perform pulmonary function testing

III. Medication delivery devices
   a. Compressor and nebulizer
   b. Metered-dose inhalers
   c. Dry-powder inhalers

IV. Pharmacotherapy of Childhood Asthma
   a. Quick relievers
   b. Controllers
      i. Cromolyn
      ii. Inhaled corticosteroids
      iii. Leukotriene blockers
   c. Treatment of moderate and severe persistent asthma
   d. Preventive maintenance

V. When Initial Treatment Fails
   a. Reviewing expectations and medication administration
   b. Unidentified triggers
   c. Concomitant illnesses
   d. Alternative diagnoses

EPIDEMIOLOGY OF ASTHMA IN CHILDREN

Prevalence, mortality, and healthcare impact

Asthma usually begins in childhood. Almost 9 million children in the United States have diagnosed asthma, including nearly 1 million under the age of 5 years; and it is suspected that many children with asthma remain undiagnosed. Although there are more adults than children with asthma, one often thinks of asthma as a pediatric disease because in most patients a diagnosis of asthma is established before age 5. In contrast to adults, among whom asthma predominantly affects women, more boys than girls have asthma.

Estimates of the nationwide prevalence of pediatric asthma in the United States vary from 5% to 16%. In New England, approximately 9% of children have active symptoms of asthma, and this number climbs to over 12% if one inquires about their ever, during their lifetimes, having had asthma. Asthma seems particularly common among children of color in our inner cities. In a detailed assessment of every child under age 13 living in a 24-block area surrounding Harlem Hospital in the Harlem section of New York City, an astounding 25% of the children were found to have asthma. Among persons of Hispanic descent, Puerto Rican children have significantly higher rates of asthma than any other group, including Mexican-American and other Latino children. Some estimates put the prevalence of asthma among Puerto Rican children as high as 30%.

Because asthma is so common, it is an everyday part of pediatric practice. Each year in the United States, children make more than 5 million routine office visits and 727,000 urgent visits (to a medical office or emergency department) for management of their asthma. The highest rates of medical utilization for pediatric asthma occur among children less than 5 years of age. Although most children who receive treatment in the emergency department will improve and be able to return home, asthma remains the third most common cause of pediatric hospitalizations in the United States, resulting in approximately 190,000 hospitalizations per year. Those who most frequently require hospital-based care for their asthma are low-income populations, minorities, and children living in the inner cities. Their burden of asthma morbidity and mortality is disproportionately high, and their potential benefit from appropriate asthma education is particularly great.

KEY POINT Asthma is the third leading cause of pediatric hospitalizations in the United States. Particularly at risk are children of color and low socioeconomic status living in our inner cities.

Fortunately, asthma mortality remains very low. Approximately 200 children die from asthma each year in the United States. Although this number is well below the approximately 5000 adult asthmatic deaths each year, our expectation is that no child should die of asthma.

In fact, there is very little published information regarding asthma mortality in children. While you might anticipate that those children with the most severe disease—treated with the most medicine—are the ones most likely to suffer fatal asthma, evidence suggests that this assumption is not correct. For example, in one study from Australia, investigators reviewed the medical records of all children who had died of asthma over a 3-year period of time. They found that 33% of these children had been judged to have a history of trivial or mild asthma and that 32% had no previous hospital admission for their asthma. They concluded that the majority of subjects in this survey could not be classified as "high risk." Factors that do put a child at increased risk for a fatal asthmatic attack include inadequate assessment or insufficient therapy of prior asthma, poor adherence with therapy, and delay in seeking help during an asthmatic attack. The good news here is that the rate of pediatric asthma deaths is leveling off in the United States after many years of steady increase, and the rate of hospitalizations for asthma is actually on the decline.

The total healthcare cost for children with asthma exceeds 3 billion dollars per year. Despite our gains in asthma care and in the prevention of asthmatic attacks, the impact of asthma on the health of our children, on the quality of their lives, and on the American economy remains substantial.

Effect on daily lives of children and their parents/caregivers

The burden of asthma on children is not just felt within the health care system. Asthma also has a tremendous impact on children in schools. Nearly half of all children with asthma miss some school time because of their asthma, and, overall, children with asthma miss more school than their classmates without asthma. On average, they miss about 10 to 14 days of school per year, three times the rate of school absences from other causes. Although 14 days may not seem like a lot of school to miss, you need to consider that the entire school year consists of only 180 days. Furthermore, those children with moderate-to-severe disease may miss as many as 30 days from school each year. Time lost from school may negatively affect a child's grades, academic achievement, self-esteem, and future life successes; and it can keep a child's care provider home from work.

The problem of school absenteeism due to asthma is the focus of a major funding initiative by the Centers for Disease Control (CDC), a government agency usually thought of as addressing medical epidemics. The CDC is bringing together several nongovernmental organizations interested in pediatric asthma (National Association of School Nurses, American Lung Association, Asthma and Allergy Foundation of America, Starlight Starbright Children's Foundation, American Academy of Pediatrics, and American Association of School Administrators) and urban school districts in seven cities (Albuquerque, Baltimore, Charlotte, Detroit, Los Angeles, Memphis, and Philadelphia). Their goal is to develop and implement policies and programs to reduce asthma episodes and related absences through asthma education and coordinated management. This is work still in progress, to which we will all *stay tuned* in the years ahead.

Surveys of both children with asthma and their parents find that one of the things bothering children and their parents most about asthma is that it interferes with activities. In one survey 48% of respondents reported that sports and recreation were limited due to asthma. While missing a baseball practice can be understandably disappointing to a child, the child's illness has the potential to disrupt the plans of other family members as well.

A wellspring of information about living with pediatric asthma comes from the recently published Children and Asthma in America survey (www.asthmainamerica.com). From among 41,000 randomly selected households across the United States, 801 children with asthma (age 4–18 years) were identified. Research assistants conducted lengthy telephone interviews with the parents of the young children with asthma in this group and with 284 older asthmatic children themselves.

This survey had many interesting findings. For instance, in the 4 weeks prior to the survey, a third of the children woke at night with asthma symptoms. We may often forget to ask about nocturnal symptoms, but coughing at night turns out to be a sensitive indicator of asthma control. When you talk to parents, their child's nighttime awakenings due to asthma are one of the most bothersome things about their child's asthma. When a child is up at night coughing, no one gets much sleep. It may be hard for the child to pay attention in school the next day due to fatigue. And as a corollary, the caregivers for these children have been found—not surprisingly—to be less productive on the job when their children are up at night sick with asthma.

KEY POINT   Waking at night with asthma symptoms is both common among children (as many as 1/3 of children in one large survey) and highly disruptive for child and parents alike.

The Children and Asthma in America survey also found that as many as two-thirds of the children had an asthmatic exacerbation in the last month, and 20% suffered exacerbations three or more times each week. Asked about sudden and severe attacks, more than half the respondents reported at least one such episode in the past year. In fact, 10% of the parents felt that their child's life had been in danger within the past year (Fig. 5-1). Although we rarely talk with parents about death due to severe asthma, the findings of this survey suggest that many parents—and likely their children—are thinking about it. Few things are as scary to children, as to adults, as feeling that you are unable to breathe. In our opinion, it is appropriate to acknowledge that even children with mild disease can experience severe and potentially life-threatening asthmatic episodes. We need to emphasize that good medical care and careful planning, including the use of asthma action plans (as discussed in Chap. 10, "Developing an Asthma Action Plan"), can reduce the risk of serious exacerbations for children with asthma. Scientific evidence supports this reassurance: for instance, studies indicate that the

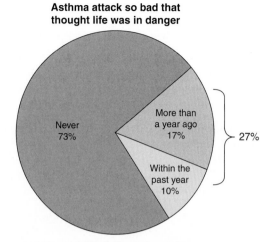

Asthma attack so bad that thought life was in danger

Q11a. (Have you/has your child) ever had an asthma attack so bad that (you/he/she) thought (your/his/her) life was in danger?
Q11c. When was the most recent time (you/your child) had an asthma attack so bad that you thought (your/your child's) life was in danger?

Unweighted N = 801

FIGURE 5-1   *The Children and Asthma in America survey of more than 41,000 households across the United States, conducted in 2004, identified 801 children with current asthma between the ages of 4 and 18. Of these, 27% had experienced an asthmatic attack that felt life-endangering, including 10% whose episode had occurred within the past year. From: www.asthmainamerica.com.*

risk of death from asthma decreases as the use of inhaled steroids, even at low doses, increases.

One of the curious findings of the Children and Asthma in America survey is that 78% of the respondents reported that their (for children old enough to provide answers to the survey questions themselves) or their child's asthma was well or completely controlled. Given the frequency of reported symptoms and exacerbations in this population, this assessment would seem excessively rosy—or perhaps a testimony to low expectations. Building on the recommendations of the National Asthma Education and Prevention Program, Dr. Mark Millard, a pulmonologist at the Baylor Asthma and Pulmonary Rehabilitation Center, developed a set of three questions to gauge asthma control, called the "Rules of Two." These three questions provide a rapid assessment of asthma control and, based on the responses, an indicator of the need for regular, preventive therapy for asthma (an asthma controller medication).

Rules of Two:

- Do you use a quick-relief inhaler more than two times a week?
- Do you wake up at night with asthma more than two times a month?
- Do you refill your asthma prescription for a quick-relief bronchodilator more than two times a year?

KEY POINT   Children with well-controlled asthma will answer "no" to all three questions related to the Rules of Two: they do not use a quick-relief inhaler more than twice per week; they do not wake at night with asthma more than twice per month; and they do not need a refill of their quick-relief bronchodilator inhaler more than twice per year.

Other simple and short questionnaires are available for assessing asthma control, including some developed with the help of pharmaceutical companies and widely distributed through medical offices and popular magazines. One such tool is the Asthma Control Test (ACT), which is supported by the American Lung Association and available on-line at www.asthmacontrol.com.

DIAGNOSIS OF CHILDHOOD ASTHMA—A CASE EXAMPLE

It is sometimes easier to think about making the diagnosis of asthma by working through a specific patient example. Here is one such case, rich with learning opportunities.

A 12-year-old young man without known asthma came to see us in clinic because of recurrent cough associated with chest tightness.

He would start to cough soon after taking to the soccer field. He managed to get through most practices, but if he had to do a lot of running, as he did during games, he would cough and feel his chest tight, making it hard for him to breathe. Although he experienced this problem for the last few seasons, it worsened this season, after he began playing on a more competitive team. He participated in practices at least twice per week and played in games most weekends. His coach was concerned about his cough and told him he could not play again until he had a note from his doctor.

When he came to the office we learned that in addition to his cough and chest tightness with exercise, he had seasonal rhinitis and eczema when younger. He did not find these latter problems troublesome. No one in his family had a diagnosis of asthma, but his older brother got bronchitis every winter and his father coughed whenever he exercised "too much." His mother mentioned that she developed nasal congestion every spring. There were no cigarette smokers at home. The family had a pet cat, which they described as an "outdoor" cat that only slept in the bedroom a few days per week.

On examination the boy appeared very comfortable, and his respiratory rate was 18 breaths per minute, within the normal range for his age. He was able to speak to us in full sentences. He was not using accessory muscles of respiration, and his nose was not flaring during inspiration. His chest had a normal configuration and was clear to auscultation with the stethoscope. He had some mild eczema on his hands. Otherwise, the remainder of his physical examination was unremarkable.

History and physical examination

This story is certainly suggestive of asthma. Exercise-induced cough and chest tightness are typical symptoms. For some children, exercise may be the only trigger of asthma and cough its only manifestation. Although we tend to label this condition as "exercise-induced asthma," what we really mean is that the child has asthma with exercise-induced bronchoconstriction. Exercise-induced asthma is asthma in which exercise is the dominant and perhaps only identified trigger of symptoms. The bronchial pathology of exercise-induced asthma is indistinguishable from any other presentation of asthma, whether allergen-induced, cigarette-smoke induced, or viral respiratory tract infection-induced.

There are other clues in the history that should make us consider a diagnosis of asthma, specifically aspects that by their presence put him at increased risk for having or developing asthma (see Table 5-1). Atopic dermatitis (also referred to as eczema) is a risk factor, particularly eczema in the first year of life. He reports having allergic (seasonal) rhinitis, another risk factor. Although there is no definite parental history of asthma, his father's cough with exercise raises some suspicion that he too may have asthma. One also wonders whether his brother's frequent bouts of "bronchitis" might represent undiagnosed asthma. A family history of asthma increases the likelihood that a child will develop asthma, especially when the mother has asthma.

KEY POINT   Risk factors for the development of asthma include the following: atopic dermatitis (eczema), a parental history of asthma, allergic rhinitis, wheezing apart from colds, and peripheral blood eosinophilia.

Neither the child nor his mother reported hearing wheezing, one of the cardinal features of asthma. Its absence should not dissuade us from considering the diagnosis of asthma. Although most children with asthma experience coughing, many will not hear wheezing. On the flip side, when patients or parents report wheezing, we need to be sure that what they are describing is the sound made by diffusely narrowed airways. Whistling sounds from the nose or throat can easily be mistaken for asthmatic wheezing, as can mucus localized in a bronchial tube. Healthcare providers define wheezing as high-pitched, musical sounds generally heard best through a stethoscope applied to the chest wall. You can listen to some good examples of wheezing on the Internet, at www.med.ucla.edu/wilkes/lungintro.htm.

TABLE 5-1

RISK FACTORS FOR DEVELOPING ASTHMA

Atopic dermatitis

Parental history of asthma

Two of the following:
• allergic rhinitis
• wheezing apart from colds
• peripheral blood eosinophilia

As you probably already know, the physical examination of a child with asthma, when he or she is well, can be completely normal. The absence of wheezing on chest auscultation does not exclude a diagnosis of asthma. Physical findings are likely to be present when airway narrowing occurs, which in this child is after exercise. When he sits calmly in a medical office, his lungs are clear. If you could examine him after exercise, you might hear characteristic diffuse, musical wheezing. You might note that compared to the duration of time spent inhaling, his duration of exhalation is prolonged. The more severe the airflow obstruction, the more prolonged the expiratory phase of respiration. Tapping on his chest (percussion) might reveal an unusually large area of resonance overlying the lungs, a sign of hyperinflation.

During a severe exacerbation of asthma, he would not feel comfortable lying down, preferring a sitting position. As the severity of the exacerbation increased, he might even assume a hunched-over sitting position with his hands supporting the torso, termed the tripod position. As he found it increasingly difficult to breathe, he might speak only in very short sentences or pause to breathe every few words. In the most severe forms of acute asthma, he might struggle for air, sweat profusely, and with respiratory failure imminent, start to breathe very slowly (bradypnea). Ominous physical findings in severe attacks include inaudible breath sounds (because breathing has become extremely shallow), cyanosis, and a change in mental status.

KEY POINT   Physical findings during a very severe asthmatic attack might include sitting in the tripod position, speech interrupted every few words for breathing, diaphoresis, a very rapid or inappropriately slow respiratory rate, the "silent chest," cyanosis, and altered mental status.

Fortunately, our patient has none of these findings. He looks perfectly fine.

Diagnostic testing

How confident are we that this young man has asthma? It helps to recall that asthma is defined as a chronic inflammatory respiratory disorder that is characterized by reversible obstruction of the airways. In the next chapter, "Pulmonary Function Testing and Peak Flow Monitoring," we will describe in detail how to test for evidence of airways obstruction and for its reversibility.

> *You decide to measure his peak flow. He follows your directions carefully and is able to blow 350 L/min on each of three efforts, a value within the normal range.*

With a clear chest and normal peak expiratory flow, you may need to reconsider the diagnosis of asthma. Certainly, a variety of other conditions can also present with cough and chest tightness (Table 5-2).

If after considering alternative diagnoses you are still favoring asthma, you could ask him to perform spirometry. Equipment that used to fill a small room can now be as small as a handheld device attached by a cable to your laptop computer. However, although the technology has improved and the cost of the device has dropped, doing spirometry in the general medical office still requires a big investment in time. It may take half an hour or longer to teach a child how to perform maximal forced exhalations that give accurate and reproducible results. However, it is well worth the investment of time and money, because spirometry has several advantages over measurements of peak flow when looking for evidence of airflow obstruction, the hallmark of asthma. Pertinent to this particular circumstance, an obstructive pattern may be found on spirometry even when the peak flow is normal.

> *You have him perform spirometry, and the results are normal.*

His normal spirometry does not confirm a suspected diagnosis of asthma, but it also does not exclude asthma. You are not deterred. You know that at this moment he is well, free of symptoms and between exacerbations. His examination and spirometry may well be completely normal, even though he has asthma (and hyperresponsive airways). At this point you may consider provocative testing.

TABLE 5 - 2

ALTERNATIVE DIAGNOSES IN CHILDREN

Acute respiratory infections
- bronchiolitis
- pneumonia

Cystic fibrosis
Vocal cord dysfunction
Gastroesophageal reflux/chronic aspiration
Tracheobronchomalacia
Vascular ring
Primary ciliary dyskinesia
Immune disorders
Habit cough

The concept of bronchoprovocative testing is that certain stimuli will provoke narrowing of the airways of persons with asthma but have little or no effect on the airways of persons without asthma. Typical of asthmatic airways is their tendency to contract "too much and too easily" in response to provocative stimuli or *triggers*. Methacholine, a derivative of the anticholinergic neurotransmitter, acetylcholine, is one such stimulus. A person with asthma will develop bronchoconstriction in response to a much lower concentration of inhaled methacholine than a person without asthma. Rapid breathing of cold, dry air will have the same distinguishing effect. In our pediatric pulmonary function laboratory, we use exercise, either on a treadmill or stationary bicycle, as our provocative stimulus. There are established protocols for the desired duration and level of exercise. Spirometry is performed before exercise and then repeated at regular intervals after exercise, evaluating for a decline in expiratory airflow (FEV_1) as an indicator of induced bronchoconstriction (see Chap. 6 for further details of bronchoprovocative testing).

He performs an exercise bronchoprovocative test. His FEV_1 declines by 20% and returns to baseline following treatment with a short-acting bronchodilator. With the information gleaned from this exercise study, you make a diagnosis of asthma and recommend treatment with a short-acting bronchodilator prior to exercise and for relief of symptoms. You schedule him for a follow-up appointment in approximately 4–6 weeks.

Your job, however, is not done. You may have made the correct diagnosis and made a good choice for his treatment, but an equally important task remains: making certain that he knows how to take his medicine. Before we consider teaching inhaler use to children and their caregivers, it is fair to ask: what if the patient were a child too young to perform pulmonary function testing? How do we make a diagnosis of asthma in very young children?

Diagnosis in children too young to perform pulmonary function testing

The diagnosis of asthma requires the demonstration of reversible airflow obstruction. In those too young to perform spirometry, we rely on typical clinical manifestations to identify airflow obstruction, such as cough, rapid breathing, prolonged expiratory phase, retractions, and wheezing and then document its reversibility (resolution of these findings) with treatment or over time. The dilemma is that many infants and young children wheeze when they have viral respiratory infections. Their wheezing may improve with the same therapies used to treat asthma, yet their problem may be recurrent bouts of viral bronchiolitis and not asthma. For many years pediatricians have used the expression "reactive airways disease" to communicate this uncertainty of diagnosis. The more precise expression is "wheezing-associated respiratory illness." Some of these children will in the end turn out to have asthma, others not. On the one hand, one hesitates to make the diagnosis of asthma because it can be a chronic, lifelong illness; on the other hand, one does not want to delay or withhold appropriate therapy that can improve the child's quality of life. It may not be possible during the first or second bout of respiratory infection to make the distinction. (In one study of children followed from birth, as many as half of all children had at least one wheezing episode prior to age 6 years.)

Features that point to a diagnosis of asthma are the occurrence of cough and wheezing in the absence of viral respiratory infections. If symptoms occur or are made worse in the presence of animals with fur, exercise, or cigarette smoke, the diagnosis is likely asthma. The presence of risk factors for asthma (see Table 5-1) weighs the odds towards a diagnosis of asthma. The *Guidelines* of the National Asthma Education and Prevention Program offer the following recommendation: make a presumptive diagnosis of asthma in a child who within the past 12 months has had three episodes of wheezing that last more than one day and affect sleep.

KEY POINT   In the first few years of life, it is often difficult to distinguish asthma from "wheezing-associated respiratory illnesses." Wheezing in the absence of other symptoms of respiratory infection suggests asthma, but in the end it may be necessary to observe the course of the child's symptoms and response to therapy, considered in the context of the presence or absence of asthma risk factors.

MEDICATION DELIVERY DEVICES

Compressor and nebulizer

Inhaled medications can be delivered to children using a compressor-driven nebulizer or a metered-dose inhaler (MDI). Nebulized medication is the easiest to take in the sense that it requires the least effort on the part of the child. The medication is put into a nebulizer cup that is attached to a compressor. The compressor forces air through the nebulizer, where the medication is transformed from a liquid into an aerosol or mist. The size of the medicine-containing droplets in this aerosol—when it finally reaches the patient—will vary depending on the speed of the gas flow from the compressor, the baffling system in the nebulizer itself, and the patient interface, being a mouthpiece or mask. The goal is to produce and then have inhaled droplets small enough to make their way down into the airways but large enough to settle onto the airways after colliding with the airway walls. The ideal size is approximately 1–5 microns.

The mist can be inhaled either through a mask or a mouthpiece. For younger children (generally under age 2), we recommend a mask. When the child is capable of making a tight seal with his or her mouth, it may be appropriate to try to use a mouthpiece. One cannot always predict which child is ready to use a mouthpiece; the only way to be certain is to observe the child using the device. A more detailed discussion of nebulizers is contained in Chap. 8, "Inhalers and Inhalational Aids in Asthma Treatment."

Metered-dose inhalers

To deliver medication from metered-dose inhalers, we recommend the use of a valved holding chamber (spacer) for children of all ages. These chambers are available either with or without attached masks. The holding chambers give you a little more time to coordinate actuation of the metered-dose inhaler with a slow, deep breath. We would emphasize that the extra time it provides is just a few seconds. Any longer and the medication droplets begin to coalesce and stick to the walls of the chamber. Some manufacturers coat the inside of their product with antistatic material in an attempt to reduce this amount of medication that is attracted to the walls (e.g., holding chambers named Vortex and Aerochamber MAX).

For younger children unable to take a slow, deep breath and hold it for 5–10 seconds, we recommend the use of a snug-fitting mask attached to the holding chamber. The mask limits entrainment of ambient air and maximizes drug delivery even at low inspiratory flow rates. When using a metered-dose inhaler with attached face mask, instead of just one deep breath, younger children take six normal, or tidal, breaths (for each puff of medication delivered into the chamber). Given the volume of air moved with each breath, even the youngest child will easily empty the chamber after six breaths.

Perhaps the greatest benefit of using a valved holding chamber is the one-way valve itself. Many children when first given any type of inhalation device have the tendency to blow into the device. The one-way valve prevents patients from exhaling into the chamber, ensuring that the medication is available for the next breath in.

We are often asked the question: which is the better delivery system, a metered-dose inhaler with valved holding chamber or compressor-driven nebulizer? In fact, both systems are far from ideal. Even with perfect technique, the metered-dose inhaler with valved holding chamber delivers to the airways only approximately 10% of the dose of medication released from the nozzle of the inhaler. Similarly, from compressor-driven nebulizers the output of medication particles of respirable size is only approximately 15%. And even these low percentages fall off further under real life circumstances. For instance, a child who is crying during a treatment administered by nebulizer with face mask receives <5% of the available dose of medication. Add a poorly fitting mask, and there will be further loss of medication. Some parents attempt to avoid the discomfort of a face mask by holding the open end of the nebulizer tubing near the child's face—a technique less frightening for some children, but also highly ineffective for medication delivery. The nose is an excellent filter and removes much of the medication from the airstream before it can reach the airways.

In the end, most important is not the decision as to which device to use for drug delivery but the investment of time to ensure that the child and caregiver are comfortable using and maintaining whichever system is chosen. The majority of time spent in our offices with a new asthmatic patient and caregiver is devoted to teaching medication administration. A skilled asthma educator is an invaluable resource in this regard. We are constantly reminded that even if we make the correct diagnosis and select the proper medications, patients won't improve unless the therapies recommended are used properly.

KEY POINT   The choice between metered-dose inhaler with holding chamber versus compressor-driven nebulizer is determined by capability in using the device properly, preferences on the part of the patient and provider, cost, and convenience. Optimal medication delivery will vary based mostly on correct and reliable use of whichever system is chosen.

Dry-powder inhalers

An increasing number of asthma medications are available in dry-powder formulations. The dry-powder inhalers have certain advantages over conventional metered-dose inhalers. First, during manufacture particle size can be carefully controlled to optimize the fraction that can be inhaled and deposited into the airways. Second, dry-powder inhalers are all breath-actuated. Once the device is readied for use, the medication stays in place until the patient breathes in. No medication is released until the patient applies his or her mouth to the mouthpiece and begins to pull air in. Third, all of the multidose devices currently on the market either display the exact number of doses left in the canister or indicate when the number of doses is getting low.

Each of the dry-powder devices (the Diskus, Turbuhaler, Twisthaler, and Aerolizer) is different from the others. You will need to familiarize yourself with the proper technique for using each device (see Chap. 8, "Inhalers and Inhalational Aids in Asthma Treatment"). In general, dry-powder devices are easier to master than metered-dose inhalers, but their use requires the ability to generate a minimal inspiratory flow rate of 30–60 L/min, generally achievable by age 5–6. They cannot be used with holding chambers (spacers) or face masks.

The most common problem with use of dry-powder inhalers typically becomes evident when you watch a child take the medication. Asked to demonstrate use of his inhaler, the child often blows into the device! Used properly, once the child places his mouth on the mouthpiece of the dry-powder inhaler, he should only breathe *in*. If he blows into the device, medication is dispersed, in part being forced into niches within the device itself, and becomes inaccessible for inhalation. Consequently, proper training and subsequent reinforcement are equally important for the dry-powder inhalers as for metered-dose inhalers.

KEY POINT   The most common error with use of dry-powder inhalers is that children tend to blow into the devices.

To test whether a young child is capable of generating the inspiratory flow needed to optimize drug delivery from a dry-powder inhaler, one can make measurements of inspiratory flow in a pulmonary function laboratory. Alternatively, one can purchase an inexpensive inspiratory flow measurement device to use in the office (e.g., a device called "In-Check Dial"). Some product-specific training devices whistle to indicate that an adequate inspiratory flow has been achieved. However, be sure to remind the child that the actual dry-powder device will not whistle, no matter how hard he tries!

After teaching proper inhaler technique, it is good practice to have the child (and caregiver) demonstrate the technique under your watchful eye. And remember, this is just the first step. Practice is essential to maintain the learned skills; and these techniques need to be reviewed at every visit. We have learned from video studies of children, their parents, and even healthcare providers just how easy it is to miss an essential step. The consequence is not just wasted drug, but also potentially the persistent risk for an asthmatic exacerbation and mis-perceived need for escalation of therapy.

PHARMACOTHERAPY OF CHILDHOOD ASTHMA

Recent studies have confirmed that the airways of children with asthma, like those of adults with asthma, show evidence of chronic inflammation. These chronically inflamed airways are hyperresponsive; they too readily respond to stimuli in the environment with excessive bronchial muscle constriction, leading to obstruction and airflow limitation. Treatment of asthma in children, as in adults, begins with the intermittent use of bronchodilators to prevent and reverse this bronchoconstriction. When symptoms are frequent or severe, we add daily therapy targeted at reducing the underlying airway inflammation.

Quick relievers

Every child with asthma needs to have a "quick-reliever" bronchodilator. Equally important, every asthmatic child (or childcare provider for an asthmatic child) needs to know how properly to use this rescue medication. Allow us to emphasize one more time: it's no good having a life preserver if you don't know how to put it on! The lessons that you, the asthma educator, teach a parent or grandparent about how to administer bronchodilator therapy to a 2-year-old toddler can prove as life-saving as the life preserver drill on-board ship.

For children up to 2 years of age, we typically prescribe albuterol (alternative: metaproterenol [Alupent]) by nebulizer with attached face mask. It might be tempting to think that albuterol syrup might be preferable—one teaspoonful of a pleasant tasting liquid versus 5–10 minutes of nebulizer treatment with a potentially restless child in one's lap. In our view—and consistent with the recommendations of the Expert Panel of the National Asthma Education and Prevention Program—the inhaled route remains preferable because: it works more rapidly, it achieves greater bronchodilation, and it has fewer side effects.

KEY POINT   Despite the greater convenience of oral syrup, quick-acting bronchodilators should preferably be given by inhalation. Inhaled bronchodilators act more quickly, provide greater bronchodilation, and cause fewer side effects than orally administered ones.

Some pediatricians have embraced the alternative quick-reliever solution for nebulization, levalbuterol (Xopenex). As discussed in Chap. 3, "Medications Used to Treat Asthma," this single-isomer formulation of albuterol was developed to reduce the side effects commonly seen among young children after treatment with albuterol, including hyperactivity, difficulty falling asleep, and a sense of agitation. Whether the drug achieves this goal or not is uncertain; there are both advocates and skeptics on either side of the debate. If the agitation caused by albuterol is a problem, it may be worth the added expense to give levalbuterol a therapeutic trial.

Both albuterol and levalbuterol come packaged in single-dose vials for nebulized administration. Albuterol is available in unit-dose vials of 0.63 mg, 1.25 mg, and 2.5 mg; levalbuterol comes in strengths of 0.31 mg, 0.63 mg, and 1.25 mg. Since it is a single isomer rather than a mixture of two mirror-image isomers, one needs half the dose of levalbuterol to achieve the same effect as albuterol. Both are recommended for administration on an as-needed basis—administer it (up to three to four times per day) when the child is symptomatic, don't use it when the child is feeling well. For children younger than 2 years of age, we recommend the 0.63 mg strength of albuterol. Levalbuterol (Xopenex) is approved for use in children over age 6 years, although it is probably equally as safe as albuterol in very young children.

Albuterol solution is also available in 10 and 20 cc bottles, where the medication can be withdrawn with an eyedropper (0.5 cc or less) and normal saline added to the nebulizer cup to create a volume of liquid of about 3 cc. One advantage over *premixed* albuterol (i.e., albuterol premixed with normal saline in unit-dose vials of 3 cc) is that albuterol can be mixed with other medications (e.g., the inhaled steroid, budesonide [Pulmicort Respules]) without having a large volume of liquid in the nebulizer cup and consequently a prolonged time for each nebulizer treatment.

In general, children between 3–5 years of age can begin to receive their inhaled beta-agonist bronchodilator by metered-dose inhaler with attached spacer (valved holding chamber). If they are capable of sealing their lips around the mouthpiece of the holding chamber and taking in a slow, deep breath (on command) to empty the chamber, the mouthpiece may be a good option. At the younger end of this age spectrum and for those unable to make a tight seal with their lips, we recommend using the metered-dose inhaler and spacer with an attached face mask. Each puff of medication is emptied from the holding chamber with six to seven regular (tidal) breaths into and out of the face mask and chamber. Even children at this age will be prescribed two puffs as the standard dose for a bronchodilator treatment.

For the child who reliably becomes symptomatic with play, especially in cold air, pre-exercise use of a quick-acting bronchodilator is an excellent strategy for prevention of asthmatic symptoms. The quick-acting bronchodilators like albuterol and levalbuterol begin to exert their effect in 3–5 minutes, have maximal effect at approximately 1 hour, and wear off approximately 4–6 hours after use. The long-acting beta-agonist bronchodilators, salmeterol (Serevent) and formoterol (Foradil), can also be used in this preventive fashion, with protection from exercise-induced bronchoconstriction lasting up to 12 hours after administration. However, the long-acting beta-agonist bronchodilators have the following drawbacks: (1) they require the ability to coordinate use of the dry-powder inhaler (generally possible only after age 5–6 years); (2) with regular (daily) use they lose their effectiveness in preventing bronchoconstriction; and (3) they carry a "black-box warning" about an associated risk of asthmatic deaths and near deaths with their regular use (discussed further in Chap. 3, "Medications Used to Treat Asthma"). We would only recommend using a long-acting inhaled beta agonist in a child already being treated with an inhaled steroid. The onset of effect for salmeterol (Serevent) is 15–20 minutes; for formoterol (Foradil) it is 3–5 minutes, just like albuterol.

KEY POINT   Use of a quick-acting beta-agonist bronchodilator prior to exercise helps to prevent exercise-induced bronchoconstriction. With *regular* use, the long-acting beta-agonist bronchodilators lose much of their protective effect given pre-exercise.

Children who develop asthmatic symptoms with exercise, needing their quick-acting bronchodilator more than twice weekly for relief, should begin regular controller therapy to reduce the frequency of their symptoms. We consider exercise as just one of numerous asthmatic triggers. When asthma is being *triggered* several times a week, it is time to think about long-term control therapy.

Controllers

CROMOLYN

In the not-too-distant past, cromolyn (Intal) was the first choice controller medication for children with asthma. It could be given as a nebulizer solution

(20 mg/vial) or dry-powder inhaler (Intal Spinhaler, 20 mg/capsule) and subsequently as a metered-dose inhaler (2 mg/puff). Its great appeal for pediatricians, parents, and patients alike was its near complete freedom from side effects (other than perhaps the irritative effect of the coarse powder released from the Spinhaler).

However, a number of drawbacks have led to cromolyn's fall from favor as an asthma controller. First and foremost is its limited effectiveness. It simply does not prevent symptoms and protect from asthmatic attacks with the same effectiveness as inhaled steroids. Second, it needs to be administered four times daily. Imagine the challenge of sitting with a child to administer nebulized cromolyn for at least 5–10 minutes four times a day—in the absence of any immediate symptomatic benefit at the time of each administration! Third, the powder released from the Spinhaler tended to leave an unpleasant residue in the throat. And during exacerbations of asthma, its irritating effect could worsen bronchoconstriction, leading to the recommendation that the medicine be withheld during asthmatic flare-ups. (The Spinhaler is no longer available in the United States.)

There remains one *niche use* for which we find ourselves occasionally still prescribing a cromolyn metered-dose inhaler. A single dose (two puffs) of cromolyn administered 20–30 minutes prior to exercise effectively blunts bronchoconstriction induced by exercise or exertion in cold air. We find that some children are so sensitive to the stimulatory effects of albuterol (jitteriness and heart racing) that they avoid its use at all costs, including for prevention of exercise-induced bronchoconstriction. With cromolyn we have an alternative to offer, one that is free of all adrenaline-like side effects.

KEY POINT   Routine use of cromolyn four times daily for control of asthma symptoms has fallen from favor, largely because of its limited effectiveness and difficulty in medication adherence. Cromolyn can still be used preventively as a single dose administered prior to exercise; it blunts exercise-induced bronchoconstriction without causing the same adrenaline-like side-effects as albuterol.

INHALED CORTICOSTEROIDS

The modern alternatives to cromolyn as asthma controllers in children, including in children under age 2, are the inhaled corticosteroids and the leukotriene receptor blockers. Inhaled steroids are the most effective controller medication available to treat persistent asthma. However, as with every medication, one needs to weigh both the risks and benefits. "Why would you even consider giving a steroid to a very young child?" you ask. Or, if not you, the parent of your very young patient certainly will ask this same question. "Won't there be harmful effects on the growth and development of the child? What about thinning of the skin, formation of cataracts, and impaired bone development? Do you want to create a generation of asthmatics of very short stature?"

These are valid, well-informed concerns that you can help to address by sharing the available medical evidence. But first, to answer the question of why one would prescribe an inhaled steroid (as *preferred therapy*, according to the Expert Panel of the National Asthma Education and Prevention Program, as shown in Table 5-3), one might begin with their proven benefits. They reduce asthmatic symptoms (including nighttime awakenings due to asthma), reduce the frequency of asthmatic flare-ups, and minimize the risk of serious asthmatic exacerbations causing emergency room care or hospitalization. The widespread use of inhaled steroids for asthmatic children has had a dramatic epidemiologic effect. In communities where their prescription and routine administration are high, asthma seems to disappear as a common medical problem from local hospitals. In short, they work well—often, dramatically well—as controller medications. Children's airways become less hyperresponsive (less *asthmatic*) and, when biopsy samples are available, they look more like normal, nonasthmatic airways.

Before addressing their potential harmful effects, we would like to emphasize two other considerations about steroids and their beneficial effects in childhood asthma. First, it is worth remembering the harmful side effects of poorly controlled asthma. These include lost nights' sleep, school absences, impaired school performance, and restricted athletic performance (which may mean sitting out gym time or outdoors free time at school). There is also often a *ripple effect* on other family members, including siblings and parents whose plans have to be modified because of the disruptive impact of the asthmatic child's illness. One other impact of poorly controlled asthma to keep in mind is—ironically—impaired growth! Children with uncontrolled asthma do not grow to be as tall as expected.

The second consideration is that side effects from inhaled steroids are dose dependent. For most children with asthma, low doses of inhaled steroids suffice to provide good control. Doses considered to be in the "low" and "medium" ranges for children are given in Table 5-4.

Now, what about the risk of long-term side effects from inhaled steroids in childhood? Skin atrophy inside the rim of the face mask is a concern when inhaled steroids are administered by nebulizer with attached face mask or metered-dose inhaler and valved holding chamber with attached face mask. However, this complication can readily be prevented by rinsing the skin with a damp face cloth after each use.

Steroids blown into the eyes might predispose to cataracts. Although there is no documented association between pediatric use of inhaled steroids and cataracts, care should be taken to minimize ocular exposure when administering inhaled steroids with a face mask attachment. Some newer face masks (e.g., the Bubbles the Fish II mask from Pari) are specifically designed to direct away from the face the medication that is not inhaled.

The greatest concern surrounding use of inhaled steroids in young children relates to their potential effect on bone growth. A number of studies have demonstrated that sufficient drug is absorbed systemically and carried to the bones to have a negative effect, and over the first year of regular use a small

STEPWISE APPROACH FOR MANAGING INFANTS AND YOUNG CHILDREN (5 YEARS OF AGE AND YOUNGER) WITH ACUTE OR CHRONIC ASTHMA

Classify Severity: Clinical Features Before Treatment or Adequate Control	Symptoms/Day Symptoms/Night	Medications Required To Maintain Long-Term Control
		Daily Medications
Step 4 Severe Persistent	Continual Frequent	■ Preferred treatment: – High-dose inhaled corticosteroids AND – Long-acting inhaled beta$_2$-agonists AND, if needed, – Corticosteroid tablets or syrup long term (2 mg/kg/day, generally do not exceed 60 mg per day). (Make repeat attempts to reduce systemic corticosteroids and maintain control with high-dose inhaled corticosteroids.)
Step 3 Moderate Persistent	Daily > 1 night/week	■ Preferred treatments: – Low-dose inhaled corticosteroids and long-acting inhaled beta$_2$-agonists OR – Medium-dose inhaled corticosteroids. ■ Alternative treatment: – Low-dose inhaled corticosteroids and either leukotriene receptor antagonist or theophylline. If needed (particularly in patients with recurring severe exacerbations): ■ Preferred treatment: – Medium-dose inhaled corticosteroids and long-acting beta$_2$-agonists. ■ Alternative treatment: – Medium-dose inhaled corticosteroids and either leukotriene receptor antagonist or theophylline.
Step 2 Mild Persistent	> 2/week but < 1x/day > 2 nights/month	■ Preferred treatment: – Low-dose inhaled corticosteroid (with nebulizer or MDI with holding chamber with or without face mask or DPI). ■ Alternative treatment (listed alphabetically): – Cromolyn (nebulizer is preferred or MDI with holding chamber) OR leukotriene receptor antagonist.
Step 1 Mild Intermittent	≤ 2 days/week ≤ 2 nights/month	■ No daily medication needed.

| **Quick Relief** All Patients | ■ Bronchodilator as needed for symptoms. Intensity of treatment will depend upon severity of exacerbation.
– Preferred treatment: **Short-acting inhaled beta$_2$-agonists** by nebulizer or face mask and space/holding chamber
– Alternative treatment: Oral beta$_2$-agonist
■ With viral respiratory infection
– Bronchodilator q 4–6 hours up to 24 hours (longer with physician consult); in general, repeat no more than once every 6 weeks
– Consider systemic corticosteroid if exacerbation is severe or patient has history of previous severe exacerbations
■ Use of short-acting beta$_2$-agonists >2 times a week in intermittent asthma (daily, or increasing use in persistent asthma) may indicate the need to initiate (increase) long-term-control therapy. |

Step down
Review treatment every 1 to 6 months; a gradual stepwise reduction in treatment may be possible.

Step up
If control is not maintained, consider step up. First, review patient medication technique, adherence, and environmental control.

Goals of Therapy: Asthma Control
- Minimal or no chronic symptoms day or night
- Minimal or no exacerbations
- No limitations on activities; no school/parent's work missed
- Minimal use of short-acting inhaled beta$_2$-agonist
- Minimal or no adverse effects from medications

Note
- The stepwise approach is intended to assist, not replace, the clinical decisionmaking required to meet individual patient needs.
- Classify severity: assign patient to most severe step in which any feature occurs.
- There are very few studies on asthma therapy for infants.
- Gain control as quickly as possible (a course of short systemic corticosteroids may be required); then step down to the least medication necessary to maintain control.
- Minimize use of short-acting inhaled beta$_2$-agonists. Overreliance on short-acting inhaled beta$_2$-agonists (e.g., use of approximately one canister a month even if not using it every day) indicates inadequate control of asthma and the need to initiate or intensify long-term-control therapy.
- Provide parent education on asthma management and controlling environmental factors that make asthma worse (e.g., allergies and irritants).
- Consultation with an asthma specialist is recommended for patients with moderate or severe persistent asthma. Consider consultation for patients with mild persistent asthma.

From: National Asthma Education and Prevention Program Expert Panel Report: Guidelines for the Diagnosis and Management of Asthma—Update on Selected Topics 2002 (www.nhlbi.nih.gov/guidelines/asthma/index.htm).

TABLE 5-4

LOW- AND MEDIUM-DOSE RANGES FOR CHILDREN UNDER AGE 12 YEARS

Drug	Low Daily Dose (mcg/day)	Medium Daily Dose (mcg/day)
Beclomethasone (Qvar)	80–160	160–320
Budesonide (Pulmicort Turbuhaler) (Pulmicort Respules)	200–400 500	400–800 1000
Flunisolide (Aerobid)	500–750	1000–1250
Fluticasone (Flovent) (Advair)	88–176 100–200	176–440 200–500
Mometasone (Asmanex)	220	440
Triamcinolone (Azmacort)	400–800	800–1200

decrease in growth occurs—on average, a loss of height of 1 cm or just under $^1/_2$ inch. But, with continuous use, there is no further slowing of growth, and at least one long-term study suggests that children catch up to their normal, predicted height before they stop growing, despite continued use of inhaled steroids. These studies are difficult to conduct: they require a stable population of asthmatic children, followed for several years, and with predictions about ultimate height based on the height of the child's parents. One needs also to factor into the equation the fact that regular, preventive use of inhaled steroids reduces the need for intermittent courses of oral steroids used to treat asthmatic attacks.

Here's how the Expert Panel of the National Asthma Education and Prevention Program summed up the evidence in 2002: "Cumulative data in children suggest that low-to-medium doses of inhaled corticosteroids may have the potential of decreasing growth velocity (resulting in a small difference in height averaging 1 cm in the first year of treatment), but this effect on growth velocity is not sustained in subsequent years of treatment, is not progressive, and may be reversible. Cohort studies following children for more than 10 years suggest that final predicted height is attained. Physicians should monitor the growth of children and adolescents taking corticosteroids by any route of administration and, if growth appears slowed, weigh the benefits of asthma control against the possibility of growth suppression or delay."

KEY POINT Inhaled steroids cause a minor decrease in growth during the first year of administration that does not progress with continued regular use. It is thought that the final height that these children achieve is normal (i.e., they "catch up" and attain their normal, predicted height).

These recommendations do not distinguish among different steroid preparations. The side effects are a "class effect," referable to all of the inhaled steroids. Insufficient data are available to suggest whether one steroid preparation is likely to cause more or fewer long-term side effects than another. The ages down to which each inhaled steroid is approved for use by the Food and Drug Administration (see Fig. 5-2) reflects the age of children recruited into the initial "pivotal" clinical trials demonstrating the safety and efficacy of the drug, rather than known lack of safety in children who are younger. Budesonide is the only inhaled steroid currently available as a liquid for nebulization (Pulmicort Respules); it is approved for administration to children as young as age 12 months. The prefilled vials should be kept at room temperature, stored in their foil packages to minimize exposure to light, and shaken gently before use. They are to be delivered by compressor-driven jet nebulizers (discussed further in Chap. 8).

LEUKOTRIENE BLOCKERS

For children with mild persistent asthma, the leukotriene receptor antagonists, montelukast (Singulair) and zafirlukast (Accolate), offer an appealing alternative to inhaled steroids. Like cromolyn (Intal), they are remarkably free of side effects. Their safety has been highlighted by the recent Food and Drug Administration approval of montelukast to treat perennial rhinitis in infants as young as 6 months of age.

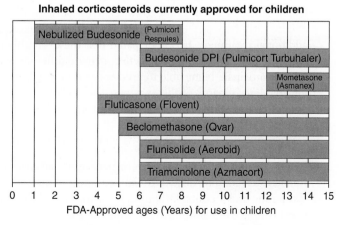

FIGURE 5-2 *FDA-approved ages (years) for use in children.*

In addition, they are administered by mouth (swallowed or chewed) rather than inhaled, and the dosing schedule can be as simple as once daily (montelukast). Montelukast (in the form of Singulair Granules) is approved to treat asthma in children as young as 1 year of age. The Singulair oral granules can be placed directly into the child's mouth or mixed with a spoonful of applesauce, carrots, rice, or ice cream. They are not meant to be dissolved in liquid. A 4-mg chewable tablet of montelukast is available for children 2–5 years of age and a 5-mg chewable tablet for children 6–14 years old. Older children are treated with the adult 10-mg dose. Zafirlukast (Accolate) is approved for administration to children as young as 5 years of age in a dose of 10 mg twice daily, increased to 20 mg twice daily for children aged 12 years and older.

Safe, convenient, and easy-to-use: what's not to love about the leukotriene blockers? Well, we haven't yet spoken about efficacy. The published experience in children mirrors that in adults: some do very well with leukotriene blocker therapy, whereas others derive little or no benefit. Overall, inhaled steroids provide more consistent freedom from symptoms and more reliable protection from asthmatic attacks than leukotriene blockers. Also, the dose of inhaled steroids can be adjusted up or down according to the severity of asthmatic symptoms; the dose of the leukotriene blockers is restricted to a single amount.

KEY POINT   Overall, inhaled steroids provide more consistent control of asthma symptoms and protection from asthmatic attacks than do the leukotriene blockers. On the other hand, the latter are easy to take and virtually free of any side effects.

In our opinion, a very reasonable approach is to prescribe a leukotriene blocker as first-line therapy in mild persistent asthma. A one-month therapeutic trial will likely suffice. If there is no improvement after one month of therapy, transition is made to an inhaled steroid; or if a serious asthmatic exacerbation occurs despite the leukotriene blocker, it is time to switch to (or perhaps add) an inhaled steroid. Some children will have striking improvement with the leukotriene blocker and need no additional treatment. It is anticipated that these variable responses to leukotriene blocking therapy will prove to reflect genetic differences in the population. Some day we anticipate being able to predict a patient's response based on analysis of the genetic determinants of the enzymes involved in his or her leukotriene metabolic pathways. In the meantime, a well-monitored therapeutic trial is necessary.

Treatment of moderate and severe persistent asthma

Children with moderate or severe persistent asthma should be treated with an inhaled steroid. The dose of the inhaled steroid may need to be escalated to bring symptoms under control, then *stepped down* to find the lowest dose that maintains good asthma control while minimizing the risk of side effects. Adding a second controller can allow continued use of a low dose of inhaled steroids or dose reduction of the inhaled steroid among those who required higher doses. As in adults, the use of a long-acting inhaled beta-agonist bronchodilator together with an inhaled steroid proves to be a particularly effective combination. The combination is made conveniently available in the dry-powder device, the Advair Diskus. The Advair Diskus has now been approved for use in children as young as 4 years of age; it is just around this age that children begin to be able to master the technique of the dry-powder inhaler. An alternative, somewhat less potent regimen is the addition of a leukotriene receptor blocker, such as montelukast (Singulair) or zafirlukast (Accolate), to an inhaled steroid. Very young children might receive budesonide by nebulizer and face mask (Pulmicort Respules) and montelukast (Singulair) as oral granules or chewable tablet. With this modern armamentarium of therapies, the vast majority of children with asthma, even those with severe asthma, can achieve good control with daily controller medications that are given no more frequently than twice daily and are generally well tolerated.

Preventive maintenance

A remarkable statistic is the observation that across the nation the vast majority of visits to the doctor for asthma are urgent visits for symptomatic flares rather than routine visits for prevention and maintenance—even though, as a general rule, less medicine is needed to keep asthma under good control than to regain control during an exacerbation. Even when things are going well, we encourage regular, follow-up medical visits for asthma. We find that children and their parents are more open and willing to discuss their asthma experiences when they are not in the midst of handling an exacerbation. We take this time not just to discuss medications but ways in which asthma impacts their lives. A comment we have often heard from parents is that a particularly frustrating aspect of asthma is its unpredictability. This opening provides an excellent opportunity to develop or review an asthma action plan (see Chap. 10, "Developing an Asthma Action Plan"). Our goal is to help parents and children feel ready to handle whatever situation may arise. We involve them in developing the plan and also work on strategies to help the children remember to take their controller medications (or the parents to give them to their children). These are also opportunities to discuss where to keep their medicines in school and even how to plan for vacations.

Treatment of serious asthmatic exacerbations will often require a short course of oral corticosteroids. Recommendation for a steroid course may be part of the asthma action plan that you develop with parent and child. Side effects from oral steroids (see Chap. 3, "Medications Used to Treat Asthma") are common and potentially severe enough to warrant discussion before the medication is needed. We are always glad to have addressed this topic before receiving the phone call reporting that the asthmatic child is acutely ill. Similarly, if a child has never needed asthma care in an emergency department, it can be helpful to take a few minutes to describe the anticipated process, including how long they are likely to wait to be seen, how emergency department triage works, and who will provide care while they are there.

KEY POINT   Routine, scheduled visits for asthma can be used to discuss asthma action plans and to anticipate elements of medical care that may be involved in managing a severe asthmatic attack, including use of oral steroids and emergency department care.

Preventive maintenance includes preparing for the change in seasons. In late summer we start talking about the flu vaccine, recommending it for all of our patients who are on long-term controller therapy. This is also a good time to raise the subject of the school environment, reminding parents to keep an eye out for potential asthmatic triggers as the school year begins. We also encourage parents to meet with the school nurse and make arrangements for keeping medicines in school. Every fall there is a virtual epidemic of emergency room visits for asthma. In part, this up-tick of asthmatic attacks each September is due to spread of viral respiratory tract infections, the most common cause of asthmatic exacerbations among children. However, it is also partly due to lack of preparedness among the parents of these children. Compared to a control group of asthmatic children not experiencing exacerbations, those with attacks were less likely to have a prescription available for their beta-agonist bronchodilator or for their inhaled corticosteroid.

Changes in the seasons also bring variation in allergen exposures. It is helpful to anticipate allergic exposures in atopic children and discuss allergy management in advance of these exposures. Children may participate in sports during certain times of the year. It may be necessary to *step up* asthma therapy to maximize asthma control during sports seasons. Some children may have learned to avoid sports or other strenuous activities so that they don't trigger uncomfortable symptoms of asthma. With careful planning and proper management, children should be able to participate in sports at every level. We remind our patients that there are many highly successful athletes with asthma, including many who participate in the Olympics and professional sports. Asthma need not be a barrier to vigorous physical activities. Whenever stepping up therapy, be sure to mention your approach to stepping down therapy. We remind parents (and ourselves) that our goal is to provide the best possible control of symptoms and to maximize lung function while using the least amount of medication.

WHEN INITIAL TREATMENT FAILS

After an initial visit for asthma—the diagnosis of asthma has been established, medications appropriate to the severity of asthma prescribed, and proper technique for administration of medications reviewed—we anticipate that our patient will do well. A good way to confirm the progress is a follow-up phone call, made within 1 week of the first visit, and then a follow-up office visit. We try to schedule the follow-up appointment in 4–6 weeks. We ask the family to bring all of the child's medication to the office with the intent of reviewing both the medications and their technique of administration.

At the follow-up visit we inquire about the child's asthma symptoms, with particular emphasis on any symptoms that disturb sleep or interfere with physical activities. When a child or parent reports that therapy is working well, we want to know the details: for example, is there improvement because the medications are working well or because the cat is being kept out of the bedroom?

Reviewing expectations and medication administration

But what if our patient does not improve? Where did we go wrong? How do we approach the patient whose initial treatment fails to bring relief? Here's where some careful detective work is needed. We ask for details about the child's symptoms, and sometimes find that misplaced parental expectations are the problem. "My child's cough goes away after nebulized albuterol, but it comes right back after 3–4 hours." Such a response, we need to explain, is consistent with the duration of action of the drug; we are on the right track. Remember too that it may take at least 1 week for anti-inflammatory therapies to start working, and you may not see their maximal benefit for a month or more.

One of the most common reasons why the child does not benefit from the prescribed inhalation therapy is that little if any of it is getting to his or her airways. In one child we observed what appeared to be well coordinated inhaler technique only to discover that she never actually actuated the metered-dose inhaler to release the spray of medication. Another patient demonstrated excellent technique in the office but casually mentioned that he usually took his inhalers while lying flat on his back in bed. Yet another patient seemed to have a good understanding of how to use her dry-powder inhaler (Diskus). Only by watching her use the device did we learn that she was trying hard to time her inhalation with *actuation* of the device (movement of the lever), as if it were a metered-dose inhaler. She would finish her inhalation before the powder was in place to inhale.

Sometimes the "devil is in the details." Check to see that the medication being administered has not passed its expiration date and that the inhaler being used is not empty of medication! Overall, the amount of time spent teaching and observing parents and children in medication administration, including opportunities for them to voice their attitudes and beliefs and to interact with each other, can be enormous. The reward may be good asthma control without adding more medicines with their associated expense, inconvenience, and risk of side effects.

KEY POINT   When a child's asthma is not improving with prescribed medication, the first *suspect* to *round up* is ineffective use of the prescribed medication, particularly poor inhalational technique with inhaled medications.

Asthma is a common pediatric illness, and many pediatricians find themselves very comfortable with its diagnosis and management. However, referral to a pediatric asthma specialist may be appropriate when the child fails to improve with standard therapy, when multiple controller medications or frequent courses of oral steroids are necessary to control the disease, or when the patient and family simply need more time to learn about asthma. They may wish the opportunity to discuss in detail trigger avoidance, use of medications, or the long-term implications of the illness. Recommendations for specialist referral from the National Asthma Education and Prevention Program are listed in Table 5-5.

After a visit to a specialist, parents often don't know whom to call if there is a problem. In general, we encourage them to coordinate their care through their primary care providers, with asthma specialists available as backup. This approach communicates an important message to parents: asthma is just one part of their child's care and must not be their only focus. At the same time we recognize that physician utilization will vary depending on the severity of the child's asthma, the specific physicians involved, and the comfort of the primary care provider in dealing with asthma. You will likely need to find the approach that works best in your particular community.

What else might the specialist have to add when confronted with a child who fails to improve with conventional asthma therapies? As noted, one resource is more time devoted specifically to the problem of asthma. He or she will likely also explore the following: Are there unidentified triggers making this

TABLE 5 - 5

INDICATIONS FOR REFERRAL TO AN ASTHMA SPECIALIST

- Child has severe persistent asthma.
- Child is under 3 years of age and has moderate or severe persistent asthma.
- Child has used long-term oral corticosteroid therapy, high-dose inhaled corticosteroid therapy, or more than two bursts of oral corticosteroids in 12 months.
- Child has had a life-threatening asthma exacerbation.
- Goals of asthma therapy are not being met after 3–6 months of treatment, or earlier if the child appears unresponsive to treatment.
- Signs and symptoms are atypical, or there are problems in differential diagnosis.
- Other conditions complicate asthma or its diagnosis (e.g., untreated sinusitis or rhinitis).
- Additional diagnostic testing is indicated (e.g., pulmonary function testing; allergy skin testing).
- Child is being considered for immunotherapy.

child's asthma particularly severe? Are there aggravating medical conditions complicating the response to therapy? Is the diagnosis of asthma correct?

Unidentified triggers

A partial list of triggers that may not have been recognized as problems is shown in Table 5-6. The time of year may provide a clue to seasonal allergies. We also ask parents to keep track of the timing of symptoms in relation to places where the child spends time. For instance, symptoms that develop after the child plays in the (damp) basement may point to mold allergy and exposure. Similarly, the time of onset of symptoms may point to exposures at school or in a friend's home.

We cared for a child who had cough and wheezing while at school, gradually improved over the weekend, and then experienced recurrent symptoms upon returning to school the following week. Although there were no pets in the child's classroom, a school-related allergic trigger was considered likely. The children in his class were asked to leave their coats on coat racks outside the classroom, thinking that animal dander might be brought into the classroom from pets at home, but the child's symptoms still did not improve. In the end, it took several weeks finally to identify the culprit: a pet rabbit kept in a classroom several doors down the corridor. Once the rabbit and its cage were removed, the child's asthma quickly came under good control.

Having changes made in a school for the benefit of one child's health may seem a daunting and perhaps presumptuous task, but remember that the law is on your side. Children and their families have the right to conditions that allow the child to breathe comfortably while attending school. These rights include adapting snacks for students with allergies and training special staff when

TABLE 5 - 6

POTENTIAL UNIDENTIFIED TRIGGERS OF ASTHMA

Allergens
- dust mites
- cockroaches
- pet (or pest) dander
- pollen

School exposures
- chalk dust
- classroom pets

Cleaning products

Cigarette smoke

Exercise, especially in cold air

Premenstrual asthma

necessary. In addition, the child should have reliable access to medication, options for physical education, and classrooms that are free of allergens and irritants. No one can be excluded or denied services just because he or she has asthma or allergies. It's the law.*

The Americans with Disabilities Act can help people with asthma and allergies obtain safer, healthier environments in which to work, shop, eat, and go to school. It also affects employment policies. For example, a private preschool cannot refuse to enroll children because giving medication to or adapting snacks for students with allergies requires special staff training or because insurance rates might go up. Likewise, a firm cannot refuse to hire an otherwise qualified person solely because of the potential need for time off from work or health insurance requirements of a family member.

KEY POINT   The Americans with Disabilities Act guarantees the legal right to a safe and healthy school environment for children with asthma and allergies.

Two other considerations should be kept in mind when sleuthing for unidentified triggers of asthma. First, remember that there may be—and often are—more than one trigger. Being atopic predisposes one to multiple allergic sensitivities; and having allergies doesn't make one immune to environmental tobacco smoke exposure and other inhaled irritants. Second, beware the late allergic response. Symptoms may not develop for several hours after an allergic exposure. For example, it is possible to develop wheezing and cough at home, 4–8 hours after encountering cat dander at day care.

Concomitant illnesses

Asthma may not be the only allergic disease troubling your patient. Often allergic rhinitis, whether seasonal or perennial, accompanies asthma. If we called asthma "allergic bronchitis," as it is in many children, we would not in the least be surprised to think that allergic inflammation of the nasal passages often exists in parallel with allergic inflammation of the intrathoracic airways. Many clinicians

*"The Americans with Disabilities Act (ADA) is a civil rights law that gives you the right to ask for changes where policies, practices, or conditions exclude or disadvantage you. Public entities and public accommodations, including schools, must ensure that individuals with disabilities have these rights. Section 504 of the Rehabilitation Act of 1973 prohibits discrimination on the basis of disability in employment and education in agencies, programs, and services that receive federal money. The ADA extends many of the rights and duties of Section 504 to public accommodations such as restaurants, hotels, theaters, stores, doctors' offices, museums, private schools, and child care programs. They must be readily accessible to and usable by individuals with disabilities, described as someone who has a physical or mental impairment that substantially limits one or more major life activities, or is regarded as having such impairments. Breathing, eating, working, and going to school are 'major life activities.' Asthma and allergies are still considered disabilities under the ADA, even if symptoms are controlled by medication." From ADA website, www.usdoj.gov/crt/ada/adahom1.htm

find that asthma comes under better control when allergic inflammation of the nose and sinuses is suppressed. Treatments may include allergen avoidance, antihistamines, nasal steroid sprays, or leukotriene blockers. With these therapies the child breathes more comfortably through his or her nose, nasal drainage into the posterior pharynx is reduced, and we often find that asthma therapy can be stepped down.

Patients with food allergy often have severe persistent asthma. On the other hand, food-triggered asthma is uncommon, occurring in fewer than 3% of children. Potential culprits are sulfites used as food preservatives (e.g., in dried fruits, prepared potatoes, bottled lemon or lime juice, and shrimp) and already diagnosed food allergens (such as milk, eggs, peanuts, tree nuts, soy, wheat, fish, and shellfish).

An infectious sinusitis can have the same effect as allergic rhinitis, making asthma control more difficult. A history of fever, facial tenderness, and purulent nasal discharge that lasts for more than 10 days makes us suspect a bacterial sinusitis. Sinus x-rays are generally not helpful in this context; and sinus computed tomography (CT) not immediately necessary. We would treat suspected sinusitis with a 2–3 week course of antibiotics and nasal decongestants and observe the child's clinical course. Often, as the sinusitis is cured, asthma comes under better control.

Another common comorbidity in children with asthma is gastroesophageal reflux. It is not entirely clear how reflux of gastric contents (containing highly acidic liquid, digestive enzymes, and possibly food allergens) into the esophagus causes worsening of asthma, but two theories are commonly offered in explanation. The reflex theory proposes that the refluxed material triggers a reflex arc via the vagus nerve. The reflex begins with sensory nerves in the esophagus and ends with bronchoconstrictor nerve pathways along the bronchial tree. This explanation derives its plausibility from the fact that the esophagus and bronchi, with their common embryological derivation, share neural pathways in common.

An alternative theory suggests that gastric contents can reflux to the level of the posterior pharynx and then be aspirated into the trachea and bronchi. It is easy to conceive of how aspirated acid and digestive enzymes would worsen airway inflammation and produce more symptoms of cough and wheezing.

Although a barium swallow is the easiest test for gastroesophageal reflux disease (GERD), it has low diagnostic sensitivity. Reflux is often missed on a routine barium swallow. More definitive—but more invasive to perform—is pH probe monitoring (using a probe at the tip of a catheter passed via the nasopharynx into the esophagus or a radio transmitting pH capsule placed endoscopically into the esophagus). Sometimes a therapeutic trial of a medicine that reduces gastric acid is preferable. Histamine-2 blockers (an example is ranitidine [Zantac]) or proton-pump inhibitors (such as omeprazole [Prilosec] and many others) are typically prescribed for a month or more to assess for a clinical response. If reflux symptoms (such as retrosternal burning, frequent burping, and postprandial regurgitation of food) are suppressed, asthma may likewise improve in parallel. When questions about the diagnosis or management of reflux remain, we would encourage referral to a pediatric gastroenterologist.

Alternative diagnoses

When the step-care approach to asthma therapy fails to bring asthma under
control—when medication delivery is optimized, environmental triggers eliminated, and comorbid illnesses treated, and still the child is troubled by respiratory symptoms—one finds oneself asking: "Am I sure that this is asthma that we
are treating?" Is it possible that what looks and sounds like asthma is something
else, mimicking asthma? Take, for example, the teenage girl who is having trouble competing in sports because of her asthma. Her exercise-induced asthma
had been well-controlled with p.r.n. albuterol when she played on the community soccer team, but now on the "traveling team," at a higher level of competition, it is interfering with her performance. After just a brief time on the field,
she develops loud wheezing and comes to the sidelines to use her albuterol-
containing metered-dose inhaler. The rescue bronchodilator has "stopped working"
for her, and she needs to have the coach take her out of the game.

The coach can see that she is having difficulty breathing. She has loud
wheezing that he can easily hear without a stethoscope, and her breathing is
labored. After just a few minutes of rest she quickly improves, but the coach is
hesitant to have her return to competition. Her parents and older sister, an
accomplished college soccer player, look on helplessly. She has had her antiasthmatic medications steadily escalated by her physician. She faithfully takes
her high-dose inhaled steroids, long-acting inhaled beta-agonist bronchodilator,
and leukotriene modifier, but nothing seems to control her exercise-induced
symptoms.

One would appropriately consider the impact on her asthma of exercising
in cold air, possible allergic sensitivity to outdoor pollens or mold, or even exercise-induced gastroesophageal reflux. At the same time, we would also encourage consideration of an alternative diagnosis besides (or in addition to) asthma.
Certain features of her story raise doubt that she has refractory asthma: the
rather abrupt worsening of her exercise-induced asthma in the absence of asthmatic symptoms at other times during the day or night; the failure of albuterol
to help control her symptoms; and especially, the brief duration of her exercise-
induced shortness of breath and wheezing. The exercise-induced bronchoconstriction of asthma typically lasts 30–60 minutes in the absence of bronchodilator
therapy, not 5 minutes or less.

Hearing this story, especially with the overlay of psychological stress
imposed by high-level athletic competition and a very successful athletic sister
with whom she will inevitably be compared, we would suspect the alternative
diagnosis of vocal cord dysfunction. Loud inspiratory and/or expiratory wheezes
can be generated when the vocal cords are inappropriately brought in close

approximation (adducted) with only a small orifice left for the passage of air. You, too, can generate an upper airway wheeze if you voluntarily bring together your vocal cords and force air through the narrowed opening. In vocal cord dysfunction, no anatomic abnormality (i.e., no polyp, tumor, or stricture) narrows the upper airway; the disorder is functional. In this example, it offers the child a means of withdrawal from the stressful competition of her soccer games, for a "medical reason." Her behavior may not be conscious and deliberate, but it does emanate from the brain, not from a disease of the vocal cords or of the lower airways.

Diagnosis of vocal cord dysfunction can be confirmed by laryngoscopy performed during a period of active wheezing. With the laryngoscope, the ear-nose-and-throat specialist can visualize the so-called "paradoxical" motion of the vocal cords and exclude alternative etiologies for upper airway obstruction. The first step in treating this disorder is its recognition and reduction of unnecessary antiasthmatic drugs. Additional treatment for vocal cord dysfunction involves relaxation techniques and breathing exercises (typically under the supervision of a speech and swallowing therapist), often in conjunction with behavioral medicine consultation.

KEY POINT   Not all that wheezes is asthma. When patients fail to improve despite appropriate therapy and good medication adherence, consider the possibility of a diagnosis other than asthma. Vocal cord dysfunction is one such example.

Other potential alternative diagnoses that can be mistaken for asthma are listed in Table 5-2 (page 173). We wish to highlight briefly two other disorders from this list. Like vocal cord dysfunction, habit cough has a psychological basis. It typically begins with the cough of an upper respiratory tract infection but then becomes persistent and habitual. The cough is frequently characterized by its loud, harsh, barking or honking nature, and it can persist for months or even years, well after the initial illness has resolved. The cough can be disruptive at school as well as at home, but it characteristically disappears when the child is asleep or distracted. Sometimes, reassurance is sufficient to stop the cough. Hypnosis has been shown to be effective therapy in many children; occasionally anxiolytic medications are needed.

A young child with cough, frequent sinusitis, and nasal polyps might be suspected of having asthma and allergic rhinosinusitis. However, allergic nasal polyposis is uncommon in childhood; and this child has frequent respiratory tract infections and a cough productive of discolored sputum. Recurrent respiratory infections more than allergic reactions seem to characterize his course, and antibiotics prove more effective treatment than antihistamines or inhaled steroids. What's your diagnosis? Consider the possibility of cystic fibrosis. Nasal polyps in a child should raise a red flag regarding possible cystic fibrosis. Although failure-to-thrive is the most common presentation in very young children, normal weight gain does not exclude the diagnosis. Frequent respiratory infections are also common in children with cystic fibrosis. Diagnosis begins with a family history, physical examination (his chest may have inspiratory crackles and signs of hyperinflation), and chest x-ray (bronchiectatic airways and surrounding inflammation may be visible on a plain chest radiograph). While spirometry in children with cystic fibrosis is initially normal, with time you see evidence of irreversible airflow obstruction. Specific confirmation of the diagnosis can be sought with a sweat test or blood test for the characteristic genetic abnormalities now known to be causative of cystic fibrosis.

We wish to end this chapter not with an emphasis on difficult-to-control asthma but with a more upbeat focus on the vast majority of children who can achieve good control of their asthma with appropriate asthma therapies. Caring for children with asthma is very satisfying. You can teach them to recognize their asthma symptoms, identify their triggers, and use their medications correctly. The result is children who can get back in the game. It helps us to think about them as well children with asthma, keeping in mind the goals of asthma therapy. Among these goals are providing the best possible control of symptoms and lung function with the least amount of medication. We try to reduce the need for urgently scheduled office visits, trips to the emergency room, and hospitalizations; and, most importantly, we strive to have asthmatic children achieve full participation in school and all activities. For some children, it "takes a village"—parents and other care providers, physician(s), school nurse, team coach, perhaps a social worker, and you, the asthma educator—to achieve these goals. The reward for these efforts is a healthy and safe child—the most valued prize of any society.

Self-Assessment Questions

QUESTION 1

Which of the following statements about the epidemiology of asthma in children is not true?

1. Asthma affects more boys than girls.
2. Asthma usually has its onset before age 7 years.
3. Asthma is the third most common cause of pediatric hospitalizations.
4. For the most part, hospitalizations for asthma are considered unavoidable.
5. The economic impact of pediatric asthma includes parental work absences.

QUESTION 2

Which of the following is a risk factor for the future development of asthma?

1. Psoriasis
2. Eczema (atopic dermatitis)
3. Nasal polyps
4. Frequent chest colds
5. Other autoimmune diseases, such as juvenile diabetes mellitus

QUESTION 3

True or false: *In a child under age 4, the absence of wheezes on examination reliably excludes a diagnosis of asthma?*

1. True
2. False

QUESTION 4

True or false: *In a child under age 15 but old enough to perform spirometry, normal pulmonary function test results (complete absence of expiratory airflow obstruction on spirometry) reliably exclude a diagnosis of asthma?*

1. True
2. False

QUESTION 5

The diagnostic label of "reactive airways disease" is often used by pediatricians to indicate:

1. Uncertainty in discriminating wheezing associated with viral respiratory tract infections from true asthma
2. Childhood asthma in the absence of associated allergies

3. Wheezing associated with environmental tobacco smoke (second-hand smoking)

4. Lingering cough following an aspiration event

5. The overlap between asthma and cystic fibrosis

QUESTION 6

You are asked to help with initiation of regular controller therapy for asthma in a 2-year-old child. Which of the following is not a suitable option?

1. Montelukast (Singulair) sprinkles

2. Budesonide (Pulmicort Respules) by nebulizer with face mask adaptor

3. Combination salmeterol-fluticasone (Advair 100/50) by dry-powder inhaler

4. Fluticasone (Flovent) 44 mcg/puff by metered-dose inhaler with valved holding chamber (spacer) and attached face mask

5. Beclomethasone (QVAR) 40 mcg/puff by metered-dose inhaler with valved holding chamber (spacer) and attached face mask

QUESTION 7

No parent likes the thought of his or her child having to take "steroids" on a regular basis. You can offer a number of reassurances to a concerned parent about inhaled steroids used to treat asthma in children. Which of the following is not a justifiable reassurance?

1. Currently available information suggests that your child will grow to his or her normal predicted height (or very close to it) despite regular use of inhaled steroids for many years.

2. Cataracts have not been found in children using regular inhaled steroids.

3. Inhaled steroids will decrease your child's need for oral steroids, which are associated with the risk of more severe side effects.

4. You can prevent skin atrophy associated with topical deposition of steroids by wiping the child's face after use of an inhaled steroid via face mask.

5. Children under age 5 do not develop oral candidiasis (thrush) because of their unique oropharyngeal bacterial flora.

QUESTION 8

Which of the following is the most appropriate use of long-acting inhaled beta-agonist bronchodilators such as salmeterol (Serevent) and formoterol (Foradil) in treating pediatric asthma?

1. Daily (a.m.) administration for prevention of school-related exercise-induced bronchoconstriction.

2. Regular use as an alternative controller therapy in children who are intolerant of inhaled steroids.

3. Regular use in combination with inhaled steroids for treatment of moderate persistent and severe persistent asthma.

4. As needed use as a long-lasting rescue bronchodilator, in place of the shorter-acting bronchodilators, such as albuterol.

5. As needed use as a long-lasting rescue bronchodilator, in addition to the shorter-acting bronchodilators, such as albuterol.

QUESTION 9

Leukotriene blockers such as montelukast (Singulair) and zafirlukast (Accolate), used alone, represent an alternative controller therapy for mild persistent asthma (instead of inhaled steroids). Which of the following statements about leukotriene blocking therapy is true?

1. Children under age 3 years cannot take this medication, because the slow-release tablets cannot be crushed for administration in applesauce.

2. Use of a leukotriene blocker is associated with fewer asthmatic symptoms and improved lung function.

3. A reasonable strategy for treating mild asthmatic attacks is doubling the dose of leukotriene blocker for a short period.

4. Leukotriene blockers should be used only in children with asthma and known aspirin sensitivity.

5. Leukotriene blockers have identical side-effects to inhaled steroids; their only advantage is oral as opposed to inhaled medication delivery.

QUESTION 10

The law is on your side if you choose to advocate for changes in an asthmatic child's school environment to ensure that allergic triggers are removed from the classroom and accommodations made for his or her medication needs. The federal law that you can invoke is called which of the following?

1. Civil Rights Act of 1964

2. Freedom of Information Act

3. "No Child Left Behind" Act

4. Equal Employment Opportunities Act

5. Americans with Disabilities Act

QUESTION 11

A 12-year-old child's exercise-induced asthmatic symptoms have changed this past year. She now reports that her quick-acting bronchodilator (Maxair Autohaler) no longer helps to prevent her wheezing and shortness of breath, and it brings only a little relief when she is symptomatic. She has had to be taken out of her soccer games early. When she comes to the sidelines, the coach can hear loud wheezing, both on inhalation and exhalation. Although she seems to improve relatively quickly (3–5 minutes), the coach is reluctant to send her back into the game. Which of the following is the most likely explanation for her difficulties?

1. Her Maxair inhaler has expired.
2. She has vocal cord dysfunction as well as asthma.
3. She has exercise-induced cardiac dysfunction (atrial septal defect with right-to-left shunting).
4. Her wheezing is due to an aspirated foreign object.
5. She has become tolerant to the effect of beta-agonist bronchodilators.

QUESTION 12

A child with asthma and any one of the circumstances listed below might benefit from intensive review of his or her care and possibly consultation with an asthma specialist. Nonetheless, which of the following is specifically a recommended indication for referral to an asthma specialist according to the National Asthma Education and Prevention Program?

1. A child under age 3 years with moderate or severe persistent asthma
2. Any emergency department visit for asthma
3. Two bursts of oral corticosteroids for asthma before the age of 8 years
4. A child with asthma, allergic rhinitis, and eczema
5. Use of a canister of quick-acting bronchodilator (e.g., albuterol) every month or more frequently

---

Answers to Self-Assessment Questions

ANSWER TO QUESTION 1 (EPIDEMIOLOGY OF CHILDHOOD ASTHMA)

The correct answer is #4. For the most part, hospitalizations due to childhood asthma are considered avoidable. Many health management organizations, insurance providers, and other medical organizations have developed asthma disease management programs attempting to reduce hospitalizations for asthma by implementation of good medical practices. The other statements about childhood asthma are true. Asthma does affect more boys than girls (until approximately the age of puberty) (answer #1). Most people with asthma are diagnosed before age 7 years (answer #2). Asthma is indeed the third most common cause of pediatric hospitalizations in the United States (answer #3). And pediatric asthma commonly causes work absences by parents needing to care for their ill child, with a consequent impact on the economy (answer #5).

ANSWER TO QUESTION 2 (RISK FACTORS FOR THE DEVELOPMENT OF ASTHMA)

The correct answer is #2; infantile eczema (atopic dermatitis) is one of the risk factors for the development of childhood asthma (along with a parental history of asthma, allergic rhinitis, wheezing apart from colds, and peripheral blood eosinophilia). Children with psoriasis (answer #1), nasal polyps (answer #3), frequent chest colds (answer #4), or autoimmune diseases such as juvenile diabetes mellitus (answer #5) are no more likely to develop asthma than children without these illnesses. We would note that finding nasal polyps in a child with respiratory symptoms should make you consider the possibility of cystic fibrosis. Finally, asthma is a disorder that involves the immune system, but it is not considered an autoimmune disease (in which the immune system makes antibodies that attack normal tissues in the body).

ANSWER TO QUESTION 3 (PHYSICAL EXAMINATION IN THE DIAGNOSIS OF ASTHMA)

The correct answer is #2 (False). Wheezing in asthma is intermittent. The absence of wheezing on chest auscultation does not exclude the possibility of intermittent airways obstruction and of wheezing present at other times (when your stethoscope is not applied to the chest). It is also possible to have a mild degree of airway narrowing without wheezing.

ANSWER TO QUESTION 4 (PULMONARY FUNCTION TESTING IN THE DIAGNOSIS OF ASTHMA)

The correct answer is #2 (False). As noted above in the answer to Question 3, the intermittent nature of airways obstruction in asthma makes a single normal spirometry test unreliable in excluding a diagnosis of asthma. On the other hand, the presence of airflow obstruction that reverses following bronchodilator administration strongly points to a diagnosis of asthma.

ANSWER TO QUESTION 5 (MEANING OF "REACTIVE AIRWAYS DISEASE")

The correct answer is #1; reactive airways disease is an ambiguous term, usually reflecting uncertainty about the diagnosis of asthma. Many young children develop wheezing in association with viral respiratory tract illnesses; only some of these children progress to the development of asthma. We prefer the term "wheezing-associated respiratory illness" to describe this finding at a time when a diagnosis of asthma cannot yet be established with certainty. Nonatopic asthma might be the term used to describe childhood asthma without associated allergic sensitivities (answer #2). We have not heard the term "reactive airways disease" applied to wheezing associated with environmental tobacco smoke exposure (answer #3), to cough following an aspiration event (answer #4), or to some combination of asthma and cystic fibrosis (answer #5). Cystic fibrosis with bronchial hyperresponsiveness might apply to this last circumstance.

ANSWER TO QUESTION 6 (MEDICATION DELIVERY TO A 2-YEAR-OLD CHILD)

The correct answer is #3. A 2-year-old child would not be expected to be able to use a dry-powder inhaler. The dry-powder inhaler requires tightening of the lips around the mouthpiece of the device and coordinating a single forceful inhalation to draw in the medicine. On the other hand, medication can be administered to children 2 years old and younger by sprinkles added to food (answer #1), by nebulizer with attached face mask (answer #2), or by metered-dose inhaler with valved holding chamber (spacer) and attached face mask (answers #4 and 5). You get extra credit if you have noted that fluticasone (Flovent) is only approved by the FDA for children 4 years of age and older; and beclomethasone (QVAR) for children 6 years of age and older.

ANSWER TO QUESTION 7 (SIDE EFFECTS OF INHALED STEROIDS IN CHILDREN)

The correct answer is #5; oral candidiasis or thrush can develop in children just as it does in adults. The risk is minimized by the use of valved holding chambers (spacers) and by rinsing the mouth after each use. The other statements (reassurances) about the use of inhaled steroids are correct. Available evidence indicates that after an initial decrease in growth velocity with institution of inhaled steroids, the decrease in growth does not progress and the ultimate height attained by the child is expected to be normal (answer #1). Cataracts are not reported in children using inhaled steroids (answer #2). Inhaled steroids protect against asthmatic exacerbations and decrease the need for bursts of oral steroids to treat such exacerbations (answer #3). Regular topical application of potent steroids to the skin can cause dermal atrophy; wiping the skin with a damp cloth after use of inhaled steroids (with a spacer and attached face mask) prevents this complication (answer #4).

ANSWER TO QUESTION 8 (LONG-ACTING INHALED BETA-AGONIST BRONCHODILATORS IN THE TREATMENT OF CHILDHOOD ASTHMA)

The correct answer is #3; long-acting inhaled beta-agonist bronchodilators *used together with inhaled steroids* are recommended in the treatment of moderate and severe persistent asthma in children. The long-acting inhaled beta-agonist bronchodilators blunt exercise-induced bronchoconstriction, but with regular use this protective effect declines significantly in as little as 1 week (answer #1). Use of a long-acting inhaled beta-agonist bronchodilator as single controller therapy is discouraged, because it is associated with an increased incidence of asthmatic exacerbations compared to an inhaled steroid (answer #2). A better approach would be to explore why the child is "intolerant of inhaled steroids" and a trial of a leukotriene blocker. The long-acting beta agonists are not recommended for rescue bronchodilator use, with or without an accompanying quick-acting bronchodilator such as albuterol (answers #4 and 5).

ANSWER TO QUESTION 9 (LEUKOTRIENE BLOCKERS IN THE TREATMENT OF PEDIATRIC ASTHMA)

The correct answer is #2; the leukotriene blockers, montelukast (Singulair) and zafirlukast (Accolate), reduce asthmatic symptoms and improve lung function (although less reliably and effectively than inhaled steroids). A "sprinkles" form of montelukast is approved for the treatment of asthma in children as young as 12 months (answer #1). There is no evidence to suggest that doubling the usual dose of leukotriene blocker to treat asthmatic flares is either effective or safe (answer #3). Aspirin sensitivity is associated with increased leukotriene production. However, aspirin sensitivity is rare in children; and many patients without aspirin sensitivity can benefit from leukotriene blocker therapy (answer #4). Leukotriene blockers are not steroids, and they do not have steroid-associated side effects (answer #5).

ANSWER TO QUESTION 10 (RIGHT TO A SAFE CLASSROOM ENVIRONMENT FOR CHILDREN WITH ALLERGIES AND ASTHMA)

The correct answer is #5, Americans with Disabilities Act. The Americans with Disabilities Act mandates that public and private schools and child care programs be usable by individuals with disabilities. For this law, asthma and allergies are considered disabilities (a physical impairment that substantially limits one or more major life activities). The other Acts do not pertain to asthma and allergies.

ANSWER TO QUESTION 11 (ASSESSMENT OF REFRACTORY ASTHMA)

The correct answer is #2. Features of her history that suggest the possibility of vocal cord dysfunction include her loud wheezing audible without a stethoscope and her rapid improvement with rest. The possibility that her Maxair inhaler has expired (answer #1) is a good consideration, but less likely (especially in light of her very rapid improvement when she rests, untreated). The cardiac abnormality described (atrial septal defect with right-to-left shunting of blood) (answer #3) is associated with hypoxemia and cyanosis, not exercise-induced wheezing. Focal bronchial obstruction due to an aspirated foreign body (answer #4) would usually cause symptoms even in the absence of exercise. Tolerance to beta-agonist use—that is, loss of bronchodilator effect because of regular or frequent use—does not occur (answer #5).

ANSWER TO QUESTION 12 (INDICATIONS FOR SPECIALIST REFERRAL)

The correct answer is #1; it is recommended that a child under age 3 years with moderate or severe persistent asthma should be referred for specialist consultation. Consultation is also recommended after a life-threatening asthmatic attack, but not after any emergency department visit for asthma (answer #2). Two steroid bursts in the past 12 months should trigger specialist referral, not two bursts before age 8 years (answer #3). Not every child with asthma, allergic rhinitis, and eczema needs specialist consultation (answer #4), only a child being considered for allergen immunotherapy. Use of a canister of quick-acting bronchodilator every month or more frequently is an indication for initiation of regular controller therapy for asthma, not necessarily consultative referral (answer #5).

II

PRACTICAL ASPECTS OF ASTHMA CARE

6

PULMONARY FUNCTION TESTING AND PEAK FLOW MONITORING

CHAPTER OUTLINE

I. Why measure lung function in asthma?

II. Spirometry
   a. How testing is performed–obtaining the spirogram tracing
   b. Pitfalls: the inadequate test
   c. Numeric results to look for
   d. What constitutes normal?
   e. The flow-volume curve

III. Obstructive pattern
   a. Reduced FEV_1/FVC ratio
   b. Reduced FVC in severe airflow obstruction
   c. Scooped appearance on the flow-volume curve
   d. What constitutes "reversible" airflow obstruction?

IV. Restrictive pattern
   a. Measuring lung volumes
   b. Reduced FVC with normal or increased FEV_1/FVC ratio
   c. Straight slope of the expiratory flow-volume curve

V. Mixed obstructive and restrictive pattern

VI. Measurement of peak flow
   a. Making the measurement
   b. Defining "personal best" peak flow
   c. Uses of home peak flow monitoring

WHY MEASURE LUNG FUNCTION IN ASTHMA?

Like you, we have often heard patients say, "I don't need to measure my lung function. I can always tell when my asthma is acting up." And often they are right. They recognize a characteristic tickle in their throat or a deep chest cough; they can feel a rattling of mucus in their chest or a band-like tightness constricting their thorax. They know that they are experiencing symptoms of their asthma and can tell you if their discomfort is mild or severe. If they are familiar with peak flow monitoring, they may even be able to predict relatively accurately what their peak flow would be, if measured, based on their symptoms.

But sometimes they cannot. Sometimes they are mistaken about the activity of their asthma, perhaps distracted by other symptoms, such as from a chest cold or seasonal allergies, or by other demands on their attention, like family stresses or job demands. We humans are often good at denial. "I don't feel that bad; it will be better by morning," we tell ourselves. In addition, some people with asthma are thought to be "poor perceivers" of their obstructed airways. Their sense of dyspnea or hypoxemia appears to be abnormally blunted.

Researchers have conducted the appropriate experiment: ask patients with asthma who are familiar with peak flow measurements to estimate their peak flow when they are having asthma symptoms, then record their actual peak flow value. Patients are frequently wrong; they either overestimate or underestimate their lung function more than half the time. The saddest observations come from investigations of deaths from asthma. Quite commonly, in the hours and days prior to a fatal asthmatic attack, persons with asthma and their families underestimated the severity of the symptoms. They did not appreciate just how sick the person with asthma actually was.

Healthcare providers do no better. In an experiment similar to the one described above, accomplished chest physicians were given the opportunity to interview and examine patients hospitalized for their asthmatic attacks, then asked to estimate the patients' peak flows. A researcher then measured the actual peak flow. Even when the estimated peak flow was considered correct if it fell within 20% of the true value, more than 50% of the estimates were erroneous—sometimes too high, sometimes too low.

The point is that we cannot know how severe a patient's asthma is based on the intensity or density of wheezing that we hear, or on the absence of wheezes. Too often, we will be fooled. We may overtreat mild asthma with a course of prednisone or undertreat a severe asthmatic flare with a course of antibiotics if we rely on history or examination alone. And the biggest risk: we may miss severe, life-threatening asthma because we "didn't think that the patient looked too bad." If you want to know how a patient's asthma is doing at the moment of your medical encounter, make a measurement. We don't estimate blood pressure based on symptoms and examination of the retina. Spirometry and peak flow measurements quantify the severity of airflow obstruction in the same way that blood pressure recording with a sphygmomanometer quantifies hypertension.

In a broader sense, we use pulmonary function testing to provide three key pieces of information: Is lung function normal or abnormal? If abnormal, is the pattern of abnormality one of *obstruction* to expiratory flow or *restriction* preventing a full, deep breath? And how severe is the abnormality? For the most part, all of this information can be obtained from spirometry, the most commonly performed pulmonary function test. The distinction as to the type of pulmonary function abnormality—obstructive versus restrictive—cannot be derived from peak flow measurement. So, we will begin this discussion of pulmonary function testing with a discussion of spirometry, then return to peak flow measurement, which—though providing more limited information than spirometry—is quick and easy to perform, inexpensive, and widely available, both in medical offices and in the home.

Like many other healthcare providers, you may associate spirometry with a meaningless babble of three-letter abbreviations and perplexing numbers. You'd rather have needles placed in your muscles for electromyography (EMG) than be asked to interpret a set of pulmonary function test results! You think that you may be allergic to spirometry, because you get slightly sweaty and itchy when someone puts a set of spirometry results in front of you and asks you to explain their meaning! Stick with us, here. The subject does not have to be made obscure; you will not be asked to make any higher mathematical calculations. If you are contemplating taking the examination to become a certified Asthma Educator (AE-C), this chapter will prove very useful to you, and all shall be made clear.

SPIROMETRY

If you have ever walked past the open door of a pulmonary function testing laboratory, you may already be somewhat familiar with the testing procedure. You may have heard an enthusiastic pulmonary function technician encouraging his or her subject: "Take a big, deep breath in, all the way, and now push out as hard and fast as you can, keep going, all the way, push, push, push, push...." Spirometry involves a maximal inspiration followed by a rapid, forceful, and complete exhalation.

It is interesting to note that when we want to assess a person's breathing, we do not simply ask him or her to breathe quietly and normally into our recording equipment. We ask him to do this maneuver—maximal breath in followed by complete and rapid breath all the way out—that one would never do in daily life. The reason, in part, is that with a mouthpiece in your mouth, if you are asked to breathe *normally*, you can't do it. Once you have been made conscious of your breathing (which is normally an unconscious act), you begin to deviate from your usual pattern, taking breaths somewhat faster or slower, deeper or more shallow than normal. On the other hand, the maximal forced expiratory maneuver of spirometry proves to be highly reproducible and rich with information about the functioning of the lungs.

Still, spirometry requires a big effort. It is without question "effort-dependent." Reliable results cannot be obtained if a patient is unable to understand the instructions, has chest pain preventing a forceful effort, or does not choose to cooperate. Nothing drives a pulmonary function technician nuttier than being asked to perform testing with a delirious or comatose patient sent to the lab on a stretcher! Successful testing requires a cooperative patient free of serious chest wall pain. Also, children under the age of 6 years are generally not able to perform an adequate test.

KEY POINT   To perform the maximal forced expiratory maneuver of spirometry, a patient must be cooperative, able to understand directions, and free of serious chest wall pain.

How testing is performed—obtaining the spirogram tracing

If you are about to have spirometry, you will be asked to sit upright in a chair. Plastic nose clips are placed on your nose to ensure that all of your exhaled air passes through your mouth, and none is lost out of your nose. You are asked to place a clean and disposable mouthpiece comfortably in your mouth between your teeth, with your lips sealed tightly around it. The mouthpiece sits at the end of collection tubing that leads to the recording device (spirometer) (Fig. 6-1). The pulmonary function technician guides you through each step of the test. In our laboratory, you would be asked first to take a few comfortable, quiet, normal breaths, then a big, deep breath in until no more air can enter your lungs. Then "blast out," forcing the air out rapidly in a steady effort until there is absolutely no more air to blow out. You might try it now (without the mouthpiece): it will take you at least 6 seconds to empty all of the air from your chest, and you will find it strange and perhaps somewhat uncomfortable to use your expiratory muscles (abdominals and chest wall intercostals) to squeeze down so tightly on your ribs. The test is typically repeated two additional times or until reproducible results are obtained. The best (largest) test result is reported as your actual values.

At one time, the recording equipment simply measured how much air you were able to force out of your lungs. The maximal amount of air that you can empty from your lungs—from all the way in to all the way out—is called (somewhat grandly) your "vital capacity." On average, your vital capacity is about 3–5 liters (about 3/4–1 1/4 gallons), varying somewhat depending on your sex, age, and height. Take a moment to think of some disorders that might reduce one's

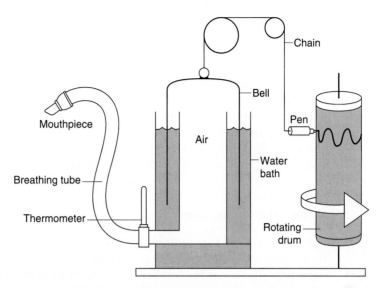

FIGURE 6-1 *Early spirometers collected exhaled air in a plastic cylinder floating on top of a tub of water. The more air exhaled, the higher the cylinder rose, and the lower the mark left by the attached marking pen. By attaching the recording paper to a rotating drum, both the volume of air exhaled and the time elapsed during exhalation could be recorded.*

vital capacity. The list is long, including things that fill up the lungs (pneumonia, pulmonary edema), that make them hard to inflate (fibrosis, lobar collapse), that surround the lungs (pleural effusion, fibrothorax), that distort the chest wall (scoliosis, ascites), or that cause respiratory muscle weakness (amyotrophic lateral sclerosis or Guillain-Barré syndrome). We will later add to the list severe asthma attacks, when the airways are so narrowed that one cannot fully empty the lungs.

In the 1950s pulmonary function recording equipment was modified to measure not only *how much* air could be emptied from the lungs, but also *how fast* the air could be emptied—and modern spirometry was launched. After many years of experience, it turned out that the most useful measure of how fast air can be emptied from the lungs is the volume of air that can be forced out in the first second. Beginning at full inspiration, you can probably get 2 1/2 to 4 liters out of your lungs in the first second of a forceful exhalation. A typical forced expired volume in 1 second (abbreviated FEV_1) is approximately 2.5–4 liters (depending again on your sex, age, and height). Note that the FEV_1 is a measure of the *speed* of exhalation. It is a certain number of liters in 1 second. The unit of "liters per second" is like "miles per hour"—it tells about how fast something is going.

KEY POINT   From spirometry we can learn *how much* air can be emptied from the lungs and also *how fast* air can be emptied from the lungs.

In the days before computer chips and microprocessors, the results of spirometry were displayed on graph paper attached to a rotating drum. A recording pen left an ink tracing of the amount (volume) of air exhaled from your lungs (on the vertical axis) while the drum rotated at a fixed speed, such that the time elapsed could be indicated in seconds on the horizontal axis of the graph paper. A normal spirometry tracing is shown in Fig. 6-2. From this graph one could calculate—ruler in hand—the total amount of air emptied from the lungs, called the forced vital capacity (FVC), and also the amount of air emptied in the first second (FEV_1). Nowadays, these data are automatically extracted and instantly displayed by computerized spirometry equipment.

Pitfalls: The inadequate test

If *spirometry* is the testing procedure and *spirometer* is the testing equipment, then a *spirogram* is the resulting graphic display of the subject's maximal forced expiratory effort. It is the test result, displayed in liters of air exhaled (vertical axis) per each unit of time (second) of exhalation (horizontal axis). Notice that a successful test results in a smooth, even spirogram curve (Fig. 6-2). Also notice that the amount of air that is forced from the lungs per second decreases with each successive second. That means, of course, that the speed of exhalation is greatest at first and progressively decreases as one continues to exhale.

A good place to start when you wish to interpret the results of spirometry is to look at the spirogram to make sure that a good test was performed. Figures 6-3

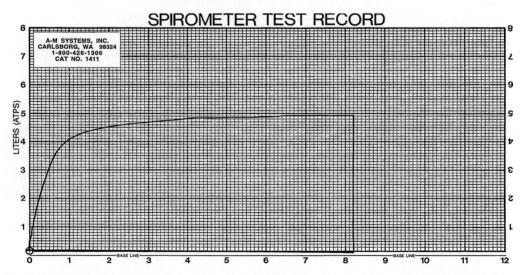

FIGURE 6-2   *The normal spirogram displays the volume of air exhaled in liters on the vertical axis and the time elapsed during the exhalation in seconds on the horizontal axis. The spirogram is a graphical volume-time display of a maximal forced exhalation.*

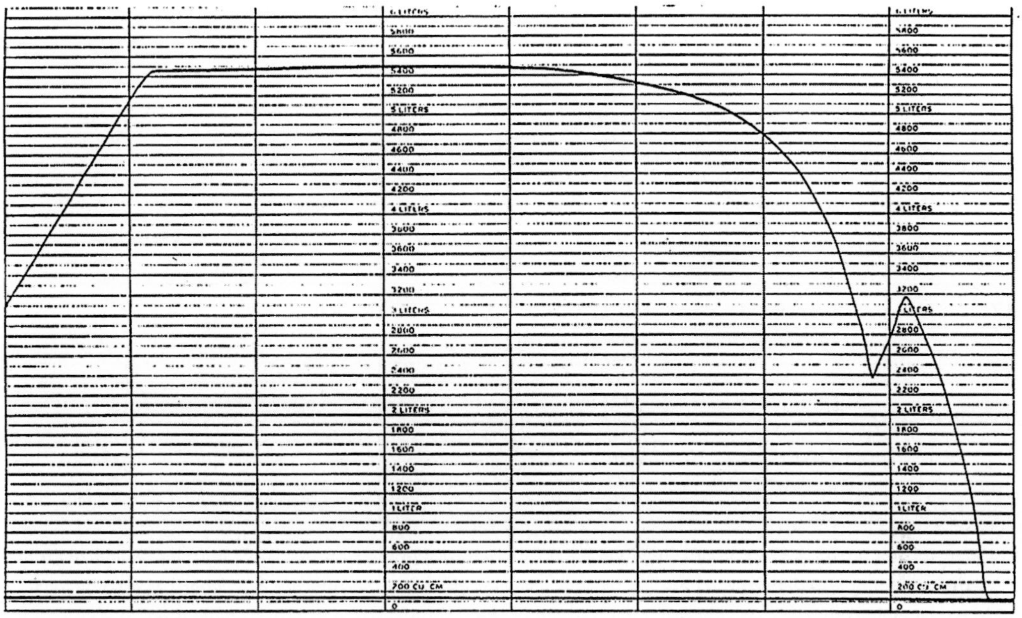

FIGURE 6-3 *The irregular spirogram curve indicates that the patient took a second quick breath in (downward deflection of the tracing) before completing the forced exhalation. (The rotation of the recording drum in this example is such that the graph is made from right to left, whereas the example in Fig. 6-2 was made from left to right.) Each vertical line represents one second.*

and 6-4 are examples of inadequate tests (despite the pulmonary function technician's best efforts). In the first example (Fig. 6-3), the subject interrupted his or her forced exhalation with a small breath in and then continued exhaling. In the second example (Fig. 6-4), the subject stopped exhaling prematurely. For satisfactory spirometry, the forced exhalation must continue for a minimum of 6 seconds. In this example, the subject stopped after only approximately 4 1/2 seconds. The numbers for FEV_1 and/or FVC derived from these tests will be erroneous, not reflecting the subject's true lung function. Management decisions made on this misinformation can be harmful. False data can be worse than no data at all, so begin your interpretation with an assessment of the adequacy of the testing procedure.

Numeric results to look for

Believe it or not, there are only three key test results that you need to view to interpret the results of spirometry, and you have already been introduced to two of them. The first is the forced vital capacity (FVC), the total amount of air exhaled from the lungs when starting at the top of a full inhalation and ending at the bottom of a complete exhalation. The result is given in liters. The second

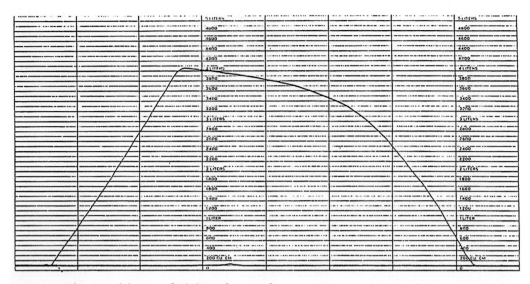

FIGURE 6-4   *The minimal duration of exhalation for a satisfactory spirometry test is 6 seconds. By recognizing that this exhalation only lasted approximately 4.5 seconds, one can identify an incomplete exhalation, with consequent underestimation of the true vital capacity. (The rotation of the recording drum in this example is again such that the graph is made from right to left, whereas the example in Fig. 6-2 was made from left to right.) Each vertical line represents one second.*

is the one-second forced expired volume (FEV_1), the amount of air exhaled in the first second of this forced expiratory maneuver. It is an amount per unit of time and so tells us a *rate* of exhalation. The result is likewise given in liters.

The third element is the ratio of these first two results. We are interested in the following measurement: what portion of the vital capacity can be exhaled in the first second? This measurement is expressed as a ratio: the one-second forced expired volume divided by the forced vital capacity (FEV_1/FVC). You can see how this measurement might be useful. What if you have a patient who has had one lung removed surgically following a traumatic injury? You are interested in assessing his lung function, and in particular in determining whether or not he has asthma. You want to find out if he can exhale air from his remaining lung at a normal speed, or whether airway narrowing slows the rate of his exhalation. You anticipate that simply because of his surgery, his vital capacity will be about half normal. In addition, the volume of gas exhaled from his lungs in the first second (FEV_1) will be half normal. If his airways and expiratory flow are normal for someone who has had a pneumonectomy, his FVC will be approximately half, his FEV_1 will be approximately half, and the *ratio* of his FEV_1/FVC will remain normal. What the measurement, FEV_1/FVC, does is to adjust the recorded expiratory flow for this particular person's vital capacity.

The FEV_1/FVC is a calculated result: it is the measured FEV_1 divided by the measured FVC. The results are typically displayed as a percentage. For instance, if your FEV_1 is 3 liters and your FVC is 4 liters, your FEV_1/FVC is 75%.

Sometimes the spirometry report lists this calculated result (the FEV_1/FVC) as the $FEV_1\%$ or $\%FEV_1$—just for the sake of confusion, we think. Then, to make matters worse, this result (say 75%) is compared with the predicted normal value for a person of your sex, age, and height. The result (your FEV_1/FVC compared to the predicted FEV_1/FVC) is also reported as a percent. Talk about taking an easy calculation and making it confusing! We find it simplest to report the ratio of FEV_1/FVC as a decimal. In your hypothetical case, we would indicate that your $FEV_1/FVC = 0.75$. Join us in this deviation from tradition, and we may start a trend of clarity in pulmonary function test reporting!

KEY POINT   The key measurements needed for interpretation of spirometry are the 1-second forced expired volume (FEV_1), the forced vital capacity (FVC), and the calculated ratio of these two measurements (FEV_1/FVC).

The pulmonary function test report that you receive for review may provide a number of other measurements derived from the spirogram, most all of which we encourage you to ignore. These include the following. The FEV_3 is left over from days gone by. It records the forced expired volume in the first 3 seconds of exhalation and adds little if anything to the now standard measure of expiratory flow, the FEV_1. The peak expiratory flow rate (PEFR) is the expiratory flow at the *moment* that it is the fastest during the entire exhalation. We will consider peak expiratory flow further when we speak of the flow-volume curve and peak flow monitoring. The test results may include the total amount of time that the patient blew his or her air out, the forced expiratory time (FET). Remember that the minimal forced expiratory time for a satisfactory spirogram is 6 seconds.

The measurement that has generated the greatest amount of confusion is the one that records the rate of expiratory flow in the midportion of the forced exhalation. Clinicians and physiologists have sought to extract additional information from the spirogram by asking about the rate of exhalation not only during the first second of exhalation (FEV_1) but also later during exhalation. You can restrict your calculation to the middle-half of the vital capacity, between 25% of the vital capacity exhaled and 75% of the vital capacity exhaled. Over this exhaled volume, you can determine the average speed of exhalation. The forced expiratory flow between 25% and 75% of the exhaled vital capacity (FEF_{25-75}) is therefore another measure of the rate of expiratory flow. It is expressed in liters per minute and in the past was also referred to as the maximal mid-expiratory flow (abbreviated MMF or MMEF).

The confusion relates mainly to the meaning placed on this test result. Some have sought to associate a reduction in the FEF_{25-75} with narrowing specifically localized to the small, peripheral airways. Perhaps a reduction in the FEF_{25-75} could point to ongoing inflammation in the small airways of persons with asthma even when expiratory flow remained normal in larger airways, leaving the FEV_1

normal. Perhaps a cigarette smoker with a normal FEV_1 and FVC could be found to have the early signs of chronic obstructive pulmonary disease (COPD) due to respiratory bronchiolitis because of a reduction in his or her FEF_{25-75}. Suffice it to say that a lot of controversy surrounds the interpretation of the FEF_{25-75}, that identifying airway obstruction predominantly localized to the small, peripheral airways is not an easy matter, and that—in our opinions— patient management should never be directed at an isolated reduction in the FEF_{25-75}. In the immortal words of Donnie Brasco (in the movie by the same name), "Forget about it."

You will also hear it said that the FEF_{25-75} belongs to the "effort-independent" portion of the spirogram, whereas FEV_1 is more "effort-dependent," meaning more dependent on how hard you try during the test. Although there is some truth to this statement, we would emphasize that: (1) the entire spirometry test is dependent on a strong and sustained effort—hence the role of the pulmonary function technician in exhorting you to "push, push, push"; and (2) in terms of reproducibility, the FEV_1 stands out as a highly reproducible test, more even than the FEF_{25-75}.

KEY POINT   You are better off ignoring the measurement of expiratory flow in the mid-vital capacity range (FEF_{25-75}) than trying to derive information about the small, peripheral airways from it or acting on an isolated abnormality of it.

What constitutes normal?

Having completed your forced expiratory maneuvers and recorded your best values, you learn that your FVC is 4 liters, your FEV_1 is 3 liters, and your FEV_1/FVC is (by simple division) 0.75. "How well did I do?" you want to know. These results only have meaning if you are also told what values you should expect for a healthy person. In children, the normal values vary mainly according to height although age and gender are also taken into account. In adults (beginning around age 18), the normal values vary by gender (larger in men), age (declining after approximately age 25 years), and height (larger in taller people).

Normal values have been assembled by researchers who made careful measurements in healthy, nonsmoking men and women of many different ages and heights. The results were tabulated and extrapolations made for persons of every age and height. As it turns out, different researchers made somewhat different observations, probably reflecting the different populations in which they made their lung function measurements. Your pulmonary function laboratory will choose one of the available sets of normal values; these are then programmed into the spirometer's computer memory and printed out with each test report.

There are racial and ethnic differences in normal lung function for people of the same sex, age, and height. The best characterized are the normal values for Cauasians and African Americans. Many computerized spirometers will provide racially corrected normal values if you enter the subject's race with the other demographic data.

As an example, imagine that you extract the following results from your spirometry report:

	Measured	Predicted (normal)	Percent of predicted
FVC	4.0	4.2	95%
FEV_1	3.0	3.2	94%
FEV_1/FVC	0.75	0.76	99%

How did you do? Well, remember that the normal value indicated for a person of your sex, age, and height represents an *average* of all the results found in healthy nonsmokers of your same sex, age, and height description. There were in fact a *range* of values recorded in these normal subjects. Some were above average, some were below average, but all were normal. So, in describing your test results, our first step is to determine whether your results are within the *normal range* or not; that is, are they normal or abnormal.

It turns out that, at least for pulmonary function test results, normal is a statistical concept. The normal range attempts to include almost all healthy (normal) individuals (with values close to the average normal value) and to exclude individuals with disease whose values are sufficiently far from the average normal value that they can be identified as abnormal. Statistically, if you are more than two standard deviations from the average normal value, you are considered abnormal.

KEY POINT   Test results will give your values and the predicted *average* normal value for a healthy person of the same sex, age, and height. We then need to determine whether your results are within the *range* of normal values around that average.

Traditionally, when interpreting pulmonary function tests clinicians have considered a result within 20% of the average normal value for FVC and FEV_1 to be within the normal range. That is, an FVC or FEV_1 80% or greater of the average normal value has been considered within the normal range. Defining the normal range for the ratio, FEV_1/FVC, is more problematic. Some physicians would say values of 95% or greater of the average normal value are within the normal range for FEV_1/FVC, but it would be difficult to find unanimity about the cut-off for the normal range of FEV_1/FVC values.

More recently, an alternative and more statistically accurate approach has been adopted by many pulmonary function laboratories, as seen on many spirometry test results. The computer will automatically calculate for you the range of two standard deviations around the average value and report this range as the 95% confidence intervals. A value outside of this range is abnormal with 95% statistical certainty. That allows the test results to include, in effect, a predicted lower limit of normal for the FVC, FEV_1, and—of particular help—FEV_1/FVC. Values above the lower end of the 95% confidence interval—that is, values above the lower limits of normal—are considered within the normal range. Here then, are your quite encouraging test results:

	Measured	Predicted (normal)	Percent of predicted	95% confidence interval (lower limit)
FVC	4.0	4.2	95%	3.4
FEV_1	3.0	3.2	94%	2.6
FEV_1/FVC	0.75	0.76	99%	0.72

Your results are normal, but they also highlight one of the shortcomings of pulmonary function testing. The results are within the range of normal values for a person of your sex, age, and height, but they are not necessarily normal for you. It is possible that 6 months ago, before you developed those strange chest symptoms, your FVC and FEV_1 were as much as 1/2 liter greater. At your best you may have had values of FVC and FEV_1 that were 107–109% of the average normal value, and now they have declined to 94–95% of that value. Unless you have had prior spirometry measurements, we cannot identify a change from your baseline; we can only make comparison with a range of values found in other healthy individuals like you.

The flow-volume curve

Nowadays, your pulmonary function test results will generally return with two different graphic displays of the results: one is the spirogram (plotting volume on the vertical axis and time on the horizontal axis); and the other is the flow-volume curve (plotting flow on the vertical axis and volume on the horizontal axis). Both tracings are derived from the same single maneuver: take a full, deep breath in, then blast it out as hard and fast as you can until you can empty no more air from your lungs. However, additional information can be derived by looking at the shape of the flow-volume curve.

Flow is volume per unit of time. It is the slope of a line placed tangentially at any point along the volume-time (spirogram) curve. The flow-volume curve displays the expiratory flow at each point of the exhaled volume, beginning with a maximal breath in and ending at completion of a full breath out. The curve (Fig. 6-5) begins at zero flow (as you are about to start exhaling), quickly increases to the maximal expiratory flow, and then progressively and steadily decreases back toward zero as you continue to blow your air out. Finally, when you have no more air to exhale, flow returns to the zero line.

There are three pieces of information to consider regarding the flow-volume curve. First, the point of maximal expiratory flow is the same as the peak expiratory flow rate (PEFR). It is this value that is measured by peak flow meters. On the flow-volume curve, the scale typically indicates flow, including peak flow, in liters/second. To compare this number with the peak flow measured by peak flow meters, which is reported in liters/minute, simply multiply the value from the flow-volume curve times 60.

Second, make note of the shape of the normal flow-volume curve. The line from peak expiratory flow to the end of exhalation is more or less a straight line. The normal curve may bulge slightly or cave in slightly, but for the most part it follows a straight line. We will contrast this appearance with the shape of the flow-volume curve in people with obstructive lung diseases. Also, a quick look at the shape and contours of the flow-volume curve will help us to judge how well the patient was able to perform the test. In that way we can avoid being fooled into interpreting numeric test results from what was an inadequate forced expiratory effort (Fig. 6-6).

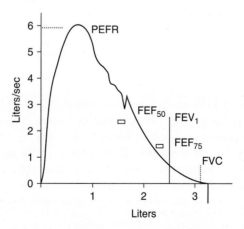

FIGURE 6-5   *The flow-volume curve plots expiratory flow on the vertical axis and volume on the horizontal axis (from full breath in on the left to maximal breath out on the right). Note the shape of the curve, with its relatively straight downward slope. (FEF$_{50}$ denotes the forced expiratory flow at 50% of the exhaled vital capacity; FEF$_{75}$ is the forced expiratory flow at the point that 75% of the vital capacity has been exhaled. The rectangles indicate the normal values for FEF$_{50}$ and FEF$_{75}$.)*

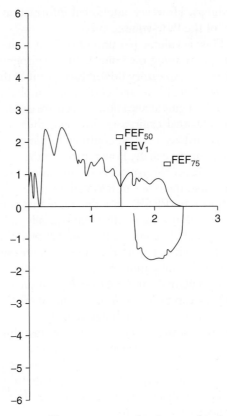

FIGURE 6-6 *This patient was unable to cooperate with pulmonary function testing. By inspecting the shape of the flow-volume curve, one knows to discount the numerical results as an inaccurate measurement of the patient's lung function.*

Third, sometimes after completing the spirometry test, at the very end of exhalation, you will be asked to inspire rapidly (through the mouthpiece and recording equipment) all the way back to a full breath in. By so doing, you inscribe an *inspiratory* flow-volume curve and, combined with the *expiratory* flow-volume curve, generate the flow-volume loop (Fig. 6-7). The size and shape of the inspiratory flow-volume curve can at times be helpful in assessing disorders of the upper airways, as we will discuss shortly.

KEY POINT   The shape of the flow-volume curve can help to distinguish normal expiratory flow from diffuse airways obstruction (as in asthma or COPD) and from upper airway obstruction.

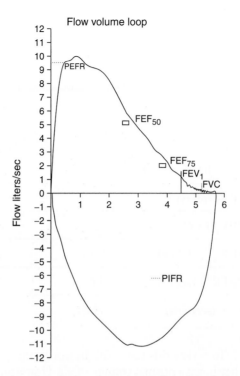

FIGURE 6-7   *The flow-volume loop displays the expiratory flow above the horizontal line and inspiratory flow below the horizontal line. Flow is displayed in liters/sec; volume is plotted on the horizontal axis in liters.*

OBSTRUCTIVE PATTERN

If one or more of the spirometric values of interest to us (FVC, FEV_1, and FEV_1/FVC) is abnormal, our next step in interpretation is to determine whether the abnormality fits a pattern of *obstruction* to expiratory flow, *restriction* to the volume of a maximal breath, or *both*. As someone interested in asthma, you can immediately see the utility of this categorization. If someone reports episodic shortness of breath, cough, and chest tightness and on spirometry has an obstructive pattern, you will strongly consider asthma in your differential diagnosis. If the same person has a restrictive pattern, a different set of diagnostic possibilities come to mind, such as heart failure, recurrent pneumonia, or inflammatory lung disease. Remember that asthma is characterized by intermittent airflow obstruction; COPD causes chronic or persistent airflow obstruction. In general, we need to demonstrate airflow obstruction on pulmonary function testing to confirm these diagnoses.

Slowing of the rate of exhalation is associated with a decrease in FEV_1, the expiratory volume in the first second of exhalation. (To reiterate: exhaled volume/second = rate of flow). The forced vital capacity (FVC) may remain normal (more on this in a moment). Reduced FEV_1 with a normal FVC gives a decreased FEV_1/FVC ratio. This is an obstructive pattern: ↓ FEV_1, normal FVC, ↓ FEV_1/FVC. Here's an example:

	Actual	% Predicted	Predicted Mean	Predicted 95% CI
FVC (liters)	2.53	101	2.51	1.7
FEV_1 (liters)	1.31	64	2.05	1.41
FEV_1/FVC	0.52	64	0.80	0.71
FEF_{25-75} (L/sec)	0.55	25	2.16	
PEFR (L/sec)	3.67	75	4.85	
FET (seconds)	11.67			

To review this test result in words, this patient was able to empty from his or her lungs a normal volume of air. However, the speed at which the air exited the lungs was slower than normal. Using the FEV_1 as our measure of expiratory flow, we would say that the speed at which air exited the lungs in the first second was 64% of the normal value for someone of this sex, age, and height. The portion of the vital capacity that could be exhaled in the first second (i.e., the FEV_1/FVC) was reduced. Normally, we would expect that, on average, 0.80 of the vital capacity could be exhaled in the first second in someone of this sex, age, and height; and that the lower limit of normal for this ratio would be 0.71. But in our example, the portion of the vital capacity that could be exhaled in the first second was only 0.52. There was obstruction to the flow of air on exhalation.

In this example we have taken the liberty of including—as you will find on most spirometry reports—the forced expiratory flow between 25% and 75% of the exhaled vital capacity (FEF_{25-75}), the peak expiratory flow rate (PEFR), and forced expiratory time (FET). You need not look at these results to interpret the results of the test (other than to confirm an adequate forced expiratory time of 6 seconds or greater). If by chance you do peak at the FEF_{25-75}, you will notice that this measure of expiratory flow is also reduced. In an obstructive pattern, the FEF_{25-75} is always reduced and always reduced to a lower percentage than the FEV_1. Noting this disproportionate reduction in FEF_{25-75} confirms an obstructive pattern, nothing more.

The spirogram tracing for this patient is shown in Fig. 6-8. A normal curve (plotting volume vs. time) for a person of this sex, age, and height is superimposed for comparison.

An obstructive pattern can be seen in asthma, COPD, bronchiolitis, bronchiectasis, and upper airway obstruction. It can be seen on occasion in diseases

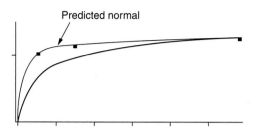

FIGURE 6-8   *In this computerized spirometry, the average normal spirogram for a person of the same age, height, and gender is automatically displayed (thin line with square boxes) along with the patient's actual spirogram tracing (heavy line). The vertical axis displays volume in liters; the horizontal axis measures time in seconds.*

that we do not normally associate with airway narrowing, such as congestive heart failure, sarcoidosis, and pulmonary embolism. Our point here is that the presence of obstruction on pulmonary function testing does not in itself make a diagnosis of asthma. It simply puts us in the broad category of obstructive disorders (and outside of the broad category of restrictive disorders).

Reduced FVC in severe airflow obstruction

Now imagine that the patient's airflow obstruction worsens. Exhalation becomes even slower; the FEV_1 decreases further from normal. Air empties from the lungs so slowly that even after 10, 12, or as many as 18 seconds of exhalation, the normal amount of air cannot be emptied from the lungs. The vital capacity becomes less that normal ($\downarrow$ FVC). The only reason for this reduced vital capacity is very slow emptying of the lungs and, at the end of exhalation, gas trapped behind narrowed or closed off bronchial tubes. The reduced FVC is not due to pneumonia or collapse or anything *restricting* a normal deep breath; it is the result of severe airflow obstruction. This patient will also have an obstructive pattern on spirometry; in this case, $\downarrow$ FVC, $\downarrow\downarrow$ FEV_1, and $\downarrow\downarrow$ FEV_1/FVC ratio. An example follows:

	Actual	% Predicted	Predicted Mean	Predicted 95% CI
FVC (liters)	1.84	65	2.80	1.98
FEV_1 (liters)	0.66	29	2.28	1.63
FEV_1/FVC	0.36	45	0.80	0.71
FEF_{25-75} (L/sec)	0.26	11	2.39	
PEFR (L/sec)	2.16	39	5.51	
FET (seconds)	7.76			

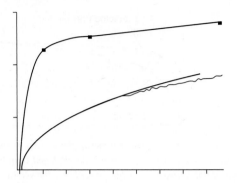

FIGURE 6-9   *Two nearly superimposed spirogram curves are displayed, one recorded before and one approximately 10 minutes after administration of a quick-acting bronchodilator. The average normal spirogram for a person of the same age, height, and gender is automatically displayed (thin line with square boxes) along with the patient's actual spirogram tracings. The vertical axis displays volume in liters; the horizontal axis measures time in seconds.*

Said in words rather than symbols, this patient has an abnormally low FEV_1 and FVC. On further inspection, the FEV_1 is markedly reduced while the FVC is less severely reduced. The portion of the vital capacity that could be exhaled in the first second, the FEV_1/FVC ratio, is decreased. The reduced FEV_1/FVC ratio indicates that for a vital capacity of this size, the FEV_1 is lower than normal: there is expiratory airflow obstruction.

The volume-time curve of spirometry helps to depict this severe obstructive pattern (Fig. 6-9). After nearly 8 seconds of exhalation, the patient was still not able to empty fully the air from his lungs, but he needed to take another breath in. The vital capacity is abnormally low because of "gas trapping," that is, more than the normal amount of gas remains in the lungs at the end of a maximal exhalation.

Here then is a major teaching point: if the FEV_1/FVC ratio is reduced, there is expiratory airflow obstruction: an obstructive pattern. If the FEV_1/FVC ratio is normal or increased, there is no expiratory airflow obstruction: no obstructive pattern. Period.

KEY POINT   A reduced FEV_1/FVC ratio indicates the presence of an obstructive pattern on spirometry. A normal or increased FEV_1/FVC ratio indicates the absence of airflow obstruction. It's that easy!

Scooped appearance on the flow-volume curve

Another way to identify expiratory airflow obstruction on pulmonary function testing (an obstructive pattern) is to look at the shape of the flow-volume curve. Airflow obstruction in asthma and COPD (and other processes widespread throughout the lungs) gives a characteristic shape to the flow-volume curve. The curve looks scooped or concave, rather than the more-or-less straight line of a normal test. The scooped appearance results from the fact that expiratory flow (shown on the vertical axis of the flow-volume curve) is reduced compared to normal and becomes progressively more abnormal in the midportion of the exhaled volume (remember that the FEF_{25-75} is always more severely depressed compared to the FEV_1 in obstructive disorders). Two examples of flow-volume curves in persons with obstructive abnormalities are shown in Fig. 6-10.

Now you know two good ways to check for an obstructive pattern when examining the results of pulmonary function testing: a reduced FEV_1/FVC ratio (less than the lower end of the 95% confidence interval or, if 95% confidence intervals are not provided, less than 95% of the predicted FEV_1/FVC ratio) and a scooped appearance to the shape of the expiratory flow-volume curve.

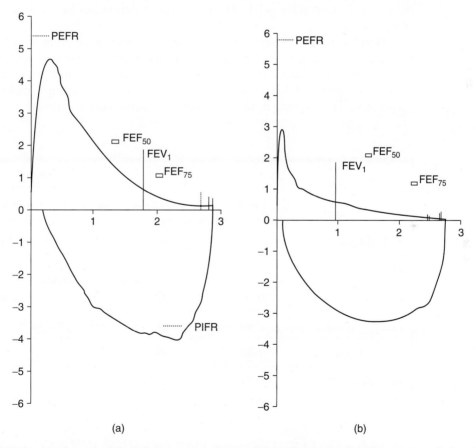

(a)   (b)

FIGURE 6-10 *The flow-volume loops from patients with (a) mild and (b) severe airflow obstruction are displayed. Flow (liters/sec) is shown on the vertical axis and volume (liters) on the horizontal axis. The scooped, concave shape of the expiratory flow-volume curve in these two examples is characteristic of diffuse airways obstruction. Normal predicated values are shown with a dotted line for peak expiratory flow rate (PEFR) and peak inspiratory flow rate (PIFR) and with rectangular boxes for forced expiratory flow at 50% of the exhaled vital capacity (FEF50) and at 75% of the exhaled vital capacity (FEF75).*

A scooped or concave appearance of the flow-volume curve is another indicator of an obstructive pattern on pulmonary function testing and can be identified simply by inspection of the shape of the flow-volume curve.

We have been careful to emphasize that the scooped appearance on the flow-volume curve is seen in obstructive disorders that diffusely involve the airways. A different pattern is found when the obstruction to expiratory flow results from a blockage or narrowing in the upper airways (trachea or throat area). Upper airway narrowing gives a characteristic flattening to the expiratory flow-volume curve, a "plateau" appearance. For a portion of exhalation, the expiratory flow is constant (hence the flat line on the graph of flow vs. volume), determined by one focal point of narrowing.

Here's a striking example of upper airway obstruction on pulmonary function testing. A young woman came to see us in consultation for her "refractory asthma." She had cough and wheezing, particularly when she lay down at night, and her symptoms didn't improve with any antiasthmatic therapy, including prednisone. The numeric results from her spirometry were as follows:

	Actual	% Predicted	Predicted Mean	95% CI
FVC (liters)	3.42	80	4.27	3.46
FEV_1 (liters)	2.39	66	3.61	2.97
FEV_1/FVC	0.70	82	0.85	0.76
FEF_{25-75} (L/sec)	2.46	61	4.02	
PEFR (L/sec)	2.80	38	7.38	
FET (seconds)	6.25			

With a low FEV_1, low-normal FVC, and reduced FEV_1/FVC, you correctly diagnose abnormal spirometry with an obstructive pattern. However, when you examine the flow-volume curve (Fig. 6-11), you are struck that its appearance is not the scooped shape of diffuse airways obstruction. It has a squared-off, table-like appearance, the plateau pattern of upper airway obstruction. Therein lay the clue to her diagnosis. A chest x-ray and then chest CT scan

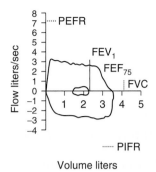

FIGURE 6-11 *The shape of the flow-volume loop, with a horizontal, relatively straight-line portion on both the inspiratory and expiratory limbs of the loop, points to an area of obstruction in the upper airway (somewhere between distal trachea and pharynx).*

were obtained for further evaluation. Cross-sectional and coronal images from her CT scan are shown in Fig. 6-12: a tracheal tumor caused this pattern of upper airway obstruction and her symptoms that mimicked asthma. She was cured of these symptoms with surgical resection of this rare, benign tracheal tumor.

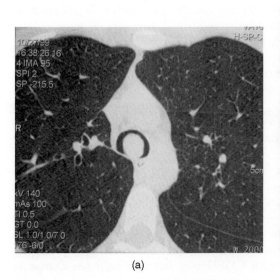

(a)

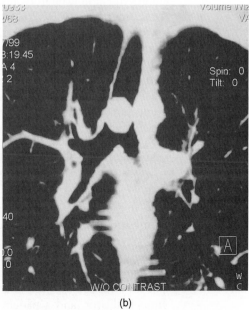

(b)

FIGURE 6-12 *The chest computed tomogram (CT) images from a patient with a tracheal tumor causing upper airway obstruction (as seen in Fig. 6-11). Near-complete obstruction of the distal trachea can be seen on the transverse (a) and coronal (b) images.*

What constitutes "reversible" airflow obstruction?

Imagine that a person with symptoms of intermittent cough, wheeze, and short-ness of breath undergoes pulmonary function testing to evaluate for possible asthma. Spirometry is performed and indicates airflow obstruction, consistent with a diagnosis of asthma. The next question that we are likely to ask is: "to what extent is this airflow obstruction reversible?" In fact, this question is short-hand for a more specific question: "To what extent does this airflow obstruction improve following administration of a medication that rapidly causes the bronchial smooth muscle to relax, a quick-acting inhaled bronchodilator such as albuterol?" As you know, characteristic of asthma is reversible airway narrowing, airflow obstruction that improves quickly in response to bronchodilator med-ication. On the other hand, little or no improvement following bronchodilator is more typical of COPD.

It is difficult to be definitive about what extent of postbronchodilator improvement in expiratory airflow is typical of asthma. Some authorities suggest a 15% increase in FEV_1 following an inhaled beta-agonist bronchodilator, others recommend a 20% increase. Like any cut-off point in medicine, where you set the value will influence the sensitivity and specificity of the test. If you insist on a 20% increase in FEV_1 following bronchodilator before you diagnose asthma with confidence, you will likely miss some patients with asthma who have a smaller improvement of postbronchodilator testing; but you will be better able to distinguish asthma from other diseases in which a smaller improvement in airflow may be seen, such as COPD or cystic fibrosis. If you choose a 15% post-bronchodilator increase in FEV_1 as your cut-off for a diagnosis of asthma, you will exclude fewer patients who truly have asthma; but you will also include more patients with other obstructive lung diseases who have some reversibility to their airflow obstruction.

In the end, asthma is not a diagnosis made on the basis of pulmonary func-tion testing. It is a clinical diagnosis, based on a characteristic medical history and physical exam, in which pulmonary function testing can provide helpful confirmation of the key feature—reversible airways narrowing—and at the same time quantify the severity of the airflow obstruction. Below is an example of a patient with asthma with dramatic improvement in expiratory flow following bronchodilator; and a patient with COPD who has no significant change in expiratory flow following bronchodilator (Fig. 6-13).

An important but somewhat different question is: How much change in expiratory flow can one expect simply from variability in test results? If you

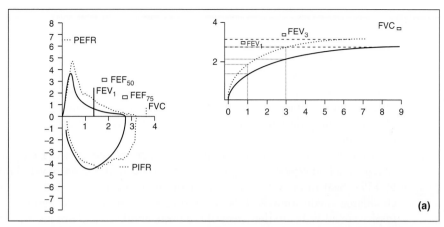

Spirometry (BTPS)		Prebronchodilator		Predicted	Range	Postbronchodilator		Percent
		Actual	% Pred	Mean	95% CI	Actual	% Pred	change
FVC	(Lts)	2.74	75	3.64	2.83	3.14	86	14
FEV$_1$	(Lts)	1.39	46	3.01	2.37	1.88	62	35
FEV$_1$/FVC	(%)	51	62	82	73	60	73	17
FEF$_{25-75}$	(L/S)	.57	17	3.24		.92	28	61
PEFR	(L/S)	3.69	56	6.55		4.75	72	28
FET	(Secs)	8.92				7.22		

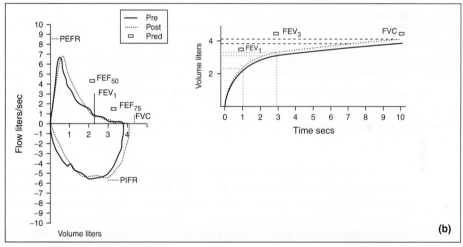

Spirometry (BTPS)		Prebronchodilator		Predicted	Range	Post bronchodilator		Percent
		Actual	% Pred	Mean	95% CI	Actual	% Pred	change
FVC	(Lts)	3.8	87	4.35	3.3	4.08	93	7
FEV$_1$	(Lts)	2.29	65	3.47	2.61	2.39	68	4
FEV$_1$/FVC	(%)	60	76	78	70	59	75	−1
FEF$_{25-75}$	(L/S)	1.13	32	3.49		1.03	29	−8
PEFR	(L/S)	6.8	79	8.52		6.87	80	1
FET	(Secs)	10.17				10.28		

FIGURE 6-13 *Spirometry results before (solid line) and after (dotted line) administration of a quick-acting bronchodilator. Example (a) shows a large reversible component to the airways obstruction, typical of asthma. In example (b) there is no significant improvement following bronchodilator.*

repeat spirometry 10 minutes after the initial study, how much might the FEV_1 increase or decrease just on the basis of repeat testing? One could perform an experiment with the same question in mind: measure spirometry, administer a placebo inhaler, and then repeat spirometry 10 minutes later. In a person with obstructive lung disease, how much might the FEV_1 increase (or decrease) on the second test?

The answer here is well studied: although *on average* the FEV_1 does not change at all on repeat testing or following placebo, the *range* of variability is up to 12%. Said in another way, only if the increase in FEV_1 following a bronchodilator medication is 12% or more, can you be 95% certain that the improvement is due to the effect of the bronchodilator and not just variability of the measurement. In persons with severe airflow obstruction, in whom the FEV_1 may be a very low number (e.g., 0.6 liters), an increase of 12% becomes a very small change (in this example, less than 0.1 liters). So, the official definition of a significant bronchodilator response—a response that can be attributed to an effect of the medication on airway smooth muscle—is an increase in FEV_1 of 12% or more and at least 200 cc (0.2 liters). Remember, however, that a *significant* bronchodilator response (a true medication effect) and an *asthmatic* bronchodilator response (a characteristically large improvement) are two different things.

KEY POINT   An increase in FEV_1 following bronchodilator that is 12% or more and 200 cc or greater can be identified with certainty as an improvement due to the medication and not due to chance variation.

One additional point: why might a person with asthma fail to have a large improvement (15–20% increase in FEV_1) following bronchodilator? Here are potential factors that might confound the results: the patient took his albuterol inhaler 30 minutes before coming for pulmonary function testing; the patient's airflow obstruction is very mild, so that the FEV_1 is only minimally reduced below normal; the patient is already on maximal bronchodilator therapy; or the patient has asthma with irreversible airflow obstruction due to "airway remodeling."

RESTRICTIVE PATTERN

Our interest in this book about asthma is airflow obstruction. We will address the topic of restrictive pulmonary function tests only briefly, mainly to clarify how an abnormality that is not obstructive might look. Many respiratory disorders might result in restriction on pulmonary function testing: anything that prevents the lungs from fully inflating with air. If you think about it for a brief time, you can probably generate a long list yourself. Our list is organized by causes of restriction: disorders filling the airspaces and making the lungs stiff (e.g., pulmonary edema, diffuse pneumonia, or pulmonary fibrosis); space-occupying lesions (e.g., large hiatus hernia or lung mass); lung collapse; disorders surrounding the lungs (e.g., pleural effusions, curvature of the spine, or pneumothorax); and respiratory muscle weakness (e.g., amyotrophic lateral sclerosis or unilateral hemidiaphragmatic paralysis).

Since restriction on pulmonary function testing means a decreased maximal volume of air contained within the lungs, spirometry is not exactly the best test to identify restriction. Remember that spirometry measures how much air you can maximally exhale from your lungs but tells us nothing about how much air is left behind within the lungs at the end of exhalation. As you know, at that point the lungs are not empty; they have not deflated totally. Even using every ounce of strength you have to squeeze air from your chest, there is still some air left behind, a "residual volume," as it is officially called. Depending on your sex, age, and height, this volume of air is normally approximately 1–2 liters.

We have already encountered the example of the patient with severe airflow obstruction. The maximal amount of air that he can exhale is reduced (↓ FVC), but the total amount of air within his lungs is normal (or perhaps even increased). The problem is that because of his severe airflow obstruction, he cannot empty a normal amount of air from his lungs. There is an abnormally large volume left behind within his lungs at the end of his forced exhalation. His residual volume is abnormally large.

Measuring lung volumes

So, a reduced FVC does not identify restriction. To determine with certainty if there is a reduced volume of air held within the lungs, one needs to measure that amount of air remaining in the lungs after a maximal exhalation, the residual volume. Then, by adding the amount of air exhaled from the lungs (FVC) and the amount left behind within the lungs at the end of maximal exhalation (residual volume, or RV), you have the total amount of air that can be held within the lungs, called the total lung capacity (TLC, not to be confused with "tender loving care!"). If the total lung capacity is reduced, there is a restrictive abnormality on pulmonary function testing. If the total lung capacity is normal or increased (as in emphysema), there is no restriction.

KEY POINT   Restriction is defined as a reduced amount of air held within the lungs after a maximal breath in. Its diagnosis requires measurement of the volume of air left behind in the lungs after a maximal exhalation (the residual volume).

How does one measure the residual volume? It involves additional testing performed in the pulmonary function laboratory—additional equipment, approximately 20 minutes of testing time, and a medical charge of several hundred dollars. Two methods for measuring residual volume and total lung capacity are called the helium-dilution technique and plethysmography. Or, on the pulmonary function testing requisition form, simply check off the box for "Measurement of Lung Volumes."

Reduced FVC with normal or increased FEV₁/FVC ratio

Still, you can *suspect* a restrictive pattern based on the findings on spirometry. If the maximal volume of air exhaled (FVC) is decreased in the absence of airflow obstruction, the likely reason is restriction. As you remember, the hallmark of airflow obstruction on spirometry is a reduced FEV_1/FVC ratio. So if the FVC is reduced and the FEV_1/FVC ratio is normal or increased above normal, there is probable restriction, as in the example below. Said in another way, restriction causes all lung volumes to be reduced, including the volume exhaled in the first second (FEV_1). Typical of the restrictive pattern is that the vital capacity (FVC) and the one-second forced expiratory volume (FEV_1) are reduced to a similar degree. This proportionate decrease in FVC and FEV_1 seen in restriction leaves the FEV_1/FVC normal or increased.

	Actual	% Predicted	Predicted Mean	95% CI
FVC (liters)	3.82	65	5.88	4.83
FEV_1 (liters)	3.36	69	4.85	3.99
FEV_1/FVC (%)	0.88	108	0.81	0.73
FEF_{25-75} (L/sec)	4.6	92	5.02	
PEFR (L/sec)	9.43	92	10.28	
FET (seconds)	6.15			

KEY POINT   Restriction can be *suspected* on spirometry when the FVC is reduced but the FEV_1/FVC ratio is normal or increased.

Incidentally, what might cause the FEV_1/FVC ratio to be increased above normal? In other words, what might make it possible to exhale more than the normal portion of the vital capacity in the first second of exhalation? How fast air is emptied from your lungs is determined by how hard you push out with your muscles, how wide open your air passageways are, and the elasticity of your lungs. As you know, fully inflated lungs are stretched like a rubber band; their elastic property makes them ready to spring back to a smaller size. The elasticity of the lungs can change in lung diseases. Emphysema causes loss of the elasticity of the lungs, contributing to the slowed expiratory airflow typical of emphysema. Other diseases, like pulmonary fibrosis, make the lung stiffer and more elastic on exhalation. In these diseases, the increased tendency of the lungs to recoil to a smaller volume causes more rapid emptying of the lungs and an increased FEV_1/FVC ratio.

Straight slope of the expiratory flow-volume curve

The speed at which air empties from the lungs decreases as lung volumes become smaller and smaller. In part, like a rubber band that is only stretched slightly, the force of recoil of the "lung spring" decreases when the initial stretch is less (at a lower lung volume). In part, less fully inflated lungs mean less widely open airways. The springiness of surrounding lung tissue contributes to pulling bronchi open to their maximal diameters. If you look at the shape of the normal expiratory flow-volume curve, you can see that expiratory flow progressively declines as lung volumes get smaller.

In restrictive respiratory abnormalities, in which lung volumes are smaller than normal, expiratory flows are reduced compared to normal, but they are preserved for any given lung volume. In the absence of any obstructive abnormality, expiratory flows stay proportional to lung volumes. And so, the shape of the curve that plots the relationship between expiratory flow and exhaled lung volume—the flow-volume curve—stays normal. An example of the flow-volume curve in a patient with a restrictive abnormality is shown below (Fig. 6-14).

KEY POINT   The flow-volume curve in restrictive abnormalities maintains the same shape as normal, just smaller.

MIXED OBSTRUCTIVE AND RESTRICTIVE PATTERN

One last point before we leave the subject of spirometry. We remind you that it is possible to have both obstructive and restrictive pulmonary function abnormalities at the same time. Some diseases can impact both lung volumes and expiratory flow:

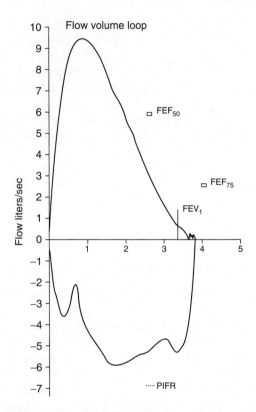

FIGURE 6-14 *In a restrictive abnormality, the shape of a normal flow-volume loop is preserved (no scooping or concavity to the shape of the expiratory limb). The curve is compressed along its horizontal axis (decreased volume of air exhaled). The horizontal axis shows volume in liters. Normal values for the forced expiratory flow at 50% (FEF50) and 75% (FEF₇₅) of the vital capacity are shown as rectangular boxes.*

diffuse bronchiectasis (as in children with cystic fibrosis) is an example. And some patients will have the misfortune of having two respiratory disorders, one causing restriction and the other causing obstruction, such as the person with emphysema who develops pulmonary fibrosis, or the person with an asthmatic attack who suffers mucus plugging and lobar collapse.

In mixed obstructive and restrictive patterns you will find a reduced FEV_1/FVC ratio and a scooped shape to the expiratory flow-volume curve (manifesting the presence of airflow obstruction). In addition, the vital capacity will be reduced, more than you might anticipate from the severity of the obstructive abnormality. The exaggerated reduction in FVC may make you suspect that restriction is also present. To be sure, you will need to order measurement of a full set of lung volumes. The finding of a reduced total lung capacity will prove the existence of the concomitant restriction.

MEASUREMENT OF PEAK FLOW

We have already encountered the peak expiratory flow in our discussion of spirometry. It is the rate of flow at the highest point of the expiratory flow-volume curve, the graphic "mountain peak." As you know, there are instruments designed to measure this single point of expiratory flow: peak flow meters. Some are rugged, highly accurate, expensive, and designed for multi-patient use (Fig. 6-15). Others, with which you are probably more familiar, are lightweight, inexpensive, designed for a single person, and appropriate for home use (see Figs. 2-4 on page 59 and 10-1 on page 374). Many different home peak flow meters are available for sale—at pharmacies, medical supply companies, and on-line—at prices in the range of $15–$30.

You also know that the peak flow, like all expiratory flows, can be reduced in obstructive disorders and in restrictive disorders. A reduced peak flow does not discriminate the cause of the abnormality. Still, it can be a very useful test, especially because of the simplicity with which the measurement is obtained. In a person whose spirometry has demonstrated an obstructive pattern, as in asthma, peak flow monitoring can be used to monitor the severity of the problem. We acknowledge that in many medical offices, peak flow measurements are used as a surrogate for spirometry. In a person with a typical history and physical exam for asthma, peak flow can be used to quantify the severity of airflow obstruction and help assess disease severity. As discussed in Chap. 2, "Diagnosing and Staging the Severity of Asthma," we sometimes use peak flow monitoring over a period of days to weeks to diagnose asthma. Variable expiratory flow is typical of asthma, whereas peak flow measurements that remain the same even as symptoms come and go argue against a diagnosis of asthma. Here we simply add the caution

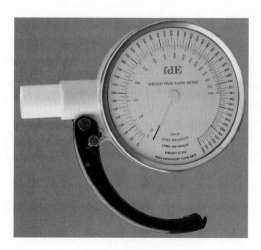

FIGURE 6-15   *Wright peak flow meter.*

that in the absence of spirometry, one can occasionally be fooled by *restriction* that comes and goes (e.g., congestive heart failure). A low peak flow does not *prove* airflow obstruction.

KEY POINT   A low peak flow does not prove airflow obstruction. Without spirometry, one cannot distinguish with certainty whether a reduced peak flow is caused by an obstructive or a restrictive breathing abnormality.

Making the measurement

Like spirometry, peak flow measurement is effort-dependent—*highly* effort-dependent. Unless one gives a strong and fast expiratory effort, one's true peak flow will be underestimated. Nonetheless, peak flow determination is easier than spirometry. It requires only a short, forceful blow, not continued exhalation until the lungs are fully emptied. A quick, hard blast out—it takes about 1 second. Most people can control their throat passage so that they can exhale directly into the peak flow meter without loss of air through the nose. If not, they can simply pinch the tip of their nose with their thumb and forefinger while doing the test. The usual procedure is to repeat the test three times. The highest result of the three determinations (*not* the average of the three) is the actual peak flow.

Patients need to be coached to perform peak flow measurements correctly and thereby to get accurate information, whether they are with you in a medical office or plan to use the peak flow meter independently at home. So, coach, you will need to ensure the following. First, the patient needs to place the mouthpiece between lips and teeth with lips tightly sealed. Next comes a deep, full breath in (peak flow will be lower from a less-than-maximal lung volume), and then a quick, hard, short breath out. (It is also acceptable to have the deep inhalation precede sealing one's lips around the mouthpiece.) The exhalation needs to be quick from the start; it is no good speeding up over a second or two. Also, you will need to be vigilant for errors that can falsely *increase* the measured peak flow. These include a spit-like maneuver that reflects emptying air from one's mouth rather than the lungs; and partially occluding the outflow passage at the other end of the peak flow meter. We encourage you to try it. Check your peak flow carefully and get an accurate recording. Then find ways to *cheat* that cause erroneous readings—too high as well as too low.

Defining "personal best" peak flow

At some point you will probably be asked, "What should my peak flow be?" or "Is that a good peak flow number for me?" There are two ways to go about answering these questions. One way is to look up the predicted peak flow on a chart of normal values (Tables 2-3 and 6-1). As for spirometry, normal peak flow values vary by height in children and by sex, age, and height in adults. The "normal"

T A B L E   6 - 1

NORMAL PEAK FLOW VALUES IN CHILDREN

Height (inches)	Peak Flow (L/min)	Height (inches)	Peak Flow (L/min)
43	147	56	320
44	160	57	334
45	173	58	347
46	187	59	360
47	200	60	373
48	214	61	387
49	227	62	400
50	240	63	413
51	254	64	427
52	267	65	440
53	280	66	454
54	293	67	467
55	307		

values shown on these tables are the predicted *average* number for a person of a certain category. As we previously discussed, normal includes a range of values, not a single number. For peak flow, the normal range in adult men encompasses values as low as 100 L/min below the average; in adult women the normal range extends to 80 L/min below average. These normal predicted values are derived from a population of healthy, nonsmoking, nonasthmatic Caucasians. They are likely to overestimate the predicted normal peak flow in African-Americans, Hispanics, Asians, and Native Americans.

The other method to answer the question posed by your patient is to determine for that particular patient what his or her peak flow is when his or her asthma is "as good as it gets." When the patient is on optimal treatment for asthma, feeling entirely well, the patient should check his or her peak flow. Or, better yet, the patient can check peak flow daily during a 2-week period of good asthma control. The best value recorded over that 2-week period is the patient's "personal best" and defines normal for him or her. Making repeated measurements over a 2-week period minimizes the chance of an error based on a single measurement.

KEY POINT Your ideal or target peak flow can be determined from a table of normal values or from measurements of your peak flow when you are feeling entirely well, "as good as your asthma gets."

The "personal best" method of determining your target peak flow has several advantages. First, it defines normal for you as an individual, not for the whole population of people of your sex, age, and height. Second, it also identifies what normal is for you using your particular type of peak flow meter. Inevitably, there will be some variability in peak flow depending on which brand of peak flow meter you use. The absolute value is less important than establishing your personal best with your own peak flow meter, then observing for changes from your best value. Third, your personal best value automatically corrects for any racial or ethnic differences not included on published tables of normal values. Fourth, and finally, if your personal best peak flow turns out to be well below the predicted normal value, you may have a component of "airway remodeling." Your bronchial tubes may have developed some degree of irreversible narrowing, present even when you feel perfectly well. In that case, your personal best peak flow sets the goal for your asthma treatment better than the published predicted normal value.

Uses of home peak flow monitoring

Imagine that a friend of yours reports respiratory symptoms whenever she enters her workplace. She experiences mainly chest tightness, particularly towards the end of her work shift. She works as a nurse in the recovery room and is convinced that there must be a problem with the air quality, especially since the recovery room is located two stories below street level. Two other recovery room nurses have reported work-related symptoms, although they have experienced primarily burning of their eyes and nasal congestion.

For further assessment you suggest that she monitor her peak flow before and at the end of each shift and make similar measurements on days when she is not at work. A reproducible fall in her peak flow of more than 20% at the end of her shift would be highly suggestive of work-related asthma. If her peak flow remains unchanged, her chest tightness probably has a different explanation. Clearly, the accuracy of the findings depends entirely on her reliability in performing the testing, but with this caveat, peak flow monitoring offers a useful screening procedure for the assessment of work-related asthma—and for the diagnosis of asthma in general.

Another brief example may help to illustrate its utility in diagnostic assessment. The coach of a junior high-school soccer team wonders whether one of her players might have asthma. The child frequently needs to be taken out of the game to rest and catch her breath, but she seems to recover quickly and is then eager to return to play. The coach worries whether it is safe for the child to start running again; is she jeopardizing the child's health by letting her compete so soon after these episodes? A peak flow meter is a useful diagnostic tool for a sport team's coach or trainer. A normal peak flow is reassuring; a reduced peak flow is a "red flag," warning that continued exercise may trigger a severe asthmatic attack. Peak flow monitoring is particularly useful when the symptoms to be investigated occur predictably at a time or location such that a visit to the doctor is not practical.

KEY POINT   Peak flow measurements can be helpful in the diagnostic assessment of asthma, particularly when measurements are needed away from the medical office. A fall in peak flow of more than 20% associated with typical asthmatic triggers and symptoms is suggestive of asthma.

We encourage almost all of our patients with asthma to have a peak flow meter available at home. We do not, however, ask them to check their (or their child's) peak flow every day or to restrict their activities whenever they find a fall in peak flow below their personal best. We do not want to create an asthma neurosis! There are, however, certain circumstances when it becomes very useful to have an objective measure of how one's asthma is doing, and to utilize a device that can perhaps detect subtle changes in lung function before they register as asthmatic symptoms.

For instance, if the doctor has suggested that your patient reduce her dose of inhaled steroid in half, this might be a good time for her to keep a close eye on her lung function at home. If her peak flow remains stable, stepping down therapy has been successful. If there is a gradual deterioration in peak flow over the next few weeks, it may be necessary to resume the higher dose of inhaled steroid again. Anytime when one anticipates that asthma control might deteriorate, monitoring for changes with a peak flow meter can be helpful. Examples might include moving into a new home, obtaining a pet animal, starting a new medication, such as a cardioselective beta blocker, or becoming pregnant.

KEY POINT   If circumstances change such that you might reasonably anticipate a possible deterioration in asthma control, peak flow monitoring provides an "early warning system" to detect change before severe symptoms develop.

When is the best time to have your patient check his or her peak flow? We generally recommend measuring peak flow in the morning before medication. Although this value may not be the highest value during the day, it best reflects overall asthma control, including the ability to suppress large diurnal variations in airways obstruction. A more detailed picture of asthma control emerges from peak flow readings made before and after bronchodilator and both morning and evening, but this sort of obsessive-compulsive data collection is psychologically unhealthy and nearly impossible to sustain. Probably most important is that one makes the peak flow measurements in the same way each time (whether before or after bronchodilator, in the morning, afternoon, or evening), so that one can "compare apples to apples" in calculating a trend over time. In many instances, one or two recordings a week will suffice to ensure stability of asthma control or to detect the lack of stability.

Another important role for peak flow measurements involves assessment of an asthmatic flare. How severe is this asthma attack? Should your patient call the doctor's office tonight or wait until morning? Is this child's cough due to a head cold, or is it his asthma acting up? We tell our patients that having a peak flow meter at home is like having a thermometer. You don't need to check your temperature every day, but when you suspect that you might have a fever, it's nice to be able to find out how high your temperature is. You will probably react differently if you find that your temperature is 104.5°F as opposed to 99.8°F.

So too, if you suffer a respiratory infection and wonder how it is affecting your asthma—"is that cough and shortness of breath due to my chest cold or a flare of my asthma?"—it is helpful to be able to measure the severity of airway narrowing. And we hope that our patients will react differently if they find their peak flow to be 150 L/min as opposed to 325 L/min. We will discuss peak flow monitoring during asthmatic flares in more detail in Chap. 10, "Developing an Asthma Action Plan," when we consider creating asthma action plans to provide patients with guidance in managing asthmatic attacks.

KEY POINT   A peak flow meter can be used like a thermometer. If you want to diagnose a fever and quantify its severity, you take your temperature with a thermometer. If you want to assess the status of asthma and measure the severity of airway narrowing, measure your peak flow.

One last benefit of home peak flow measurement: it provides an extremely useful tool for patient-provider communication during telephone triage. When our asthmatic patients call to say that they are feeling poorly, short of breath, coughing, or tight in the chest, we find ourselves asking them, "have you checked your peak flow?" and, if not, "can you go do it now?" We are aware that the information provided is not always accurate, either because the test was not done correctly or the peak flow meter was not functioning properly. But in the context of the current symptoms and the patient's past asthma history, we can often use the information about peak flow to help give better telephone advice. In addition, we and our patients are less likely to overlook or downplay dangerous airflow obstruction when confronted with numerical data. For example, when the patient returns to the telephone to report—breathlessly—that the measured peak flow is only 30% of his or her personal best, we will know that major intervention is needed, quick!

Self-Assessment Questions

QUESTION 1

Spirometry, correctly interpreted, can help you to do all of the following except:

1. Distinguish obstructive from restrictive respiratory abnormalities
2. Distinguish allergic from nonallergic asthma
3. Quantify the severity of airflow obstruction in asthma
4. Distinguish normal from abnormal lung function
5. Quantify the reversibility of airflow obstruction in asthma (measured before and after bronchodilator)

QUESTION 2

The vital capacity measures the amount of air that you can empty from your lungs, from "breathe all the way in" to "breathe all the way out." On spirometry, this value is referred to as the forced vital capacity (FVC). Which of the following conditions would not be expected to cause the FVC to be reduced?

1. Respiratory muscle weakness (e.g., Guillain-Barré syndrome)
2. Kyphoscoliosis
3. Pulmonary edema
4. Pulmonary fibrosis
5. Acute bronchitis

QUESTION 3

Accurate spirometry requires which of the following?

1. Forced exhalation for a minimum of 6 seconds
2. Patient in a standing position
3. Testing performed with the patient N.P.O. (nothing to eat for 4 hours prior to testing)
4. Patient at least 10 years of age
5. Patient able to hold his or her breath for at least 10 seconds

QUESTION 4

Measurements that give information about the rate at which air empties from the lungs (the speed of exhalation) include all of the following except:

1. FEV_1 (L)
2. FVC (L)

3. FEV_1/FVC

4. FEV_3 (L)

5. FEF_{25-75} (L/sec)

QUESTION 5

Although it is derived from the same forced expiratory maneuver as the spirogram, the flow-volume curve can provide additional useful information, including:

1. Distinguish asthma from emphysema

2. Distinguish obstructive from restrictive abnormalities

3. Distinguish upper airway obstruction from the intrathoracic obstruction typical of asthma

4. Eliminate need to calculate FEV_1/FVC

5. Eliminate need for additional, more expensive testing, such as measurement of lung volumes and diffusing capacity

QUESTION 6

Features typical of an obstructive pattern, as may be seen in someone with asthma (or COPD or other obstructive lung diseases), include all of the following except:

1. Reduced FEV_1

2. Reduced FEV_1/FVC

3. Normal FEV_1/FVC with FEV_1 and FVC reduced proportionately

4. Scooped, concave appearance to the flow-volume curve

5. Reduced FEF_{25-75}

QUESTION 7

Significant improvement in lung function following bronchodilator administration is defined as:

1. Visibly detectable separation of the spirographic and flow-volume curves obtained before and after bronchodilator

2. Increase in FEV_1 of at least 12% and at least 200 cc

3. Increase in FEV_1 of at least 20% and at least 500 cc

4. Doubling of FEV_1

5. Increase in the FEV_1/FVC ratio of 15%

QUESTION 8

A 60-year-old man comes for evaluation of shortness of breath of approximately 6 months' duration. He has no prior history of asthma or allergies and has never smoked cigarettes. Based on the results of his pulmonary function tests shown below (which you are asked to interpret), which of the following diagnoses is most likely?

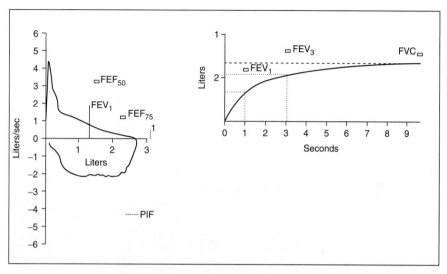

Spirometry (BTPS)

		Prebronchodilator		Predicted	Range
		Actual	% Pred	Mean	95% CI
FVC	(Lts)	2.7	87	3.09	2.04
FEV$_1$	(Lts)	1.33	52	2.54	1.68
FEV$_1$/FVC	(%)	49	59	82	74
FEF$_{25-75}$	(L/S)	0.61	22	2.77	
PEFR	(L/S)	4.44	68	6.47	
FET	(Secs)	9.64			

1. Asthma
2. Pulmonary fibrosis
3. Pleural effusion
4. Morbid obesity
5. Deconditioning

QUESTION 9

Much to your surprise, the younger sister of the patient described in Question 8 comes to the office the following week. She too has been short of breath over the last 6–12 months, with a nonproductive cough. Based on the results of her pulmonary function tests (shown below), which is the most likely diagnosis?

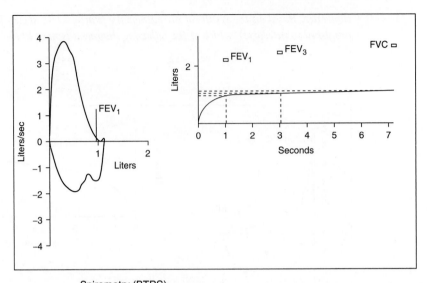

Spirometry (BTPS)

| | | Prebronchodilator | | Predicted | Range |
		Actual	% Pred	Mean	95% CI
FVC	(Lts)	1.13	42	2.65	1.84
FEV$_1$	(Lts)	0.97	43	2.22	1.58
FEV$_1$/FVC	(%)	86	103	83	74
FEF$_{25-75}$	(L/S)	1.72	68	2.5	
PEFR	(L/S)	3.85	71	5.37	
FET	(Secs)	7.18			

1. Asthma

2. Emphysema

3. Chronic bronchitis

4. Bronchiolitis (diffuse inflammatory disease involving the small airways)

5. Pulmonary fibrosis

QUESTION 10

A 45-year-old woman with asthma undergoes pulmonary function testing, with the results as shown below. You explain to the patient and to the nursing student who accompanies the patient that the results indicate severe airflow obstruction. The nursing student, who has been studying pulmonary function testing, wonders why—if your assessment is correct—the vital capacity (FVC) is reduced. You explain that it is probably reduced because:

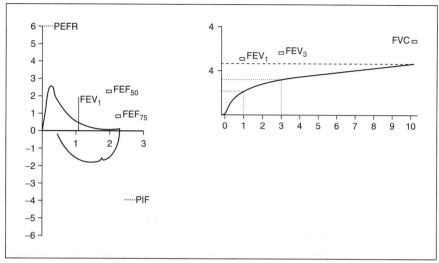

Spirometry (BTPS)

		Prebronchodilator		Predicted	Range
		Actual	% Pred	Mean	95% CI
FVC	(Lts)	2.32	69	3.33	2.52
FEV$_1$	(Lts)	1.1	43	2.52	1.88
FEV$_1$/FVC	(%)	47	66	71	62
FEF$_{25-75}$	(L/S)	0.31	14	2.16	
PEFR	(L/S)	2.6	43	6.03	
FET	(Secs)	10.13			

1. Long-standing asthma has led to permanent, irreversible airways obstruction (airway remodeling).

2. Severe obstruction can lead to "gas trapping" with a large volume of gas left in the chest even after complete exhalation.

3. She most likely has asthma and pulmonary fibrosis combining to give severe airflow obstruction and a simultaneous restrictive abnormality.

4. The vital capacity must always be reduced somewhat as part of an obstructive abnormality on pulmonary function testing.

5. The FVC is reduced because the FEV$_1$/FVC ratio is so low.

QUESTION 11

Which of the following statements about home peak flow measurements is correct?

1. To be useful, peak flow measurements need to be made daily, preferably in the morning.

2. Peak flow measurements give the same information as spirometry, only less expensively.

3. Unlike spirometry, peak flow measurements do not require a full breath in followed by a maximal expiratory effort.

4. An accurate peak flow measurement requires a forced exhalation of at least 6 seconds.

5. A 20% or greater fall in peak flow measured repeatedly at the end of a work shift compared to the beginning would be typical of work-related asthma.

QUESTION 12

A young mother asks your advice about measuring her son's peak flow at home. He is 9 years old and has recently been diagnosed with asthma. You indicate that:

1. He is still too young to perform reliable peak flow measurements.

2. It would be useful to establish his "personal best" peak flow by measuring his peak flow for several days when he is feeling perfectly well.

3. Peak flow measurements should be avoided in the morning because they might trigger bronchospasm before he goes to school.

4. Peak flow measurements are only useful if measured before and after bronchodilator.

5. For his safety, peak flow measurements should be checked routinely before he goes to school or out to play.

Answers to Self-Assessment Questions

ANSWER TO QUESTION 1 (INFORMATION THAT SPIROMETRY CAN PROVIDE)

The correct answer is #2. Spirometry can identify an obstructive pattern such as is seen in asthma, but it cannot distinguish among the many causes of an obstructive pattern. On a single spirometry test, allergic asthma, nonallergic asthma, COPD, and a viral bronchiolitis will all look alike. Spirometry proves useful in distinguishing disorders that cause expiratory airflow obstruction from disorders that cause restriction to the amount of air held in the chest (answer #1). Spirometry can also indicate how severe airflow obstruction is (answer #3); distinguish normal from abnormal lung function (answer #4); and, in those with an obstructive pattern, quantify how much of the airflow obstruction can be reversed toward normal with administration of a quick-acting bronchodilator (answer #5).

ANSWER TO QUESTION 2 (CAUSES OF A REDUCED VITAL CAPACITY [FVC])

The correct answer is #5 (acute bronchitis). If one thinks of those things that might prevent the lungs (and all the millions of alveoli within the lungs) from fully filling with air, disorders that come to mind include weakness of the respiratory muscles (answer #1: e.g., Guillain-Barré syndrome), deformity of the ribs and spine preventing expansion of the lungs (answer #2: kyphoscoliosis), edema fluid filling the alveoli (answer #3: pulmonary edema), and scarring (collagen tissue) filling the alveoli and stiffening the fabric of the lungs (answer #4: pulmonary fibrosis). Acute bronchitis refers to inflammation, generally infectious in etiology, involving the large bronchial tubes. It does not prevent taking a full, deep breath and generally has no significant impact on one's measured lung function.

ANSWER TO QUESTION 3 (REQUIREMENTS FOR AN ACCURATE SPIROMETRY TEST)

The correct answer is #1 (forced exhalation for a minimum of 6 seconds). Standards established by the American Thoracic Society insist on a minimum of 6 seconds of exhalation to ensure complete emptying of air from the lungs. Testing is performed in the seated position, not standing (answer #2). Although a very large meal consumed immediately before testing would not be ideal, there is no need for patients to be kept N.P.O. prior to pulmonary function testing (answer #3). In general, children who can hold their breath under water for several seconds also have the breath control to perform pulmonary function testing. This developmental task is typically achieved at approximately age 6, well before age 10 (answer #4). Breath-holding for at least 10 seconds is not required for spirometry (answer #5).

ANSWER TO QUESTION 4 (TEST RESULTS INDICATING EXPIRATORY FLOW)

The correct answer is #2. FVC is a *volume*; this measurement gives no information about the *speed* at which this volume is exhaled. Although reported in liters (L), both FEV_1 (answer #1) and FEV_3 (answer #4) are measures of the rate or speed of exhalation. These measurements include in their definitions units of time (forced expiratory volume *in one second* [FEV_1] or forced expiratory volume *in three seconds* [FEV_3]. Volume per time (liters per 1 second or liters per 3 seconds) gives a measure of speed of exhalation. The FEV_1/FVC (answer #3) gives information about the speed at which air can be emptied from the lungs because we know that normally about three-quarters or more of the vital capacity can be emptied in the first second. If the FEV_1/FVC ratio is less than approximately 0.75, it indicates slowing of the rate of exhalation (evidence for an obstructive abnormality). FEF_{25-75} (answer #5) measures the speed of exhalation between 25% and 75% of the vital capacity and is reported in liters/second.

ANSWER TO QUESTION 5 (ADDITIONAL INFORMATION THAT CAN BE DERIVED FROM EXAMINATION OF THE FLOW-VOLUME CURVE)

The correct answer is #3. Airflow obstruction that results from a single point of narrowing in the upper airways gives a straight horizontal line or "plateau pattern" on the flow-volume curve, easily distinguishable from the concave, scooped appearance of airflow obstruction that results from thousands of bronchial tubes narrowed inside the thorax, as in asthma. Neither the pattern on a spirogram (volume on the vertical axis; time on the horizontal axis) nor flow-volume curve (flow on the vertical axis; volume on the horizontal axis) distinguishes asthma from emphysema (or other intrathoracic obstructive abnormality) (answer #1).

Both the spirogram and flow-volume curve have different patterns for obstructive and restrictive abnormalities (answer #2); for this purpose, no *additional* information is obtained from examination of the flow-volume curve. Display of the flow-volume curve does not eliminate need to measure FEV_1/FVC (answer #4); nor does it provide the information that may be needed from measurement of lung volumes and diffusing capacity (answer #5).

ANSWER TO QUESTION 6 (FEATURES TYPICAL OF AN OBSTRUCTIVE PATTERN ON PULMONARY FUNCTION TESTING)

The correct answer is #3. If the FEV_1/FVC ratio is normal, there is no evidence present for airflow obstruction. A normal FEV_1/FVC with FEV_1 and FVC both reduced proportionately would be a finding suggestive of a restrictive abnormality. On the other hand, in obstructive abnormalities one finds a reduced FEV_1 (answer #1); reduced FEV_1/FVC (answer #2); scooped, concave appearance to the flow-volume curve (answer #4), and reduced FEF_{25-75} (answer #5).

ANSWER TO QUESTION 7 (DEFINITION OF "SIGNIFICANT IMPROVEMENT" IN LUNG FUNCTION FOLLOWING BRONCHODILATOR ADMINISTRATION)

The correct answer is #2. If the FEV_1 measured after bronchodilator administration is $\geq 12\%$ and ≥ 200 cc larger than the FEV_1 measured before bronchodilator, the improvement is considered significant (and more than one would expect to see simply due to variability of the measurement itself). Smaller increases (e.g., enough to cause a visible separation of the spirographic and flow-volume curves recorded before and after bronchodilator [answer #1]) may be due to chance variation alone. When the increase is at least 12% and at least 200 cc, one can be 95% certain that the improvement was due to administration of the bronchodilator and not due to chance variation alone. An increase in FEV_1 of 20% and at least 500 cc (answer #3) and a doubling of FEV_1 (answer #4) are increases in FEV_1 greater than are needed to be 95% certain that the improvement following bronchodilator is not due to chance variation alone. When a bronchodilator causes significant improvement in lung function, it may cause both the FEV_1 and the FVC to improve. If both FEV_1 and FVC improve a comparable amount, the FEV_1/FVC ratio will not change. Therefore, changes in the FEV_1/FVC ratio (answer #5) are not reliable in assessing the significance of a response in lung function to bronchodilator administration.

ANSWER TO QUESTION 8 (PULMONARY FUNCTION TEST INTERPRETATION)

The correct answer is #1 (asthma). The spirometry results indicate a pattern of expiratory airflow obstruction. The FEV_1/FVC ratio is reduced, indicating obstruction. The expiratory portion of the flow-volume loop is concave and scooped, typical of an obstructive pattern. Of the potential diagnoses listed, asthma is the one most likely to be associated with an obstructive pattern on pulmonary function testing. Pulmonary fibrosis (answer #2), pleural effusion (answer #3), and morbid obesity (answer #4) would most likely cause a restrictive pattern. Physical deconditioning (answer #5) can cause shortness of breath on exertion, but it would not be expected to cause any abnormality on pulmonary function testing.

ANSWER TO QUESTION 9 (PULMONARY FUNCTION TEST INTERPRETATION)

The correct answer is #5 (pulmonary fibrosis). These spirometric and flow-volume curves are suggestive of a restrictive pattern, such as would be seen in pulmonary fibrosis. The FEV_1/FVC ratio is normal (therefore, no obstruction is present) and the flow-volume curve has a normal shape, not the concave and scooped appearance seen in obstruction. Confirmation of the restrictive pattern could be obtained with measurement of lung volumes. One would expect to find a reduced total lung capacity (TLC), diagnostic of restriction. One would anticipate an *obstructive* abnormality on pulmonary function testing in someone with asthma (answer #1); emphysema (answer #2); chronic bronchitis (answer #3); or bronchiolitis (answer #4).

ANSWER TO QUESTION 10 (EXPLAINING WHY THE FVC MAY BE REDUCED IN SEVERE AIRFLOW OBSTRUCTION)

The correct answer is #2. In severe obstructive abnormalities—in the absence of any restriction—the vital capacity can be reduced. The explanation relates to the very slow speed at which air empties from the lungs. The patient cannot exhale for a long enough time to empty her full (normal) vital capacity; extra gas is left behind at the end of exhalation (gas trapping). Sometimes in severe obstruction, bronchial tubes narrow to the point of closing, physically trapping air behind blocked off tubes. This is another mechanism for gas trapping and a reduced FVC in severe obstruction. Permanent, irreversible airways obstruction (airway remodeling) (answer #1) can be mild, moderate, or severe and may or may not manifest with a reduced FVC. The combination of obstruction and restriction (e.g., asthma and pulmonary fibrosis) could also cause a reduced FVC (answer #3), but this combination of diagnoses seems far less likely. Measurement of lung volumes, including total lung capacity (TLC) and residual volume (RV) would help to distinguish explanations #2 and #3. Severe obstruction with gas trapping would be associated with a large residual volume and normal total lung capacity. Asthma with pulmonary fibrosis would cause a reduced total lung capacity (typical of restrictive disorders) and a normal or reduced residual volume. The vital capacity is not usually reduced in mild obstruction (answer #4). A very low FEV_1/FVC implies a very low FEV_1 and does not explain a low FVC (answer #5).

ANSWER TO QUESTION 11 (PEAK FLOW MEASUREMENTS)

The correct answer is #5. Peak flow monitoring in a reliable patient can be useful in assessing work-related asthma. A "cross-shift" fall in peak flow of $\geq 20\%$, if found repeatedly, suggests a workplace stimulus that is triggering worsened airway narrowing. Peak flow measurements can be useful even if made only intermittently (answer #1) (e.g., to assess the severity of airways obstruction during an asthmatic attack). Peak flow measurements do not contain as much information as the results of spirometry (answer #2). For instance, using only a peak flow meter, one cannot distinguish between obstruction versus restriction as the cause of a reduced peak flow. Like spirometry, peak flow measurements do require a full breath in followed by a maximal blast of air out (answer #3). However, the exhalation for a peak flow measurement is shorter, only a second or two, compared to spirometry (a minimum of 6 seconds of exhalation) (answer #4).

ANSWER TO QUESTION 12 (HOME PEAK FLOW MONITORING)

The correct answer is #2. Although one can look up an *average* normal value for this child on a table of normal peak flow values, it would be best to determine his individual best value or "personal best" by making measurements of his peak flow when he is feeling at his best with respect to his asthma. This personal best peak flow (which may be above or below the *average* normal value) can then be used to make comparisons when he is not feeling well. Reliable peak flow measurements can usually be made by ages 5 or 6 (answer #1). Peak flow measurements infrequently trigger bronchospasm (answer #3). If they do, the resulting bronchospasm is generally mild and brief (lasting only a few minutes). Although informative, it is not necessary to measure peak flow before and after bronchodilator (answer #4), a practice that would prove very time consuming. It is possible to overdo home peak flow monitoring, such as not letting a child go to school or out to play without first checking peak flow (answer #5).

CHAPTER

7

IDENTIFYING ALLERGIC SENSITIVITIES AND PROMOTING ALLERGEN AVOIDANCE

C H A P T E R   O U T L I N E

I. Asthma and Allergies
    a. Defining atopic diseases
    b. Evidence that links asthma and allergies
    c. Not all asthma is allergic

II. Identifying Allergic Sensitivities
    a. History taking
        i. Distinguishing allergic from nonallergic reactions
    b. Allergy skin tests
    c. Blood tests for allergy

III. Common Allergic Triggers of Asthma and Their Avoidance
    a. Dust mites
    b. House pets
    c. Indoor mold
    d. Cockroaches and other indoor pests
    e. Pollens and outdoor mold
    f. Nonallergic, irritant exposures
    g. Finding an overall strategy that is practical

IV. Interventions That Work
    a. Multidimensional interventions
    b. Home visits

ASTHMA AND ALLERGIES

Asthma and allergy are closely linked. For some people, asthma is their "allergic bronchitis," accompanying their allergic rhinitis and conjunctivitis and their allergic (or atopic) dermatitis (also called eczema). And if you have already read Chap. 1 of this book ("Understanding and Teaching the Mechanisms of Asthma"), it is easy to understand why there is such a strong association: these conditions share a common biologic mechanism. People with allergies of this sort make immunoglobulin E (IgE) antibodies that recognize allergens as foreign substances and initiate a complex sequence of chemical events seemingly designed to "fight them off," although in fact the allergens (like dust mites and cat dander) are harmless to our bodies.

The body can make a variety of types of biologic reactions in response to foreign substances, all described as "allergic." For example, the generalized skin eruption, red and slightly raised (maculopapular rash), in reaction to an antibiotic such as amoxicillin is an immune reaction involving immunoglobulins, but it is unrelated to asthma or allergic rhinitis. It occurs no more or less commonly in people with asthma than in people without asthma. So too, the pneumonia-like reaction in the lungs caused by an immune reaction to inhaled pigeon antigens ("pigeon-breeders' lung disease") is an allergic reaction very different from asthma. In response to these inhaled antigens, the body makes granulomas in the walls of the alveoli, a type of reaction called hypersensitivity pneumonitis in the United States and extrinsic allergic alveolitis in England. It too has no relation with asthma or allergic rhinitis.

Defining atopic diseases

The specific type of allergic response that characterizes asthma, involving immunoglobin E and mast cells and typically involving the presence of eosinophils, has been called the Type I immune response or immediate hypersensitivity reaction. Certain types of proteins (allergens) tend to elicit this specific response. Certain people are genetically programmed to make this type of allergic reaction when they encounter these allergens. People with this genetic make up are said to have atopy. Their atopy may manifest as one or any combination of multiple atopic diseases: asthma, allergic rhinitis, allergic conjunctivitis, atopic dermatitis, hives, food allergies, and anaphylaxis.

KEY POINT   A specific immunologic mechanism links the allergic diseases of asthma, allergic rhinitis, allergic conjunctivitis, allergic (atopic) dermatitis (also referred to as eczema), food allergies and anaphylaxis. This type of allergic reaction is characterized by involvement of immunoglobulin E, mast cells, and eosinophils.

When the immediate hypersensitivity reaction—with release of multiple inflammatory chemicals from mast cells and eosinophils—takes place in the eyes (or, more specifically, along the lining of the eyes), the consequence is allergic conjunctivitis. The lining along the whites of the eyes (the sclerae) become red-streaked with swollen blood vessels. Fluid can collect under these membranes, causing the eyes to swell; and clear fluid drains at the corners of the eyes. Red, itchy, swollen, watery eyes—maybe you've had a similar experience if a foreign body (like a piece of sand) got caught in your eye (in the conjunctival sac under your eyelid). In allergic conjunctivitis the offending substance is microscopic and otherwise harmless. It is the body's allergic reaction that causes all the misery.

Similar symptoms can develop in the nose from allergic reactions there: swelling of the membranes lining the nasal passageways; a clear, watery nasal drainage; and itching and sneezing. For some people, it's the swelling that pre-dominates. They are unable to breathe comfortably through their nose and become "mouth breathers." As you know from your experiences with a stuffy nose during viral upper respiratory tract infections, this is particularly uncom-fortable at night, when you wake with a dry, caked mouth and tongue. Other people are troubled mostly by the mucoid nasal drainage. At times the clear fluid seems to run from the nose "like a faucet." "I never can go anywhere without my box of tissues," patients may say. At other times the same fluid drains down from the back of the nose into the back of the throat (from the nasopharynx into the hypopharynx). The patient with this postnasal drip may be constantly clearing his throat or coughing to rid himself of the mucoid drainage.

When nasal symptoms are brought on only during certain seasons by out-door pollens, the condition is referred to as seasonal allergic rhinitis. "Hay fever" is the popular expression for allergic rhinitis and conjunctivitis in late summer and fall, triggered by ragweed pollen. An old-fashioned expression for seasonal allergic rhinitis and conjunctivitis in the springtime is "rose fever." When allergens that are present year-round (like dust mites) cause symptoms throughout the year, the condition is described as perennial allergic rhinitis.

It takes only a small leap to see asthma as an allergic disease of the bronchial tubes. Swelling of the tubes and clear, watery mucus secreted from the walls of the tubes lead to analogous symptoms: difficulty breathing through a narrowed sys-tem of tubes and cough to clear out these mucoid secretions. For some asthmatics, cough may be the dominant symptom; others experience mainly shortness of breath and chest tightness. Some people experience their symptoms of asthma only during certain seasons, others have year-round asthmatic symptoms.

Evidence that links asthma and allergies

Several lines of evidence support the close relationship between asthma and allergy.

- In children, 80% or more of asthmatics show evidence of allergic sensitiv-ities (e.g., by manifesting allergic reactions on skin testing). In adults the number falls to approximately 50–60%.

- In a large population-based study of children and adults, the risk of having asthma was shown to correlate directly with the blood level of immunoglobulin E (Fig. 7-1).

- In children genetically at risk for asthma (because of having allergic parents), exposure to allergens in the home (particularly dust mite, cat, and cockroach) predisposes to the development of asthma.

- Asthmatic persons with allergic sensitivities living in environments where they are exposed to those allergens have more severe, poorly controlled asthma; and allergen avoidance can improve their asthma control.

- In laboratory animals such as mice, asthmatic-like reactions and asthmatic-looking bronchial tubes can be created by repetitive exposure to allergens.

KEY POINT   The vast majority of children with asthma under age 16 are allergic. On the other hand, as many as 40–50% of adults with asthma show no signs of atopy.

Sometimes when we evaluate patients for persistent cough (despite their never having smoked cigarettes and having a normal chest x-ray), we are able to tell them—after an extensive work-up—that they do not have asthma. We are then occasionally asked, "Well, if it's not asthma, do you think that my cough could be due to allergies?" The answer is no. Allergy of the bronchial tubes is asthma. (We recognize that allergic rhinitis with postnasal drip can sometimes cause cough; and an allergic-type hypersensitivity pneumonitis can likewise

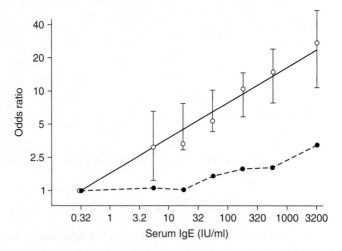

FIGURE 7-1   *The likelihood of asthma (solid line connecting open circles) is directly related to the level of immunoglobulin E (IgE) in the blood. The relationship between hay fever and serum IgE (dashed line connecting solid circles) is less strong. Reproduced with permission from Burrows B, et al., Association of asthma with serum IgE levels and skin-test reactivity to allergens. N Engl J Med 1989; 320:271–7. Copyright 1989 Massachusetts Medical Society. All rights reserved.*

manifest with cough. The point is that among the atopic diseases, the allergic lung disease is asthma.)

Not all asthma is allergic

It would be easy to conclude from this discussion that asthma is an allergic disease, but the truth is not that simple. Many people with asthma have no allergies at all. They have no hay fever, eczema, or hives. Their blood level of immunoglobulin E is normal. Their skin tests are all negative. And yet they have asthma that—other than for the absence of allergic sensitivities—behaves in every way like allergic asthma. The symptoms of asthma are the same, the nonallergic triggers are the same, bronchial hyperresponsiveness if measured is the same, and the bronchial tubes on biopsy look the same. If we want to come someday to understand fully the causes and mechanisms of asthma, we will need to explain both allergic and nonallergic asthma. In the meantime, our terms remain descriptive: atopic and nonatopic asthma or, in what is now mostly discarded terminology, extrinsic and intrinsic asthma.

KEY POINT   Many people with asthma do not have allergies. They have no personal or family history of atopic diseases. Yet in every other way, their asthma behaves the same as allergic asthma.

The remainder of this chapter focuses on efforts to identify among our patients with asthma which ones are atopic, what their asthmatic allergic sensitivities are, and what can be done to help them avoid exposure to those allergens. It is worth remembering at the outset that not all of the patients whom you see have allergic asthma. When a patient asks you, "Is it worth my while getting those allergy-proof wraps for my mattress and pillows?", you need to stop and think before answering. Does this patient have allergic asthma? And if so, is he or she allergic to dust mites? If not, wrapping the mattress and pillows to minimize exposure to dust mite allergen will be a waste of money and effort.

IDENTIFYING ALLERGIC SENSITIVITIES

Perhaps you have had a conversation with an adult asthmatic patient that went somewhat like this one:

Provider: *"Do you know what sets off your asthma? What your triggers are?"*

Patient: *"Yes, I'm allergic to just about everything: cats, dogs, dust, mold, grasses and trees, cigarette smoke, and changes in the weather."*

Provider: *"Have you ever had allergy skin testing?"*

Patient: *"Yes, many years ago. They tested me up and down my back, and I reacted to everything."*

Provider: *"It sounds as though you are allergic to life!"*

Patient: *"Yeah. I've wondered if I'm allergic to my husband!"*

History taking

Often patients with asthma know exactly to what they are allergic. "Every time I get near a cat, my eyes water, I start sneezing, and my chest tightens right up," one patient may say. Another patient may note that whenever she or he dusts and vacuums at home, the cleaning brings on asthmatic symptoms. In the work environment, more than 100 different inhaled substances have been identified as potential causes of occupational asthma. One workplace allergen of particular interest to healthcare workers is latex. But outside of these specific occupational exposures, only a limited number of allergens trigger asthma in the home (or school or office). These include seasonal allergens, such as pollens and outdoor mold spores, and year-round (perennial) allergens, including dust mites, furry pets, cockroaches, mice and rats, and indoor mold (Table 7-1).

Given this relatively limited number of key environmental allergens, it is easy to take a history inquiring about sensitivity and exposure in the asthmatic patient.

Have you noticed that your asthma is worse in certain seasons, such as in the spring when the trees are all blooming or in the early fall when it's ragweed season [at least in New England]?

Do you get asthmatic symptoms when you are around cats or dogs, either your own animals or your friends'? Do you have any pets at home?

Does your asthma get worse when you dust or vacuum at home? Do you have carpeting at home? In your bedroom?

Have you had any infestations at home? Cockroaches, mice, or rats?

Do you find that damp, moldy places bother your asthma? Do you have any such places at home? For instance, a basement where the rug may have got wet during flooding and you can smell the mildew when you enter the room?

KEY POINT   With a limited number of questions, one can inquire about allergic sensitivities and exposures to the common allergens important in asthma: pollens, pet animals, dust mites, cockroaches and other pests, and mold.

This might also be a good time to clarify for your patient the distinction between allergens and irritants. Cigarette smoke is a common trigger of asthma. As you know, people with asthma have *twitchy*, highly irritable airways, and cigarette smoke—with its combination of chemicals and particulate matter—can set off an asthmatic reaction with bronchoconstriction. But it does not elicit an

TABLE 7-1

COMMON ALLERGENS IMPORTANT IN ALLERGIC ASTHMA

Seasonal

   Tree pollen
   Grass pollen
   Weed pollen
   Outdoor mold spores

Perennial

   Dust mites
   Animal dander
   Cockroach
   Indoor mold spores

Occupational (examples)

   Flour dust (baker's asthma)
   Plicatic acid (sawdust from western red cedar)
   Latex

allergic reaction; humans do not make IgE antibodies to any of its components. So too with hot, humid weather, a sudden change in barometric pressure, or ingestion of alcoholic beverages: none acts as an allergen. It may be equally worthwhile for your patient to avoid these nonallergic triggers of asthma, but they do not fall under the category of allergen avoidance. You cannot test for these irritant sensitivities with allergy skin tests, you cannot desensitize to them with allergy shots, and you cannot modify reactions to them with the novel anti-IgE monoclonal antibody therapy, omalizumab (Xolair).

Allergy skin tests

There is no perfect blood (or skin) test that answers the question: does inhalation of a particular allergen make my asthma worse? For example, your patient may tell you: "We've had a dog in our family for years, and I've never been allergic to pets. You don't think that our dog could be the reason my asthma has been so trouble-some, do you?" The definitive answer to this question would require a specialized test that is rarely if ever done clinically, called an allergen inhalation challenge. You would have to prepare a sterile solution containing dog antigen (preferably from the patient's own dog) and measure the patient's lung function before and after inhalation of gradually increasing amounts of the antigen. The development of air-flow obstruction in response to the inhaled dog allergen would be evidence of aller-gic sensitivity of the bronchial tubes. If no airflow obstruction were to develop, you could say with certainty that he was not allergic to dogs. (You may have thought of another potential test to offer this patient: find another home for your dog and see if your asthma gets better. It's a good idea, but less conclusive—if his asthma doesn't get better, it will not prove that dog allergy is not one of multiple factors contributing to his severe asthma—and it will be a "tough sell" to your patient.)

What we can offer is an *indirect* assessment of allergic sensitivity of the bronchial tubes, utilizing the skin as our assay. If we apply a small amount of dog antigen beneath the surface of the skin, will we elicit an allergic reaction typical of atopy: a hive? In general, people without allergy to dogs will not make a hive-like reaction when dog antigen is introduced into their skin. People who do make a hive-like reaction in *their skin* demonstrate that they are capable of making atopic reactions and have the potential for such reactions *in their bronchial tubes.* The correlation between skin test reactivity to allergens and bronchial reactivity to the same allergens is not perfect. Still, it is reasonable to conclude (in a patient with asthmatic symptoms) that, in most instances, if dog allergen applied to the skin initiates the allergic cascade there, the same immunologic apparatus will be present in the bronchi, waiting to react when that same allergen is inhaled.

KEY POINT With allergy skin testing we acquire indirect evidence to answer the question: if a particular allergen is inhaled into the bronchial tubes, will it likely elicit an asthmatic reaction in that individual?

The advantages of allergy skin testing over direct allergen inhalation challenges are numerous. With skin testing, multiple allergens can be tested at once; asthmatic attacks are very rarely induced; and far less equipment and patient effort is needed for the testing procedure. At our Asthma Center, our routine practice is to test for approximately 20 common allergens in every patient undergoing allergy skin testing, using a standardized panel of commercially-available allergen extracts. We administer these antigens on the forearms of children and adults in two parallel rows on each arm. For each allergen tested, a single drop of the extract solution is placed on the surface of the skin and then the pin-like tip of a lancet (Fig. 7-2) is pierced through the drop, carrying antigen to superficial layers of the skin (approximately 2–3 mm below the surface). This method of allergy skin testing is called the "prick test."

If one fears a very strong allergic reaction (e.g., in a patient with a history of anaphylactic reactions to certain allergens), a "scratch test" allows introduction of an even smaller amount of antigen into the skin. In the scratch test method, a drop of allergen extract is placed on the surface of the skin and then the lancet is simply scratched lightly along the surface of the skin through the allergen. At the other extreme, if one strongly suspects allergic sensitivity but has not demonstrated it with the prick test method, one can proceed to an "intradermal" skin test. Here a larger amount of antigen is used to provoke an allergic response. The test is done with a technique identical to purified protein derivative (PPD) skin tests for tuberculosis. One-tenth of 1 cc of allergen extract is injected intradermally, and then one observes for an immediate wheal and flare reaction at the site.

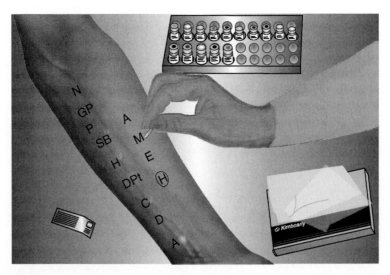

FIGURE 7-2 *Allergy skin testing using a lancet to perform prick tests on the subject's forearm.*

An allergic response results when IgE antibodies affixed to the surface of mast cells located within the skin recognize the allergen, bind to it, and then trigger explosive release of chemical mediators from the mast cells. Within a minute or two the patient may experience itching in the area of the allergic reaction. Then within approximately 10–20 minutes a hive develops. It may initially look like the reaction to a mosquito bite, but, depending on the intensity of the allergic reaction, it can grow quite large (up to a few centimeters in diameter) and assume irregularly-shaped extensions (pseudopods). Edema fluid and inflammatory cells create this bump in the skin. At the same time superficial blood vessels around this hive-like reaction dilate, causing surrounding redness of the skin (erythema). In official parlance, the hive is called a "wheal" and the surrounding erythema a "flare" (Fig. 7-3).

As noted, allergy skin tests are not perfect. False negative results (suggesting lack of allergic sensitivity when one actually does exist) can result if the patient has recently taken an antihistamine (that blocks the allergic reaction in the skin), if the allergen extract is faulty, or if the person performing the test fails to pierce the skin properly with the lancet. False positive results (suggesting allergic asthmatic sensitivity when one does not really exist) can occur when the patient's allergic response is limited to the skin (and possibly eyes and nose) but does not involve the lungs. In this case, the patient could accurately be said to have an allergy to the substance tested, but the allergen would not cause asthmatic symptoms when inhaled. Some people have skin that reacts to the physical trauma of every lancet prick with a wheal and flare reaction (dermatographism). In this instance a positive reaction is not specific for the allergen chosen.

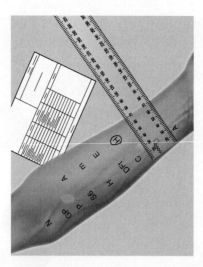

FIGURE 7-3   *Wheal and flare reactions to allergen prick tests.*

Control skin tests are used to detect some false negative and false positive results. Allergy skin testing usually includes pricking through a droplet containing histamine (positive control) and a droplet of normal saline (negative control). It is anticipated that everyone will make a cutaneous reaction to histamine; failure to do so might indicate faulty technique or prior use of antihistamines. At the other extreme, saline pricked into the skin should elicit no reaction. If one occurs, the patient has unusually sensitive skin and other positive skin test reactions do not give meaningful information about specific allergic sensitivities.

Despite its limitations, allergy skin testing can offer valuable information to the asthmatic patient (and his or her care provider). As one goes through life with an abnormal sensitivity of the bronchial tubes (asthma), it is a reasonable and common desire to want to know what the allergens are that can worsen one's asthmatic inflammation and can trigger one's asthmatic symptoms. No further detective work is needed when, for instance, every time the patient is around a cat, he develops chest tightness and wheezing and has to reach for his quick-relief bronchodilator. Other sensitivities, however, can be more subtle. "How can I be sure if I'm allergic to dust?" your patient asks. "Where I live, dust is everywhere." Another patient may have had allergic reactions to cats as a child but more recently has not experienced any asthmatic symptoms when visiting a friend with a pet cat. "Maybe I've outgrown my allergy to cats," she wonders. Allergy skin testing can help to answer these questions.

Allergy skin testing offers another, often powerful message: the visual image of seeing your own body reacting to a tiny amount of allergen with swelling, itching, and redness. The impact of watching your arm puff up within minutes of applying cat antigen just below the surface of the skin is probably far greater than general advice from your healthcare provider telling you that you are an atopic person and shouldn't risk bringing a cat into your home. "Imagine this reaction occurring throughout your bronchial tubes," we tell our patients. "The swelling would leave little room for the passage of air." The visual feed-back can be very compelling—a teachable moment achieved!

KEY POINT Prick tests can be used to assess allergic sensitivity to 20 or more allergens in one ses-sion. Watching an allergic, hive-like "wheal and flare" reaction emerge on your own skin—and feeling the associated pruritus—can provide a powerful message about the importance of similar allergic reactions potentially taking place in your bronchial tubes.

Adverse reactions to allergy skin testing are rare, but they do occur. Intense allergic reactions at the testing site can cause considerable itching and discom-fort. Very rarely, patients are so severely allergic that in response to minute amounts of allergen introduced into the skin, they develop a generalized, sys-temic reaction: anaphylaxis. It may manifest as light headedness, wheezing, or throat swelling. Treatment includes the immediate administration of epinephrine and may include antihistamines and systemic corticosteroids. It is our practice to obtain informed consent for allergy skin testing and to perform the testing in a setting where administration of epinephrine is immediately available.

Medications that interfere with skin test results (and need to be stopped in advance of testing if accurate results are to be obtained) include antihistamines and beta-blockers. We also avoid performing skin testing in those with wide-spread skin conditions, including severe eczema, that involve the testing site (usually the forearms).

Blood tests for allergy

As informative as allergy skin testing can be, it would be far simpler if one could just send one's patient for a blood test to determine his or her allergic sensitivities. If one reflects on the process, allergy skin testing seems quite primitive: grinding up cockroaches (for example), extracting and purifying the relevant antigen, preparing a solution containing the cockroach antigen to be placed in a droplet onto the skin, and then poking a needle through the liquid and watching for an allergic reaction to emerge in the skin. "Isn't there just some blood test that I can have?" A blood test would save on the costs of the skin testing procedure (staff, equipment, and allergen extracts) and avoid the risk, though rare, of a serious systemic allergic reaction resulting from the skin test itself. For many practitioners, it would bypass the need for referral to an allergist for the sole purpose of skin testing.

We can—and often do—measure in the blood the total level of IgE anti-body and the percentage (on the white blood cell differential count) or absolute number of eosinophils in the peripheral blood. Elevated IgE blood levels are common in allergic asthma, and some people with allergic asthma will have an elevated percentage and absolute number of eosinophils in the blood. The problem is that we are unable to measure what we would really like to know: the presence of IgE antibodies bound to mast cells and of eosinophils in the walls of the bronchial tubes. These proteins and cells circulating in the peripheral blood mirror only very loosely their presence in the tissues of the lungs. Normal blood levels do not exclude allergic sensitivities and the possibility of allergic reactions in the bronchi (or eyes, nose, or skin). At the same time, elevated blood eosinophil levels can be seen in other, nonatopic conditions: for instance, in certain infections, inflammatory conditions, cancers, and commonly in drug reactions.

Still, when we see an asthmatic patient with increased levels of IgE or with peripheral blood eosinophilia, we think allergy. But to what? Can blood testing tell us if the IgE proteins found in the blood have been formed in response to dogs, cats, mold, or dust mites? The answer is yes. With modern, highly sophisticated immunologic techniques, we can test the blood of our patients for the amount of IgE protein specific for cat allergen, the amount directed at dust mite allergen, and so on. Instead of a panel of skin tests to multiple allergens, we can request a panel of blood tests, each test looking for IgE proteins generated to a specific allergen.

The technique used for this blood testing is called a radioallergosorbent test and is abbreviated RAST. When compared with allergy skin tests, RASTs lack the same sensitivity. A patient may exhibit allergic reactions when assessed by skin tests that are not detected by RAST. With this drawback (and perhaps also their expense), they represent a simplified alternative to allergy skin testing and a very useful initial screening procedure. Negative results can be followed up with allergy skin testing, if there remains sufficient suspicion of allergic sensitivity.

KEY POINT   Blood tests (RASTs) are available that measure the amount of IgE protein in the blood directed at specific allergens. Though not as sensitive as skin testing, these blood tests are simpler to perform and carry none of the risk (though small) of adverse reactions involved with allergy skin tests.

COMMON ALLERGIC TRIGGERS OF ASTHMA AND THEIR AVOIDANCE

Allergens are potent triggers of asthma. We have had asthmatic patients who went from feeling perfectly healthy to desperately short of breath and riding in an ambulance on the way to the local emergency department within minutes of exposure to a dog or cat. Even more drastic evidence of the power of allergens comes from studies of fatal asthma. Scientists investigating a series of deaths from asthma in the

Midwest found that outdoor mold exposure (to the spores of Alternaria, common in the Midwest) had been the most likely triggering event in many of the cases.

And yet it would be an oversimplification to view the harmful effects of allergen exposure in the allergic asthmatic patient as being limited to setting off asthmatic attacks, like exercise or inhalation of smoke from a wood-burning stove. As discussed in Chap. 1, "Understanding and Teaching the Mechanisms of Asthma," allergens are also inciters of asthmatic inflammation, causing the airways to become more twitchy and swollen. Over time, chronic allergen exposure causes more severe asthma—perhaps in the absence of identifiable asthmatic attacks. For the cockroach-allergic child, living in a cockroach-infested home will probably not mean that he experiences an asthmatic attack each time that he enters the home. But it will mean, in the long run, that his asthma is likely to be more severe: he will suffer more asthmatic symptoms, require more medications to treat his asthma, miss more days from school, and have more disturbed nights' sleep than if he lived in a cockroach-free environment.

KEY POINT   Allergens not only trigger asthmatic attacks in allergic patients, they also stimulate worsened inflammation of the bronchi. The consequence can be worsened asthma control and need for more anti-asthmatic medications.

This particular example regarding cockroach allergy is relevant to the problem of inner-city asthma, as was made evident from the results of the National Cooperative Inner-City Asthma Study. As you know, children (and adults) living in our inner-cities have the highest rates of asthma morbidity and mortality in the nation. This multi-city research study of children between age 4–9 years, living in inner-city urban environments, explored potential reasons for this observation, based on allergen exposures in their homes. The investigators found that approximately 37% of the children had allergic sensitivities to cockroaches (by allergy skin testing). Of these cockroach-allergic children, approximately half lived in homes with high cockroach allergen content (as measured in samples of dust vacuumed from their bedrooms). And it was these children—with allergic sensitivity and high levels of allergen exposure—who had the most severe asthma in the study. They had the most days with asthmatic symptoms, the most unscheduled visits to their healthcare providers for asthma, the most hospitalizations for asthma, and the highest rate of canceled plans for their parents because of their asthma.

The implications of this study—as important as they are for managing asthma among inner-city residents—extend far beyond cockroach allergy. One could just as well substitute into the equation cat sensitivity and cat exposure or dust mite sensitivity and dust exposure. The lesson is that on-going exposure to allergens to which an asthmatic patient is allergic fuels worsened asthma. The message to the cat-allergic cat-lover is no less clear than to the parents (and landlord) in the cockroach-infested apartment. Allergen avoidance will not only lessen your exposure to a trigger of asthmatic attacks; it also has the potential to improve your asthma control overall.

Dust mites

It would be easy to dismiss dust as a common irritant, like smoke or air pollution, something that merely irritates hypersensitive airways. But in temperate climates there live within house dust tiny, microscopic creatures known to entomologists as *dermatophagoides* (most vividly translated to mean "skin eaters") and known more commonly as house dust mites. You may have seen photomicrographs of these minute creatures; magnified greatly, they appear quite fearsome (Fig. 7-4). In fact, they are, of course, invisible to the naked eye, approximately 1/3 mm in length. You would have no way of knowing that each night you are sharing your bed with millions of these microscopic critters.

The remarkable fact is that throughout the world, human beings with atopy commonly make IgE antibodies directed at a protein produced by these

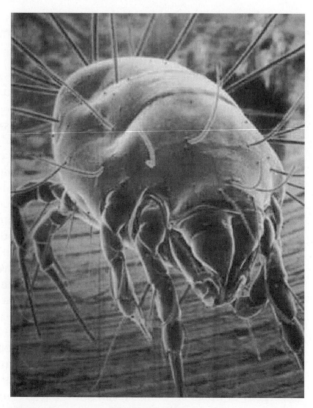

FIGURE 7-4 *Microscopic image of house dust mite.*

house dust mites. To be precise, we humans make allergic reactions to a protein within the fecal droppings of house dust mites. Why this is so is unknown— there is nothing harmful to us about this protein—but it has been speculated that the protein bears sufficient similarity to one made by a common parasite that our bodies simply confuse the two. This is the essence of allergy: a biologic *misfiring* of an immune system response effective against worms and parasites misdirected at harmless substances in our environment.

Because allergy to this protein is so common, medical providers have taken an interest in the otherwise obscure topic of the "life and habits" of the house dust mite. Here is what we know. Mites feed on human (and pet) scale (sloughed skin). As a result, they can be found in particular abundance in places where we leave behind the dead, most superficial layer of our skin: in our mattresses, pillows, box springs, carpeting, and upholstered furniture. No surprise, then, that the highest concentrations of dust mite antigen are found in the dust from our bedrooms, a place where children (and most adults) spend 8 or more hours each day. Other dust and dust mite collectors are stuffed animals, curtains and drapes, and of course those "dust bunnies" that build up in corners over time. Dust mites thrive in warm, humid air. They are less prevalent at high altitude (where the humidity is low), in the desert, or in climates cold all year round. An interesting observation is that asthma becomes more prevalent when people move from rural to urban environments. One corollary of this migration is sleeping on mattresses, having carpeting on the floors, and spending more time indoors—that is, greater exposure to house dust mites.

KEY POINT   Dust mites are living creatures that collect in places where we leave our sloughed superficial skin (especially in mattresses, pillows, box springs, and carpeting). They thrive on relatively high humidity.

Dust mite antigen is relatively heavy; it settles out of the air quickly and accumulates on surfaces. In a room left undisturbed, there is relatively little dust mite antigen in the air. But shuffle across the carpet, plop down onto the mattress, or start sweeping with a broom, and allergen soon fills the air. Of course, very young children and toddlers do this best—shuffle along at an altitude of just 2–3 feet above the carpeting. This observation that dust mite allergen settles quickly out of the air has been offered as one explanation why the use of room air filters, including the highly-effective HEPA (high-efficiency particulate air) filters, fail to alter dust mite allergen exposure in the home.

The single most effective intervention to reduce exposure to dust mite allergen in the home appears to be the use of zippered, allergen-impermeable wraps for the pillows, mattress, and box springs. These tightly-woven synthetic fabrics are impermeable to the dust mite and dust mite antigens. Now when you lie down on the mattress, the offending antigen is sealed inside. The fabric used for these mattress and pillow covers is relatively soft and pliable; it does not at all feel like "sleeping on plastic." In addition, conventional sheets and pillow cases are used over the allergy-proof wraps. More human scale and consequently dust mites will collect on the sheets and pillow cases, but by washing them regularly (e.g., weekly) in hot water (recommended washing temperature is >130°) the mites will be killed and the offending allergen destroyed.

Allergy-proof mattress encasings cost approximately $30–$40. They can be found at some large departmental stores and at any of a number of online allergy supply companies. Many medical insurance plans will cover the cost of these items if they are prescribed along with a letter indicating their medical necessity.

At one time, recommendations for dust mite management included treating carpeting with a powder to kill the dust mites (benzyl benzoate [Acarosan]) or with a solution of tannic acid to render the dust mite antigen inactive. Although commercial products are still available for this purpose, there routine use is no longer recommended. Their effectiveness has been called into question; frequent applications are needed; and some patients experience worsened asthmatic symptoms in response to these chemicals. The best option, if available, is the removal of carpeting and use of small area rugs, if needed.

As noted, dust mites require relatively high humidity to grow. In wintertime, the ambient humidity falls as the air temperature falls. Many people feel that the dry air is uncomfortable and wonder if it would be better for their asthma if they ran a humidifier during the winter months. The answer is no. Keep the relative humidity less than 50% to inhibit dust mite growth. For the thoroughly compulsive patient, devices that measure ambient humidity, called hygrometers, are widely available. We view running a humidifier like regular feeding of dust mites and discourage it among our dust-mite allergic patients. If the patient complains of intolerably dry nasal passages with crusting, it is better for him to use a nasal saline spray rather than to humidify an entire room or house. In the summertime, air conditioners and dehumidifiers help to reduce the indoor humidity.

Frequent vacuuming would seem to offer useful protection to the dust-mite allergic patient, but there is a catch. Conventional vacuum cleaners use vacuum bags that are relatively porous; dust mite antigen is suctioned up, passes through the collection bag, and is blown into the air via the vacuum's exhaust system. What is needed is a vacuum bag that traps the antigen inside. These are commercially available via allergy supply companies. Probably most effective are the vacuum cleaners equipped with HEPA filters, which trap particles as small as 1–2 microns in diameter (1 micron = 1/1000th of a millimeter), including dust mites and dust mite antigen. If your only option is dusting and sweeping, use a wet cloth and wet mop to reduce the dispersion of allergen into the air. Some people wear a filtering medical face mask when cleaning.

One other trick: keep your child's stuffed animals dust mite-free by periodically either washing them (if washable) or putting them in the freezer compartment for a day or two! The latter effectively kills the mites, but it does not immediately remove the allergen.

Methods for dust mite avoidance include allergy-proof encasings for the mattress, pillows, and box springs; minimizing use of carpets in the house; maintaining relatively low indoor humidity; vacuuming with special filtering vacuum bags; and washing or freezing a child's stuffed animals.

House pets

Pet cats and dogs are everywhere in our society. More than half of all American households own a cat, dog, or both. And it's a rare parent whose children have not pleaded—ever so convincingly—that without a pet cat or dog of their own, their lives will be empty and unfulfilled. From this desperate desire among children and adults alike to bring a lovable, furry pet into the home come many myths about pet ownership—all false. "We'll always keep the cat or dog outside." "How about a hairless cat? It won't cause allergies because it doesn't have fur." "I'm only allergic to long-haired dogs; a short-haired dog won't bother me." "We'll get a bichon; I was told that that's a nonallergenic breed." "I've read somewhere that having lots of cats at home is good for asthma."

The relationship between cats in the home and the development of asthma in the children of atopic parents (who are genetically at risk for developing asthma) is complex and a matter of on-going medical research. Some evidence suggests that while having one cat in the house may increase the risk of a child's going on to develop asthma, having multiple cats may actually decrease this risk. What is certain is that if a child or an adult already has allergic asthma, having a cat in the house is a risky business. The chance of being or becoming allergic to the cat is high, and cat allergen is one of the most potent of all stimuli of allergic reactions, as any cat-allergic patient will tell you. We frequently hear stories of allergic reactions to cat antigen from exposure in rooms which haven't seen the cat for days, or reactions to antigen brought to school on the clothing of cat-owning classmates.

The protein to which we humans make allergic reactions is produced by cats primarily in the oil-secreting sebaceous glands of their skin; it is also found in their saliva (which is then licked all over their bodies) and in their urine. It is a *sticky* allergen that clings to furniture, clothing, and carpeting. Measurements of cat allergen have been made in homes where a cat was kept as a pet but no longer resides there. The question was: how long does the cat allergen remain detectable? In carpeted homes, cat allergen was found for as many as 6 months later. In addition, once disturbed from surfaces, cat allergen stays airborne for hours. As you recall, this property is different from the behavior of dust mite allergen, and it makes cat allergen a potential target to be removed from the air with room HEPA filters.

Our advice to allergic individuals who are considering obtaining a pet cat is: don't. Even if you are not allergic to cat allergen now, there remains the possibility that with repeated exposure you will develop sensitivity over time. And it is emotionally far more difficult to separate from a beloved pet than not to form a strong relationship in the first place.

Our advice to those with allergic asthma who already own a cat is predictable: try to find another home for your cat. It's good advice that is rarely heeded. No longer do we recommend bathing the cat weekly to reduce the amount of allergen on its fur. Washing the cat leads to only modest reductions in the amount of detectable allergen; the benefit is short-lived and likely inconsequential; and the cat-bathing experience is traumatic to the cat and human alike. When a pet cat enters a room, the amount of allergen in the room increases several-fold. Therefore, keeping the cat (or dog) out of the bedroom can help a little bit, as can a room HEPA filter used to remove cat allergen when it is airborne.

Although, in general, cats seem to cause more trouble for asthmatics than dogs, animal sensitivity is highly variable from one individual to another; and dog allergen can send a person to the hospital with a severe asthmatic attack just as readily as cat allergen. The offending protein has been less well characterized for dogs than for cats. It is found in dog dander (the material collected when one brushes the surface of your pet). It is present in all breeds of dogs, large and small, with fur or hair, short-haired and long-haired, without significant differences from one breed to the next. There is no such thing as a nonallergenic or hypo-allergenic breed of dog; it is wishful thinking. As for cats, the best advice is that if you have allergic asthma, don't get a dog. If you have a dog, keep it out of the bedroom (or out of the house) and use a HEPA filter in your bedroom and living areas to reduce allergen exposure. And remember: gold fish, iguanas, and pet turtles are all nonallergenic!

KEY POINT   A nonallergenic breed of cat or dog does not exist.

Indoor mold

We've all seen mold growing in our homes. It appears on too-old bread and decaying fruits and vegetables. It stains moist wallpaper, grout between tiles in the shower stall, and leather products left in a dark closet. We recognize it by the discoloration that it causes and by its musty smell. "Mildew" is a popular expression for mold. Mold is a category of plant life with many different species, including aspergillus, actinomyces, cladosporium, penicillium, and alternaria. These microscopic plants—a subcategory of fungi—grow into visible colonies, and they release spores (as other plants release seeds) for the purpose of propagation. It is these airborne mold spores that elicit allergic reactions.

Recently, much interest (and some paranoia) has focused on "black mold." In fact, many different types of mold can grow into black-colored colonies; those with black color are no more toxigenic or allergenic than any other type. Our schools and places of employment are frequently buildings with centralized ventilation systems for heating and air-conditioning. Mold growing within the ventilation tubing can release spores that are then blown repeatedly into our classrooms or work spaces. In our experiences, this is a potential but very rare cause of asthmatic exacerbations or worsened asthma control. (By contrast, a study of allergic sensitivities to *outdoor* molds, especially alternaria and cladosporium, conducted among more than 1000 adults across three continents, found that the presence of mold allergy was associated with more severe asthma.)

Mold thrives on moisture. To reduce mold growth in one's home, one needs to reduce the indoor humidity and avoid areas of standing water. Air conditioners and dehumidifiers help to keep down indoor humidity. Areas to check for trapped water include under the kitchen sink, in bathrooms, and in underground basements. A big offender is the basement that periodically becomes flooded with water during heavy or prolonged rains. The carpeting gets wet and even after its surface dries, moisture remains trapped under the carpeting (especially over a cement floor). Water from a leaky roof can get trapped behind walls; north-facing walls are the most common offenders because they get the least amount of (drying) sunshine. A quick check of the pipes above the furnace will provide adequate assessment regarding mold growth in the forced hot-air ventilation system of one's home. In the absence of visible mold growth, no additional investigation is necessary.

KEY POINT   Indoor mold thrives on moisture. Keeping the indoor relative humidity low with dehumidifiers and air-conditioners helps to discourage mold growth.

To rid the home of mold, one will need to take up and clean the carpeting from the once-flooded basement. Check to see that the filter on your furnace or air conditioner is free of mold contamination. Visible mold on the floor, in the bathroom, or underneath the sink can be readily killed using a solution of dilute bleach (bleach mixed 1:1 with water). Take the time to fix those leaky faucets or roof tiles, and maintain a low indoor humidity. For additional information about indoor air quality in general and indoor mold exposure in particular, a useful website to review is maintained by the Environmental Protection Agency at www.epa.gov/iaq/ (see www.epa.gov/mold/moldresources.html).

Cockroaches and other indoor pests

Cockroaches in the home are a fact of modern life, particularly in urban settings (Fig. 7-5). What has emerged in recent years is evidence that the more exposure that one has to cockroach antigen in the home, the more likely one is to develop allergic sensitization to the antigen (as demonstrated by positive skin tests or measurement of specific IgE in the blood); that repeated exposure appears to be a risk factor for the development of asthma in persons who have become sensitized;

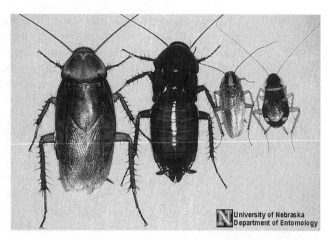

FIGURE 7-5 *From left to right, American, Oriental, German, and brown-branded cockroaches. Reproduced with permission from the Department of Entomology, University of Nebraska-Lincoln (http://entomology.unl.edu/images/cockroaches/cockroaches.htm).*

and that in people with established asthma and cockroach allergy, living in a home with high cockroach antigen levels leads to worse asthma control and more frequent and severe asthmatic attacks. All of these observations may seem intuitively obvious, but in fact it was not until the early-1960s that techniques were developed to measure cockroach antigen. Evidence of the importance of cockroach antigen emerged in the decade thereafter. Prior to this time, the role of cockroach allergy in asthma development and asthma severity was unknown. This fact raises the possibility (and even likelihood) that other environmental allergens of importance are yet to be discovered.

The cockroach seems to be as hardy an insect as it is an unappealing one. It survives on our untidiness: food left on kitchen surfaces and crumbs on the floor. Other food sources include paint, wallpaper paste, and book bindings. Its water sources include sweating pipes, standing water, and any moist items or areas in the home. Cockroaches find hiding places in cracks and crevices, cardboard boxes, stored newspapers, and grocery bags. Reliable evidence for cockroach infestation is the patient's report of sighting of the insects in the home. For every one seen, many hundreds are present in hiding places.

Even after the last cockroach has been killed, cockroach antigen is left behind. It is found in their shed outer coverings (cuticles), urine, feces, and eggs. It can be measured in our house dust and bedding. We have previously mentioned the National Cooperative Inner-City Asthma Study. In order to participate in this study, families had to reside in a census tract in which at least 20% of the households had incomes below the federal poverty level. Dust samples were collected from the homes of children with asthma living in these inner-city environments. The results were dramatic: what were considered high levels of cockroach antigen were found in the bedroom dust of 50% of the homes (and detectable antigen in 85%).

KEY POINT   Cockroach allergy is associated with poverty and is common among residents in the inner cities. Teaching about and helping with cockroach extermination is part of the role of asthma educators working with inner-city populations.

Ridding the home of cockroaches is a formidable task. Most successful is the application of pesticide by professional exterminators. Successful treatments lead to measurable decreases in the cockroach population within 2 weeks, maximal benefit at 1 month, and eradication that typically lasts for at least 3–6 months. For more minor infestations, baited traps are sold commercially and can be set out safely in the kitchen and other highly-trafficked rooms. Once the cockroaches have been eliminated, the challenge is removal of the residual antigen; extensive cleaning and vacuuming are necessary. At the same time, it is worthwhile discouraging their return: cleaning counters, tables, and floors after food preparation and eating; discarding rather than storing papers, boxes, and paper bags; and eliminating obvious water sources, including bottles left open and puddles on the floor.

The National Cooperative Inner-City Asthma Study also addressed allergy to rats and mice among children living in our inner cities. In this study caregivers for the children were asked about mice or rats in their homes; an astounding and dismaying 40% reported having seen either mice, rats, or both. We know from the experiences of animal handlers working in medical research laboratories that regular exposure to mice and rats can be a powerful sensitizer. People without any prior history of asthma can develop mice or rat allergy and the new onset of asthma after months or years of repeated exposure (a form of occupational asthma). It is plausible that less intense but daily exposure in the home would cause atopic children to develop allergy to mice and rats. In fact, approximately 20% of the children had positive skin test reactions to mouse antigen, and a similar percentage was sensitized to rat antigen. Of these two, rat allergy combined with exposure to rat allergen in the home correlated with increased asthma symptoms and asthmatic attacks. It is apparent that for the nation's poor living in the inner city, asthma management begins with creating healthy living environments and asthma advocacy begins to merge with calls for social and economic justice.

Pollens and outdoor mold

You know some asthmatic patients whose symptoms vary dramatically according to the seasons. "Every spring," they say, "when the flowers and trees start blooming, that's when my asthma gets bad." Or, "Autumn is my worst season. I can't wait until the first frost; that's when my asthma will quiet down again." Histories such as these suggest allergic sensitivities to pollens and outdoor mold, which have strong seasonal variation in their presence. You can follow the pollen and mold spore counts as they rise and fall between March and

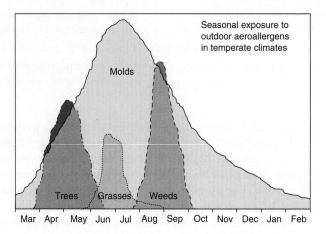

FIGURE 7-6   *Seasonal pattern of plant pollination in New England.*

November on various websites (such as one maintained by the American Academy of Allergy, Asthma, and Immunology: www.aaaai.com, click on "Pollen Counts") and many news broadcasts. The accompanying figure gives a broad overview of exposure in climates like New England (Fig. 7-6). In the spring, think tree pollens; in midsummer, grass pollens; and in the fall, weed pollens. Outdoor mold spores are produced from March until November, peaking in midsummer.

Many trees, grasses, and weeds propagate by producing pollen granules that are carried by the wind to fertilize the female plants of the species. At times pollen production and release can be so prolific that we find surfaces, outdoors and in, covered with a thin layer of green powder. It is said that one ragweed plant can make a billion pollen granules each season, leading to millions of tons of ragweed pollen produced across the North American continent each year. Other plants, like flowering plants in our gardens, have their pollen carried from one plant to the next by bees and other insects. As a result, humans in general do not become allergic to roses, lilies, phlox, and the like.

There is a diurnal variation to pollen counts in the air. They are highest first thing in the morning (5–10 a.m.) and lowest in the afternoon or after a rain. Dry, hot, windy days are best for distributing pollen grains, worst for pollen allergy sufferers.

Outdoor mold, to which allergic sensitivity is common, is found wherever living plant material is left to decay. Mold has an important role in the "circle of life," promoting the decomposition of dead and dying plant material, whereby it returns to become a part of the soil. It is present widely throughout nature, found in any wooded area, on the fallen leaves of autumn, in brown spots on our plants, and in our mulch and compost piles. Between June and early fall, the release of mold spores into the air is at its peak (Fig. 7-7).

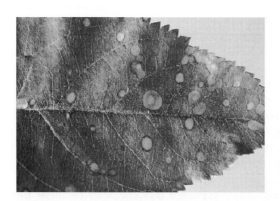
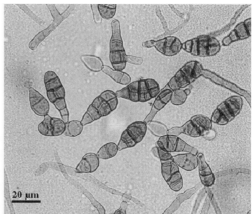

FIGURE 7-7   *Mold colonies growing on plant leaves (left) and photomicrograph of a mold spore (right). Left image: photograph by Turner B. Sutton; reproduced with permission from Mid-Atlantic Orchard Monitoring Guide, NRAES-75, published by NRAES, the Natural Resource, Agriculture, and Engineering Service, Cooperative Extension, 152 Riley-Robb Hall, Ithaca, New York 14853–5701, U.S.A. Right image: reproduced with permission from Mycology Online, Department of Molecular and Biomedical Science, The University of Adelaide, Australia (www.mycology.adelaide.edu.au/gallery/ photos/alternaria02.html).*

KEY POINT   Plant pollen and outdoor mold spores are causes of seasonal allergies. In the Northeast, tree pollens peak in the spring; grass pollens in midsummer; and weed pollens in the fall. Outdoor mold exposure is highest in midsummer and continues until late fall.

As previously mentioned, mold allergy and mold exposure (the latter is inevitable with life outdoors) is associated with more severe asthma and has been implicated as a contributing factor in a series of deaths from asthma. The same is not true for allergy to plant pollens. For some reason, pollen is a much greater troublemaker for those with seasonal allergic rhinitis and conjunctivitis than it is for asthma. It may be that the size of the pollen grains is such that they are primarily filtered out by the nose and pharynx before they can reach the bronchial tubes.

A curious exception to this rule was discovered when scientists sought to understand the sudden increase in asthmatic exacerbations observed after thunderstorms in some parts of the world. It seems that moisture causes release of fractured particles of ryegrass pollen and that wind conditions during thunderstorms favor distribution of these particles at ground level. The sudden peak in asthmatic exacerbations after thunderstorms is thought to be the result of allergy to ryegrass pollen. There's a bit of asthma trivia for you!

Complete avoidance of pollens and outdoor mold is impossible; we do not recommend living indoors from first bloom to first frost with the windows and doors all closed! Things that can be done to reduce exposure might include the following: avoid exercising outdoors in the early morning, take your daily walk or run in the afternoon or early evening instead; after being outdoors for a long time, shower and change clothes, because pollen will stick to your hair and clothing; if available, use air conditioning in your home and car, it will allow you to keep the windows closed and to filter the outdoor air; dry your clothes in the dryer, not on an outdoor clothesline; and use a room air filter (HEPA filter) to help remove pollen and mold spores from the indoor air.

Nonallergic, irritant exposures

In this chapter we have focused on identifying allergic sensitivities and on ways to help our asthmatic patients avoid allergens to which they are sensitive. At the same time, we do not wish to downplay the importance of nonallergic, irritant exposures and the benefits that can result from their avoidance as well. Cigarette smoking is a perfect example of the latter, and a shockingly common one. In some studies of inner-city asthma, as many as 30% of adults with asthma smoke cigarettes. Likewise second-hand smoke exposure is a common problem for children growing up with asthma. In the National Cooperative Inner-CityAsthma Study, 48% of the households in which the participating children lived had at least one cigarette smoker. And of course cigarette smoking is by no means confined to minority populations or the inner cities. When in doubt, ask if your patient or anyone living with him or her smokes cigarettes.

KEY POINT   Ask if your patient or someone living with him or her smokes cigarettes. Environmental tobacco smoke can aggravate asthma—unnecessarily.

There is some evidence that growing up in a household with cigarette smokers increases a child's risk of developing asthma. For a child with established asthma, environmental tobacco smoke exposure (as "passive smoking" or second-hand smoke exposure is now called) clearly worsens asthma control. Here a simple intervention can have a significant impact. If the adult caregiver quits smoking (not simple) or limits smoking to outdoors only, the child's asthma will tend to improve. And for the adult asthmatic who smokes, the dangers are myriad: worse asthma control, development of irreversible obstructive lung disease (emphysema), and all the other well-known and disastrous potential consequences such as lung cancer, throat cancer, heart attacks and strokes, and the like.

Some have suggested that inhaling marijuana might be therapeutic for asthma, causing airway smooth muscle—and just about everything else—to relax. However, marijuana often carries with it impurities from the soil, including fungi such as aspergillus. As asthma specialists, we view marijuana use as a risk factor for the development of allergic bronchopulmonary aspergillosis (a complication of asthma previously mentioned in Chap. 4, "Treating Asthma in the Ambulatory Setting"). And while we are on the topic of illicit drug use and airway irritants, crack cocaine may top the list in terms of potential for severe airway reactions. Whether due to cocaine itself or impurities mixed with it, inhaled cocaine can cause severe airway injury (as well as lung hemorrhage). Emergency physicians and intensivists are familiar with severe bouts of respiratory failure requiring intubation and mechanical ventilation due to cocaine-induced severe asthmatic attacks.

Indoor air pollutants for our asthmatic patients to avoid include smoke from fireplaces or wood-burning stoves; fumes from cleaning agents, oil paints, and other chemicals; and dust from sanding or other household construction projects. Preventive strategies include: staying away; ensuring good ventilation; and wearing a surgical face mask when particulate matter is in the air. Some patients find that strong odors and scents from perfumes and colognes aggravate their asthma; avoidance and a strong measure of diplomacy are recommended.

Outdoor air pollution—which contains a mixture of potentially harmful components, including ozone, nitrogen dioxide, and very small particulates—poses a concern to people with asthma. It is an easy target when trying to explain the rise in asthma prevalence and severity in recent decades—but probably incorrect. Federal clean air acts and automobile emission control standards led to improvements in air quality at a time when asthma cases increased substantially in this country. Still, on a smog-filled summer's day, as ozone levels rise, so do emergency room visits and hospitalizations for asthma. The irritant gases and particulates in air pollution can stimulate inflammatory reactions in the airways, and they may act synergistically with allergen exposure. That is, some evidence indicates that inhaled allergens may precipitate more severe reactions in persons whose airways have already been inflamed by irritant gases. Children and athletes may be especially vulnerable. They are most likely to increase their level of ventilation with running and sports, thereby bringing larger amounts of air pollutants to the lower airways.

Finding an overall strategy that is practical

As a well-informed asthma educator, you have come to know a lot about allergens and techniques for allergen avoidance, and perhaps more about the living habits of the house dust mite and cockroach than you had ever thought desirable! This knowledge can prove highly valuable to your patients. Many of them will turn to you for help with their asthma, seeking a solution that does not involve their taking more medication. There must be something, they suspect, in their home or workplace or school that is causing their asthma to be so active, and they are ready to work hard to make things better for themselves or their children with asthma. "Should I change my diet?" "Would exercise help?" "Maybe if I dusted and vacuumed more often."

Armed with the information in this chapter, you can steer your patients in the right direction. "No," you can tell them, "that sugar-free diet or yeast-free diet that you heard about from a friend will not likely be helpful for your (or your child's) asthma." "Regular exercise is good for you—in many ways—but you should not expect it to cause your lung function (peak flow) to improve."

And "Dusting and vacuuming regularly can help if you or your child is dust-mite allergic; and I have some suggestions for how to clean your house without putting more dust into the air."

We also want to emphasize that you need to make "real-world" recommendations, suggestions that fit with the lifestyles of your patients. Remember that you are an asthma educator, not an allergen-avoidance missionary. We need to temper our zeal for helping others with the realization that our patients live complicated, multifaceted lives. They often have many other demands on their time and mental energy, whether financial constraints, psychosocial stresses, work-related demands, family crises, or other medical problems. In this context, for example, showering and changing clothes after coming indoors during the summer months may not be a high priority for the pollen-allergic patient. Taking up the carpeting in the child's bedroom and fixing the floor beneath may not be feasible, despite his or her dust mite allergy.

KEY POINT   Be careful not to overwhelm your patient with recommendations for too many or too complex changes to make in their homes and in their lifestyles. Like you, they lead complicated, multifaceted lives, of which asthma is only one aspect. Strategize with your patient and select key issues on which to focus for maximal gain.

To have the greatest impact, it may be worthwhile strategizing together with your patient. What is doable; what is not? Prioritize together, starting with the major allergic exposures and the interventions likely to have the biggest impact. If cockroach infestation is the key concern, you may have to become a public health and housing advocate. If getting rid of the pet cat is not a possibility—any more than sending off one of our children to live elsewhere would be—then move on to other options: keeping the cat out of the bedroom and perhaps obtaining a free-standing HEPA filter for the bedroom and main living area. In the end, remember that we work in a "helping profession" and need to find a way to be helpful without being confrontational or overwhelming. We need to bring support with our allergy-avoidance advice, not criticism or discouragement—and so ends this homily!

INTERVENTIONS THAT WORK

"Show me the data," you say (appropriately). "I admit that it *sounds* like a good idea, but where is the evidence that all of this time and money spent reducing allergen and irritant exposures in the home make a difference? Is there any convincing evidence that I can share with my patients?"

Multidimensional interventions

Until recently, many of the reports published in the medical literature were quite discouraging. A controlled trial of allergy-proof encasings for the mattress and pillows showed no benefit in terms of asthma control compared to control (conventional cotton) materials. HEPA filters failed to reduce dust mite allergy symptoms. Cockroach extermination and allergen removal seemed an insurmountable task in multiresident dwellings. All of this pessimism evaporated, however, with the report of the federally-funded Inner-City Asthma Study in 2004, which appeared in the *New England Journal of Medicine*. This group of investigators evaluated the effectiveness of a multifaceted, home-based, environmental intervention for children with asthma living in the inner-city. Their study, a randomized, controlled clinical trial, dramatically demonstrated the worth of the intervention. It is worthwhile reviewing the study in detail.

KEY POINT   Yes, there is evidence that a systematic effort at reducing allergic exposures in the home can improve asthma outcomes, even in the most challenging (poor, inner-city) homes. It is worthwhile knowing one particular study, called the Inner-City Asthma Study, in detail.

For this large-scale trial, the investigators recruited 937 atopic children with asthma, aged 5 to 11 years, from seven major cities across the U.S. Children were randomly assigned to an intervention group or a control group. The intervention, which lasted for 1 year, included both an educational component and help reducing exposure to indoor allergens and environmental tobacco—the work of asthma educators! In the intervention group, an intervention team taught the child's caregiver about the importance of allergens and irritants in aggravating the child's asthma. They then introduced an "environmental intervention plan," an important part of which was the creation in the child's home of an environmentally-safe sleeping zone.

Supplies that were made available as part of the intervention were:

- allergen-impermeable covers to be placed on the mattress, box spring, and pillows of the child's bed;
- a vacuum cleaner equipped with a HEPA filter;
- a free-standing room HEPA filter for the child's bedroom, if the child was exposed to environmental tobacco smoke, had a cat or dog with evidence of allergy to it, or had allergy to mold;
- professional pest control for children allergic to and exposed to cockroaches.

This package of interventions worked. The amount of dust mite antigen in the children's beds and bedroom floors declined; less cockroach antigen was found on the children's bedroom floors. These improvements correlated with fewer complications of asthma: fewer hospitalizations and fewer unscheduled visits for asthma. As is often the case in clinical trials such as this one, the children in the control group also improved over the course of the study. Perhaps being told that your child is participating in a study regarding the importance of allergens and cigarette smoke on his or her asthma is enough to lead some caregivers to make changes in their homes for the better. However, as shown in the accompanying figure (Fig. 7-8), the group of children assigned at random to the intervention group did better than the children in the control group, and significantly so. They had fewer days with asthma symptoms, fewer nights with lost sleep, fewer days of school missed due to asthma, and fewer unscheduled asthma-related visits to an emergency department or clinic.

Perhaps most remarkable, many of the observed benefits extended for the full 2 years of the observation period, even though the intervention team was only active in the homes during the first year. This finding suggests that the intervention, once made, is sustainable through the efforts of the families alone. During the 2-year period, children living in homes receiving the environmental modification intervention would have had, on average, 34 fewer days with wheezing compared with children in the control group. Of interest, this magnitude of improvement is similar to what one might find if one group had been randomly assigned to receive inhaled corticosteroids and the other not.

The authors of this report speculated as to why their efforts at environmental control had succeeded whereas those of others had not. They credited two particular

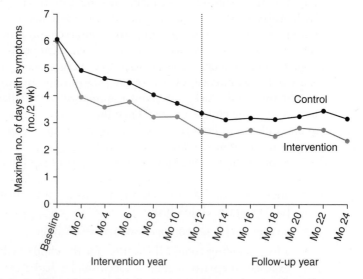

FIGURE 7-8   *In this randomized trial of a systematic intervention to reduce allergen exposure in the homes of children living in our inner-cities, the intervention achieved a significant reduction in the number of days with symptoms (compared with the control group, which received no such environmental control measures). The benefit from the intervention persisted during the subsequent year of follow-up. Reproduced with permission from Morgan WJ, et al., Results of a home-based environmental intervention among urban children with asthma.* N Engl J Med 2004; 351:1068–80. *Copyright 2004 Massachusetts Medical Society. All rights reserved.*

aspects of their intervention. First, it was multifaceted, not limited to a single allergen or asthmatic trigger. Allergy-proof dust mite covers may fail to improve asthma as a single intervention if other aspects of dust mite control are not addressed and if other important allergic and irritant exposures are not simultaneously modified. Second, an effective model was used to affect behavioral change. Members of the intervention team modeled the desired behaviors for the asthmatic children's caregivers, had the caregivers rehearse the behaviors, and then verified that the caregivers had successfully mastered these behaviors. They offered encouragement about reasonable outcomes to expect and their ability to achieve them.

As a minor footnote, we would note that the stand-alone air filters chosen for this study were HEPA filters, not ozone-generating electrostatic precipitators or ionizers. The latter, including the enormously popular Ionic Breeze filter, are of limited effectiveness; and their release of ozone into the indoor environment is potentially harmful. Their use has been discouraged by the California Air Resources Board and Consumers Union, among others.

Home visits

An integral aspect of home allergen remediation in the Inner-City Asthma Study was the home visit. The asthma educators (intervention team) visited the subjects' homes and made assessments of allergen and irritant exposures in person. They did not rely solely on the reports of allergen exposure from the children's care providers. Although not of proven utility based on randomized, controlled clinical trials, home visits are believed by many practitioners to add great value to asthma disease management initiatives. "One inspection," one might argue, "is worth a thousand words."

The U.S. Environmental Protection Agency makes available on its website a guide to initiating a program of asthma home visits, called "Implementing an Asthma Home Visit Program: 10 Steps to Help Health Plans Get Started." To quote from this document, "Home visits are one way to give enrollees the tools they need to address their asthma effectively as part of a comprehensive disease management program incorporating medical and environmental management techniques." The guide was developed "with input from seven health care organizations that offer asthma home visits as part of their comprehensive asthma management programs. It incorporates their experiences establishing and operating home visit programs, and reflects their belief in the value, both to the enrollee and to the health insurer, of such programs." This document can be found at the website, www.epa.gov/asthma/publications.html.

Self-Assessment Questions

QUESTION 1

In which of the following patients would you anticipate a greater likelihood of asthma compared to the general public?

1. Allergy to penicillin
2. Sensitivity to aspirin (because of a history of bleeding ulcers)
3. Having "hay fever" (seasonal allergic rhinitis and conjunctivitis)
4. History of farmer's lung disease (hypersensitivity pneumonitis to moldy hay)
5. Angioedema in response to the angiotensin converting enzyme inhibitor, captopril

QUESTION 2

Atopy refers to the tendency to make allergic reactions characterized by immunoglobulin E production and mast cell activation. Which of the following diseases is not part of the spectrum of disorders seen in atopic individuals?

1. Asthma
2. Eczema
3. Allergic rhinitis
4. Hives
5. Chronic bronchitis

QUESTION 3

Which of the following statements regarding the association of asthma and allergy is correct?

1. "By definition, having asthma means being allergic to something in the environment."
2. "Most children with asthma have positive allergy skin tests to one or more allergens."
3. "Most infants with atopic dermatitis (eczema) go on to develop asthma."
4. "Allergic sensitivities are uncommon among adult asthmatics over age 30 years."
5. "Asthmatics who have not developed allergy to animals by age 12 won't develop allergy subsequently."

QUESTION 4

A 15-year-old asthmatic patient reports to you that every time she pets the cat at her friend's house, she develops sneezing and a "drippy nose." She also gets small hives at the site where the cat licks her. She wonders whether her asthma would get worse if she adopted a cat into her home and asks you about skin testing to help clarify the matter. Which of her following assumptions about allergy skin testing to cat allergen is correct?

1. A positive skin test reaction will give evidence of her allergy to cats but will not prove that her asthma will get worse with cat exposure.
2. A negative skin test reaction means that she is not allergic to cats.
3. A negative skin test reaction means that although she is allergic to her friend's cat, she is not allergic to all cats.
4. She can use the size of the skin test reaction to cat allergen to assess how allergic to cats she is.
5. The skin test will be positive regardless of her own allergic sensitivity to cats because she has been around cats during the week before testing.

QUESTION 5

Blood tests (RASTs) can be used to test for allergic sensitivities. They can measure:

1. The amount of a particular allergen (e.g., dust mite allergen) in the blood.
2. The amount of immunoglobulin E antibody directed at a particular allergen (e.g., dust mite allergen).
3. The amount of any antibody (IgG, IgM, or IgE) directed at a particular allergen (e.g., dust mite allergen).
4. The percentage of allergy cells (called eosinophils) formed to react to a particular allergen (e.g., dust mite allergen).
5. All of the allergens to which an individual is sensitive.

QUESTION 6

Which of the following statements about allergy skin testing is true?

1. Transmission of viral infections such as hepatitis and human immunodeficiency virus (HIV) may result from piercing the skin with contaminated needles.
2. Anaphylactic reactions have been reported after introducing even minute quantities of allergen under the skin.
3. Skin testing has been replaced in the modern era by blood testing, which can measure sensitivities to the very same allergens.
4. Patients can protect against adverse reactions from skin testing by taking an antihistamine (e.g., loratadine) 1 hour before testing.
5. Without skin testing, one cannot establish a diagnosis of allergic asthma.

QUESTION 7

A 45-year-old woman with asthma reports that whenever she dusts or vacuums at home, she experiences tightening in her chest and a nonproductive cough that lasts for a few hours. She recalls that as a child she had multiple positive skin test reactions, including to house dust mite. You advise her to consider the following action:

1. Ask her doctor about intensifying her antiasthmatic regimen of medications.
2. Use her quick-acting bronchodilator immediately before house cleaning.
3. Obtain a vacuum cleaner with built-in HEPA filter.
4. Hire a house-cleaning service.
5. Restrict her house-cleaning to once monthly.

QUESTION 8

Following her second asthmatic exacerbation this year treated in the emergency department of her local hospital, your 26-year-old patient wonders what she should do to reduce her risk of recurrent attacks. She makes it clear that under no circumstances will she give up her two pet cats. Despite her strong attachment to the cats, you advise her as your first recommendation that she find another home for her cats. If she can't do that, you suggest that she:

1. Obtain a free-standing room air HEPA filter for the bedroom
2. Change clothes when entering and leaving the house
3. Bathe the cats weekly in warm, soapy water
4. Shave the cats' fur
5. Change the "kitty litter" at least once daily and, preferably, have someone else do it

QUESTION 9

Evidence about the importance of cockroach allergy in inner-city asthma has emerged over the last few decades. It is now known that:

1. Detection of any cockroach allergen in the home, regardless of the amount, is associated with more severe asthma.
2. Cockroach antigen in the air causes respiratory symptoms even in those without a history of asthma.
3. High levels of cockroach antigen found in the bedroom causes worsened asthma even in children without specific cockroach allergy.
4. Cockroach extermination and antigen removal with cleaning cannot lead to better asthma control in persons living in multi-resident urban apartment buildings.

5. In the cockroach-allergic asthmatic, high levels of cockroach antigen exposure in the home are associated with more frequent emergency room and unscheduled provider visits for asthma.

QUESTION 10

Your 17-year-old patient (and high-school softball player) from Lowell, Massachusetts complains that every spring (in April and May), her asthma seems to worsen and she develops itchy eyes and a watery nose. By early June she improves, just as the softball season at her school ends! You suspect that she is allergic to:

1. Latex
2. Outdoor mold
3. Ragweed
4. Tree pollens
5. Cleaning agents used in the locker room

QUESTION 11

You are concerned that the 22-year-old mother of a 5-year-old boy with asthma continues to smoke inside their apartment. You control your anger, and suggest to her politely and with conviction that:

1. Her son's asthma is likely to improve if she quits smoking and no one smokes inside their apartment any more.
2. Unless she quits smoking, her son has a high risk of developing emphysema when he grows older.
3. Her smoking is the likely cause of her son's asthma.
4. Her cigarette smoking puts her son at risk for developing multiple allergic sensitivities that he would otherwise not likely develop.
5. All of the above.

QUESTION 12

Of the following, which intervention was not part of the "environmental intervention plan" employed in the Inner-City Asthma Study? This study gave proof that a multidimensional intervention within the home environment could lead to improved asthma control, even among impoverished, inner-city residents.

1. Vacuum cleaners equipped with HEPA filters
2. Cockroach extermination
3. Structured smoking cessation counseling programs
4. Allergy-proof wraps for the pillows, mattress, and box springs
5. Free-standing room air HEPA filters

Answers to Self-Assessment Questions

ANSWER TO QUESTION 1 (DISTINGUISHING ATOPIC FROM OTHER TYPES OF ALLERGIC AND NONALLERGIC REACTIONS)

The correct answer is #3 (having "hay fever" [seasonal allergic rhinitis and conjunctivitis]). Like allergic asthma, hay fever is an atopic disease. People with one atopic illness (and therefore evidence of the tendency to make this particular type of allergic reaction) are more likely to have other atopic diseases. Allergy to penicillin (answer #1) is not an atopic disease; it is not more common among people with asthma and hay fever than those without these conditions. The reaction described in answer #2 (bleeding ulcers in response to aspirin) is not an allergic reaction at all. It is a consequence of the effect of aspirin on gastric mucosal cells and on platelet function. The immune response described in answer #4 (hypersensitivity pneumonitis) involves immunoglobulin G (IgG) and granuloma formation and is unrelated to atopic reactions. Angioedema (answer #5) can be part of an atopic reaction (e.g., throat swelling during an anaphylactic reaction), but the idiosyncratic drug reaction to angiotensin converting enzyme (ACE) inhibitors described in answer #5 is unrelated to allergic angioedema or to asthma.

ANSWER TO QUESTION 2 (IDENTIFYING ATOPIC DISEASES)

The correct answer is #5 (chronic bronchitis). Chronic bronchitis refers to the daily cough and sputum production that occurs in long-term cigarette smokers. It is part of the spectrum of chronic obstructive pulmonary disease (COPD). The other choices (answers #1–4) are all part of the spectrum of atopic diseases. They can all be caused by allergic reactions involving IgE and mast cells.

ANSWER TO QUESTION 3 (THE ASSOCIATION BETWEEN ALLERGY AND ASTHMA)

The correct answer is #2 ("Most children with asthma have positive allergy skin tests to one or more allergens."). It is estimated that 80% or more of children with asthma have evidence for allergic sensitivities. However, not all people with asthma have allergies (answer #1). Infantile eczema is a risk factor for the subsequent development of childhood asthma; however, only a minority of children with infantile eczema goes on to develop asthma (answer #3). It is estimated that 50% or more of adults with asthma will have some allergic sensitivities; they are not uncommon after age 30 (answer #4). The new onset of allergies after age 12 happens quite routinely. The absence of allergies in childhood is no protection against their development later in life (answer #5).

ANSWER TO QUESTION 4 (EVIDENCE OF ALLERGY BY PATIENT HISTORY)

The correct answer is #1. A positive skin test reaction gives evidence of allergy (such as to cats), but it does not indicate with certainty that this reaction will take place in the airways (as in asthma). It is possible that the patient's allergic reactions will be limited to her nose and skin. Given her strong history of allergic reactions to cats, a negative skin test would be interpreted—in light of this history—as a false negative (answer #2). Skin testing as routinely practiced cannot distinguish allergy to individual animals of a species; that is, it cannot answer whether the patient is allergic to one cat versus another (answer #3). Skin test reactivity correlates poorly with the *degree* of sensitivity to a particular reaction; they are usually interpreted simply as negative or positive reactions (answer #4). Regular or routine exposure to allergens (such as cats) does not predict with certainty allergic sensitization to these allergens. Those who are not atopic will not make IgE antibodies to these allergens, despite intense exposure (answer #5).

ANSWER TO QUESTION 5 (BLOOD TESTS FOR ALLERGIC SENSITIVITIES [RASTS])

The correct answer is #2 (measures the amount of IgE antibody directed at a particular allergen, such as house dust mite). We cannot measure allergens in the blood, and for the most part these substances are limited to the surface of body tissues (e.g., conjunctivae, nasal membranes, skin, and bronchi) and do not enter the bloodstream (answer #1). The allergy blood tests such as RASTs measure only IgE antibodies to allergens; other antibodies, such as IgG and IgM, are of more interest in studying reactions to infection (answer #3). Eosinophils do not bear receptors on their surfaces that target specific allergens (answer #4). They are nonspecific inflammatory cells that can be attracted into tissues such as the airways in response to many different signals, including atopic reactions. There exists no comprehensive blood test panel that tests for all known human allergies (answer #5).

ANSWER TO QUESTION 6 (ALLERGY SKIN TESTING)

The correct answer is #2; rarely patients can experience an anaphylactic reaction after a minute amount of allergen is pierced into the skin (and bloodstream). Disposable needles are used for skin testing; no blood-to-blood transmission of viruses takes place (answer #1). Even in the age of allergy blood tests such as RASTs, allergy skin testing continues to play an important role (answer #3). Skin tests are more sensitive than blood tests and can provide important immediate visual feedback about the importance of one's allergic reactions. Antihistamines need to be avoided in the days prior to allergy skin testing, lest they block all skin test reactions and cause false negative results (answer #4). A strong history of asthmatic reactions and/or positive blood tests (RASTs) to common allergens can establish a diagnosis of allergic asthma even in the absence of allergy skin test results (answer #5).

ANSWER TO QUESTION 7 (DUST MITE ALLERGY AND ALLERGEN AVOIDANCE)

The correct answer is # 3. Her history strongly suggests that she is allergic to house dust mites, and the proposed intervention (obtain a vacuum cleaner with built-in HEPA filter) will help to reduce her exposure to dust mite antigen lifted into the air via the exhaust of a conventional vacuum cleaner. The other potential actions may be helpful, but they do not specifically help with her dust mite allergy. In our opinion, it would be a preferable approach to try to decrease her allergen exposures rather than have her take more antiasthmatic medications (answer #1). A bronchodilator taken before dust exposure (answer #2) may succeed in minimizing bronchoconstriction (with chest tightness and cough) caused by dust mite allergen inhalation, but it won't address the allergic inflammatory reaction that the allergen causes in the airways. A house-cleaning service (answer #4) sounds appealing, but it is probably an option that she would have pursued without your advice were it readily available to her. Once-monthly house-cleaning (answer #5) may lead to troublesome allergen accumulation in the weeks between cleaning.

ANSWER TO QUESTION 8 (CAT ALLERGY AND ALLERGEN AVOIDANCE)

The correct answer is #1 (obtain a free-standing room air HEPA filter for the bedroom). Unlike for house dust mites, where allergen-containing particles float in the air only briefly, animal danders remain airborne longer and are more amenable to clearance via room air filters. Changing clothes when entering and leaving the house (answer #2) will not reduce exposure to cat allergen in the home environment. Bathing the cats weekly (answer #3) has been abandoned as a recommendation to cat-allergic cat owners because of its limited and temporary benefit and the potential danger from a very angry cat. Shaving the cats' fur (answer #4) will not eliminate cat antigen, which is found in a cat's saliva and oil-making (sebaceous) glands of its skin. Likewise, changing the "kitty litter" frequently (answer #5) will not address the major sources of cat allergen.

ANSWER TO QUESTION 9 (COCKROACH ALLERGY AND ALLERGEN AVOIDANCE)

The correct answer is #5. High levels of cockroach antigen exposure in the home have indeed been found to be associated with more frequent asthmatic exacerbations in asthmatics who are cockroach-allergic. Low levels of cockroach antigen in the home do not provoke the same frequency and severity of asthmatic symptoms (answer #1); allergic reactions are to some degree dose-dependent. Cockroach allergens in the air do not cause respiratory symptoms in healthy, nonasthmatic people (answer #2). In the absence of cockroach allergy, cockroach antigen in the bedroom, even high levels, will not provoke any symptoms (answer #3). The results of the Inner-City Asthma Study give evidence that cockroach extermination and antigen removal with cleaning can successfully reduce cockroach antigen exposure in the home (and contribute to better asthma control), even in asthmatic children living in multi-resident apartment buildings (answer #4).

ANSWER TO QUESTION 10 (SEASONAL ALLERGENS)

The correct answer is #4 (tree pollens). In temperate climates such as New England, tree pollens fill the air from March through June. Outdoor mold spores (answer #2), while present to some degree year-round, are at their highest levels between June and September. Ragweed pollen (answer #3) (and the pollen from other common weed plants) peak between August and October. Cleaning agents used in the locker room (answer #5) sound like a pretty farfetched explanation for her symptoms!

ANSWER TO QUESTION 11 (ROLE OF ENVIRONMENTAL TOBACCO SMOKE EXPOSURE IN CHILDHOOD ASTHMA)

The correct answer is #1. Evidence from clinical trials indicates that symptoms improve in children with asthma when smokers in the home either quit smoking or smoke only outdoors. It is not true that environmental tobacco smoke causes emphysema (answer #2). Although it is possible that his mother's cigarette smoking was a contributing factor to his development of asthma, it would be erroneous (and impolitic) to say that it was the *cause* of his asthma (answer #3). Environmental tobacco smoke is not known to predispose to the development of allergic sensitivities (answer #4). Consequently, not all of the answers are correct (answer #5).

ANSWER TO QUESTION 12 (THE INNER-CITY ASTHMA STUDY AND ITS MULTIDIMENSIONAL "ENVIRONMENTAL INTERVENTION PLAN")

The correct answer is #3. Although smoking cessation was encouraged, no formal smoking cessation counseling program was incorporated as part of the intervention plan. All of the other interventions listed (answers 1, 2, 4, and 5) were part of the intervention plan used in this study of home-based environmental modifications among children living in inner-city homes (in seven major U.S. cities). Cockroach extermination took place in homes where a child had cockroach allergy and was exposed to cockroaches. Free-standing room air HEPA filters were provided for the child's bedroom if the child was exposed to environmental tobacco smoke, had a cat or dog and was allergic to it, or had an allergy to mold.

C H A P T E R

8

INHALERS AND INHALATIONAL AIDS
IN ASTHMA TREATMENT

C H A P T E R   O U T L I N E

I.   General Principles

II. Metered-Dose Inhalers
     a. Inhalational aids, including spacers
     b. Breath-actuated metered-dose inhaler
     c. HFA propellant-driven metered-dose inhalers
     d. Determining if a metered-dose inhaler is empty
     e. Cleaning the inhaler

III. Dry-Powder Inhalers
     a. Diskus
     b. Turbuhaler
     c. Twisthaler
     d. Aerolizer
     e. Handihaler

IV. Nebulizers

GENERAL PRINCIPLES

It has long been recognized that the preferred method to deliver medications to the airways is by inhalation. Far smaller amounts can be administered than when medicine is swallowed into the stomach, often achieving quicker onset of action, fewer side effects, and—with respect to bronchodilators—more potent results. The inhaled route of administration avoids issues of gastrointestinal metabolism, food and medication interactions, and stomach upset. Inhaled medications can be continued in the patient who is "N.P.O." (*nil per os*, or nothing by mouth) because of gastrointestinal disease or impending procedures or surgery.

The challenge for manufacturers of drugs and medical devices has been to find ways to get medications into particles of the proper size to deposit onto airways. If too big (and heavy), the medication-containing droplets will continue in a straight line, settling onto the mouth and pharynx rather than making the turn down to the larynx and airways. If too small (and light), they can be carried into the lungs and back out again (like a gas), never depositing onto the walls of the bronchi. The optimal size of these so-called "respirable particles" is said to be a diameter of 1–5 microns. Other factors influence the output from devices meant to deliver medication to the bronchi, including the speed at which a spray is released from the device and the impact of water evaporation on the size of aerosol droplets. In the end, only about 10–15% of medication released from modern inhalational devices actually makes its way to the airway surface, even with the best of patient coordination.

Inhalational therapy for asthma has a colorful history, including use of "asthma cigarettes," bulb nebulizers, and hooka-like steam pipes (Fig. 8-1). You can imagine how variable and uncertain was the actual dose of medication delivered with each treatment. A major advance in the technology of inhalational therapy occurred in 1956, when 3M introduced the metered-dose inhaler (MDI) (Fig. 8-2). Multiple doses of medication could be contained within a pressurized metal canister, and with each actuation exactly the same amount of medicine was

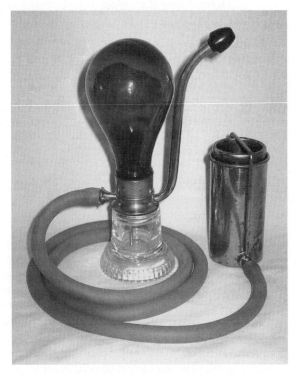

FIGURE 8-1 *Antique bulb nebulizer. Reproduced with permission from: www.inhalatorium.com.*

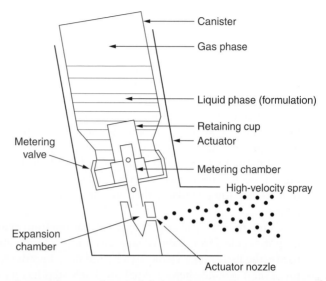

FIGURE 8-2   *Schematic diagram of metered-dose inhaler. Reproduced with permission from Newman SP. Principles of metered-dose inhaler design.* Respiratory Care 2005; 50:1177–88.

released from the device's nozzle. The spray released from the MDI contains a large percentage of particles of the desired *respirable* size.

Nonetheless, as you know, a major barrier exists between medication released from an inhalation device and medication deposited onto the airways: namely, human error. Murphy's law applies to the ability of people to coordinate the metered-dose inhaler and other inhalational devices: "anything that can go wrong, will go wrong." Whereas swallowing tablets or liquids is a skill acquired almost universally at a young age, inhaling medicine can be a complicated and unfamiliar process involving relatively sophisticated hand-breathing coordination. Compliance is predictably poor. There often exists a huge gap between the healthcare provider's prescription and the patient's effective use of the medication. Enter the asthma educator. With proper patient instruction, a seemingly ineffective asthma medication can be made effective—not by changing the dose or frequency of administration but by having it reach its intended target, the airways. Many physicians have limited familiarity with the various inhalational devices used to treat asthma. They will often rely on you—consciously or not—to make their prescription a practical reality.

KEY POINT   Inhalation is the preferred route of administration for bronchodilators and for corticosteroids used for maintenance therapy. However, the effectiveness of these medicines is fully dependent on the ability of our patients to inhale them properly onto the airways.

METERED-DOSE INHALERS

At the present time, virtually everyone with asthma over the age of approximately 5 years will have a metered-dose inhaler for administration of a quick-acting bronchodilator. "Can you show me how you use your inhaler?" is a wonderful opening gambit for an asthma educator. Even patients who have had asthma for many years will generally appreciate the opportunity to review their inhalational technique with an expert. And you will thereby have the chance to witness errors in technique that you hadn't imagined, from failure to remove the cap to holding the device upside down, from actuating the device only after a full inhalation to actuating it twice, then holding the spray in the mouth like a breath freshener!

Our goal in teaching proper inhalation from metered-dose inhalers is to keep it simple. The essential steps are three: (1) actuate the inhaler as you start to breathe in; (2) take a slow, steady, and deep breath in; and (3) hold your breath for several seconds before exhaling. Each step has its rationale. Timing of the actuation of the spray at the start of the breath in makes the medicine available to be carried to the airways with the airflow of an inhalation. Actuate the inhaler too late after the start of inhalation, and one has not enough breath left to pull the medicine into the lungs. Actuate it too early, and much of the medicine impacts on the mouth and throat before the remainder is pulled into the lungs. A slow and deep breath in helps to distribute the medicine along the thousands of airways with bronchial muscles. By contrast, a rapid, short *gasp* causes most of the medicine to settle on the trachea and more proximal bronchi, limiting its usefulness. Finally, a brief breath hold before exhalation allows time for particles carried deep into the lungs to *rain out* onto the bronchial walls rather than to be carried back out of the lungs during exhalation.

Our advice for using the metered-dose inhaler goes like this:

- Remove the cap.
- Shake the device before each spray.
- Close your lips tightly around the mouthpiece or position the mouthpiece 1–2 inches from your open mouth.
- As you start to breathe in slowly, press down on the canister to release the medication and continue a slow, steady, deep breath in.
- Hold your breath for 5–10 seconds, then relax and exhale.

Our procedure does not ask patients to exhale fully before actuating the device and beginning inhalation. You may well have been taught to include this step, and there is nothing wrong in doing so. By exhaling first, one maximizes the size of the breath available to pull in the medication. However, in our minds, doing so also complicates the process too much, and it poses some risk of inducing cough and bronchoconstriction if patients fully empty their lungs. A limited, gentle exhaling before actuating the inhaler and beginning inhalation is fine.

Debate over the open-mouth versus closed-mouth technique strikes us as a bit obsessive. Advocates of the open-mouth method (hold the mouthpiece of the canister about two fingerbreadths from your open mouth) can point to experiments demonstrating better medication deposition onto the airways (because there is more time for the spray to slow its speed before entering the airstream and more time for evaporation of water, leaving more particles of the respirable size). Advocates of the closed-mouth technique (seal lips and teeth around the mouthpiece) can rightly note that errors of aim can be avoided this way. At least the medication can be guaranteed to enter the mouth. The closed mouth technique more closely parallels the method for using dry-powder inhalers; and many patients will need to learn use of both types of devices. In our opinion, in terms of efficacy, the difference between the two methods is small, and the choice can be left to individual preferences (yours and/or your patient's). There is no one *right* way.

KEY POINT   In teaching use of the metered-dose inhaler, keep the instructions as simple as possible. The choice between the "open-mouth" and "closed-mouth" techniques is mostly a matter of style and personal preference.

It is one thing for the patient to be able to demonstrate proper technique using a metered-dose inhaler in the medical office; it is another matter to retain that skill uncoached at home. Even the patient who has learned proper technique under your tutelage will likely need reinforcement at follow-up visits. And some patients will simply be unable to master its proper use, including the very young, some elderly or arthritic individuals, and others for whom lack of motor skills or anxiety gets in the way. In these circumstances, inhalational aids such as spacers can help.

Other aspects of inhaler technology about which you may wish to know are "creaming," "priming," and "tail-off." Creaming refers to the tendency of components of suspensions to separate when left undisturbed for a period of hours to days, like cream rising to the surface of an old-fashioned bottle of nonhomogenized milk. Patients are encouraged to shake their MDI dispenser before use to mix medicine and propellant into a uniform suspension, ensuring a consistent dose of medicine. A quick shake for 2–3 seconds suffices. Likewise, after nonuse for a day or more, the first spray released from the metered-dose inhaler contains less medicine (e.g., 50–75%) than subsequent sprays. Some providers encourage their patients to waste a dose (actuate the device and release the medicine into the air) before inhaling their next puff; that is, to *prime* their inhaler. We encourage priming with two wasted sprays when the inhaler is first used. However, in our own opinion the consequence of the reduced concentration of medicine in the first puff is small and generally does not justify the expense of multiple wasted doses with each subsequent use of an inhaler that has sat untouched for a day or two.

Finally, "tail-off" refers to the progressive decrease in medicine contained in each puff of medicine as the canister approaches empty. After the promised number of doses (e.g., 200 puffs contained within an albuterol canister), the concentration of medicine in each puff rapidly decreases to zero even though some mist continues to be released for several more actuations. The rapidity of tail-off varies among different devices, but the principal is the same: don't continue to use inhalers after the promised number of puffs/canister, or you will rapidly find yourself using a "placebo" inhaler. Creaming, priming, and tail-off do not apply to dry-powder inhalers.

Inhalational aids, including spacers

Holding chambers (spacers) are based on a simple concept, although their design may be aerodynamically quite sophisticated (Fig. 8-3). The idea is to create a chamber into which the spray released from a metered-dose inhaler can be held as an aerosol for up to a few seconds prior to inhalation. Attach the metered-dose inhaler (cover off!) to the spacer, actuate the metered-dose inhaler, and then inhale the medication from the opposite end of the spacer. Valved holding chambers (popular models include Aerochamber, Optichamber, and Vortex) contain a one-way valve to prevent escape of medication except during patient inhalation and dilution of medication during exhalation (the exhaled breath is vented from the mouthpiece to the surrounding air without entering the chamber).

The use of valved holding chambers with attached face masks (attached to the mouthpiece at the end opposite the metered-dose inhaler) has revolutionized medication delivery to young children. It makes possible delivery of medication from metered-dose inhalers to children too young to use a mouthpiece or time their breathing to actuation of the inhaler. With normal breathing (the routine in and out of quiet respiration called *tidal* breathing), a young child can empty the chamber of medication after approximately six

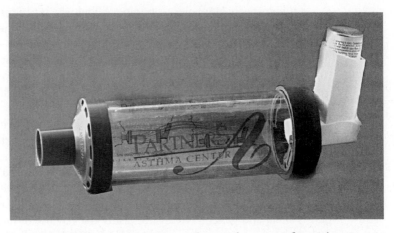

FIGURE 8-3 *Valved holding chamber or spacer. Photograph courtesy of Kenneth M. Bernstein.*

breaths. The metered-dose inhaler with spacer and attached face mask can be held away from the child's face when actuated, then brought quickly to cover nose and mouth while the child breathes in and out. Use of a metered-dose inhaler with valved holding chamber and attached face mask dramatically expands the range of medications that can be offered to young children.

KEY POINT   With attached valved holding chamber and face mask, medications marketed in metered-dose inhalers can be administered to very young children.

This is not to say that use of spacers with face masks in young children is easy. Parents and other care providers need lots of coaching and practice. The best method to teach its use will depend on the age of the child and will vary from child to child—and from one parent-child pairing to another. Getting the child to rest comfortably in the parent's arms or lap is a good start. Introducing the spacer and face mask without medication can be helpful; the child can be kept contented with familiar objects or interesting distractions. Meanwhile, the care provider needs to be able to hold the metered-dose inhaler-spacer-face mask unit in a free hand, shake the unit (thereby shaking the metered-dose inhaler prior to actuation), actuate the inhaler, and bring the face mask to the child's face. As you might imagine, learning and practicing these skills can be a major portion of the time spent in a medical visit for pediatric asthma. The role of a skilled asthma educator is invaluable.

Two additional points about medication delivery using spacers with attached face mask: First, variable mask sizes are available; they are generally sold in small, medium, and large sizes. Plastic cut-outs in the shape of the mask are available from manufacturers and can be used to identify the optimally-sized mask for an individual child. As the child grows, a larger size may become needed. It is usually at approximately age 5–6 years (or at approximately the time that a child masters the ability to hold his breath underwater) that the child can be transitioned from the face mask to sealing his lips around the mouthpiece of the spacer.

Second, just as we ask our adult patients to rinse their mouth with water after use of an inhaled steroid, we need to ask the parents of young children using an inhaled steroid by metered-dose inhaler with attached spacer and face mask to rinse both the inside of the child's mouth and outside of the face around the nose and mouth with a moist facecloth. One of the concerns about repetitive application of a potent corticosteroid to the skin is dermal atrophy, with permanent changes in the structure and—most importantly—the appearance of the skin. This complication is prevented by simply rinsing clean the skin surfaces underneath the area of the face mask after each use of an inhaled corticosteroid.

Although we have emphasized so far the role of valved holding chambers (or spacers) in medication delivery to young children, we would too note their value in older children and adults. They offer two main benefits: improved medication

delivery to the airways and reduced oropharyngeal deposition of medication. In
those who—despite your best efforts—cannot master proper coordination of the
metered-dose inhaler, adding an attached spacer will often overcome the imped-
iments to effective inhalation of the medicine. It is no wonder why: first, instead
of the strong blast of medication being released from the MDI nozzle and
immediately striking the back of one's throat, now the medication is captured in
the chamber and is pulled out of the chamber at the speed of the patient's inhalation. And second, the perceived stress of split-second timing between actuation
of the inhaler and the beginning of inhalation is eliminated. The patient's breath
in can be delayed for a second or two after the medicine is sprayed into the holding chamber. During that time most of the medication remains airborne and
available for a calm inhalation.

Except in special circumstances, older children and adults will use the
mouthpiece of the spacer rather than an attached face mask. And they should be
taught to empty the holding chamber with one or two slow, deep breaths (rather
than with tidal breathing). As noted above, a slow, steady inhalation maximizes
medication delivery to the smaller, more peripheral airways. Some spacers come
with a small, built-in whistle that emits its sound during a rapid inhalation. It is
meant as a warning that the inhalation was too fast; an appropriately slow breath
in does not cause the whistle to sound.

The second major advantage to the use of a spacer with a metered-dose
inhaler is reduction in the amount of medicine left behind in the mouth and
back of the throat—an advantage of some significance when using an inhaled
steroid. In experiments using radiolabeled medication to track the site of deposition of medicine released from metered-dose inhalers, one finds that the percentage of medicine settling onto the oropharynx is decreased from approximately 75% to approximately 10% by attaching a spacer. In effect, the larger
and heavier particles contained in the MDI spray settle in the holding chamber
rather than in the oropharynx; the smaller and lighter (respirable) particles continue in the airstream to their intended target along the bronchial tubes. Less
steroid deposited in the oropharynx means less risk for oral candidiasis (thrush)
and less medicine available to be swallowed, absorbed out of the stomach into
the bloodstream, and distributed systemically. By reducing systemic absorption
by approximately half, spacers can decrease concerns about long-term potential
side effects from inhaled steroids.

KEY POINT Spacers have two major advantages: they improve medication delivery to the airways in
those who have difficulty coordinating use of metered-dose inhalers; and they minimize
the amount of inhaled corticosteroid that deposits on the oropharynx (and thereby
becomes available for systemic absorption).

Among adults with asthma, why shouldn't every patient given a metered-dose
inhaler also be asked to use a spacer with it? We offer two reasons to consider.

First, there is the matter of inconvenience and social discomfort. Don't underestimate the embarrassment that your patient may feel about using his or her metered-dose inhaler in public; this discomfort will only be magnified by the more conspicuous attached spacer. It is one thing to carry a metered-dose inhaler with you in your pocket or purse; it is another matter to transport a valved holding chamber everywhere you go. Second, a patient *with good inhalational technique* gets no advantage for using his or her quick-acting bronchodilator with a spacer compared to without one. The bronchodilator effect is identical.

For many of our adult patients, this dilemma is easily resolved. We ask them to leave their steroid-containing metered-dose inhaler attached to a spacer at home in the medicine cabinet for regular use once- or twice-daily (in the privacy of their own home), and carry with them their bronchodilator metered-dose inhaler—without a spacer—for use as needed. Other patients, aware that they cannot effectively use their metered-dose inhaler without a spacer, will need to carry the spacer with them.

One manufacturer of an inhaled steroid emphasized the importance of use of an attached spacer by building a small-volume spacer into the plastic holding device sold with each canister of medicine. When pulled opened, the device containing the inhaled steroid, triamcinolone (Azmacort), expands into the shape of an "L" with the nonvalved spacer coming off at a right angle from the nozzle of the metered-dose inhaler. When the canister is depressed and the spray actuated, the patient inhales from the mouthpiece at the end of the spacer (Fig. 8-4). After use, the spacer is straightened 90° into a straight line with the canister and then collapsed back to its original size.

The built-in spacer of the Azmacort inhaler is simply a hollow plastic tube, and it raises the question of the ideal shape and size for a spacer. Many different

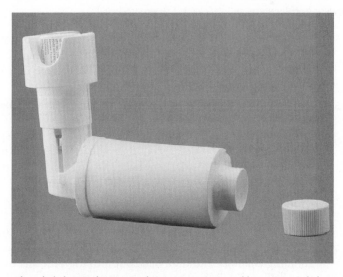

FIGURE 8-4 *The inhaled steroid, triamcinolone (Azmacort), is sold as a metered-dose inhaler with built-in spacer. Photograph courtesy of Kenneth M. Bernstein.*

devices are available, and one might wonder whether adapting the cardboard center from a roll of toilet paper wouldn't suffice! In fact, a larger volume proves desirable (despite the convenience of "mini-spacers"), and devices with one-way valves to direct exhalation away from the medication in the chamber have added value. Some valved holding chambers are made of metal or antistatic polymer rather than plastic (Vortex and Aerochamber MAX). Unlike the plastic spacers, these chambers are free of electrostatic cling, so that medication will not adhere. The noncling surface is meant to maximize medication availability for inhalation to the airways. One can reduce the electrostatic cling of conventional plastic spacers by coating the inner surface with a thin layer of liquid detergent or initially filling the chamber with multiple doses of medication, but neither of these practices is particularly practical nor widely employed.

An important teaching point for patients is that they cannot *load* multiple doses of medication into the spacer prior to inhalation. For effective medication delivery, each spray from the metered-dose inhaler gets its own inhalation from the chamber. On the other hand, it is fine to use one spacer with multiple different metered-dose inhalers. Simply pull one metered-dose inhaler from its attachment at the end of the spacer and replace it with another. Spacers can be cleaned by washing with soapy water, rinsed, and allowed to air dry. Valved holding chambers can be periodically disassembled for more thorough cleaning, then reassembled. The one-way valve should remain flexible and functional for a year or more.

KEY POINT   Multiple doses of medication should not be loaded into the holding chamber. Teach patients to complete inhalation of the first dose prior to spraying a second puff of medicine into the chamber.

The cost of a valved holding chamber is approximately $20–$25; and of a valved holding chamber with face mask, approximately $35. Most health plans will cover the cost of these inhalational aids; some may require a letter of medical necessity emphasizing its need.

An inhalational aid of unique design is the InspirEase holding chamber. It has two components: an accordion-like collapsible holding chamber and an attached pipestem-like mouthpiece (Fig. 8-5). The two parts are easily attached at one end of the holding chamber; the other end of the holding chamber has no opening. The InspirEase device is not used with the entire metered-dose inhaler but only with its metal canister, which needs to be pulled from the plastic holder. The nozzle of the metal canister is then seated into a well in the pipestem-like portion of the InspirEase device. When the canister is depressed and medication released, the spray is directed into the collapsible holding chamber. With lips sealed around the mouthpiece, the patient breathes in from the holding chamber and then back out into it. With this tidal breathing, the chamber collapses and then reexpands. After one or two cycles, the chamber is emptied of medication.

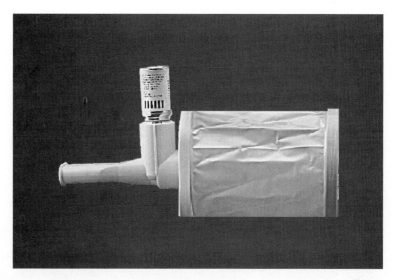

FIGURE 8-5   *The InspirEase holding chamber. Photograph courtesy of Kenneth M. Bernstein.*

The big appeal of this device is that one can watch the chamber collapse and then reinflate. A parent can confirm that the child is correctly using the device and getting a full dose of medication. A built-in whistle sounds if the child inhales too fast. Drawbacks to the device are the following: one needs to disassemble the metered-dose inhaler in order to withdraw the metal canister from its plastic holder; the chamber is difficult to wash and its thin, flexible plastic sides tend to crack over time, necessitating replacement as often as every few weeks; and the relatively small size of the holding chamber makes it inappropriate for older children and adults with large tidal breaths, whereas very young children will be unable to seal their lips around the mouthpiece. It is probably most appropriate for use in children between the approximate ages of 5 and 10 years.

KEY POINT   The InspirEase holding chamber provides visual confirmation of medication use; the reservoir bag collapses and expands during tidal breathing. No attachable face mask is marketed with this device.

One other inhalational aid is worth mentioning, although it pertains to a very selected group of patients with asthma (or other obstructive lung diseases) and arthritis involving their hands. Especially patients with rheumatoid arthritis, who may develop joint displacement (subluxation) at the base of the thumb and weakness in thumb-finger apposition, can have great difficulty in generating

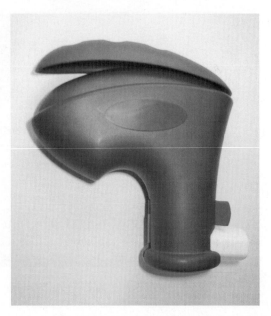

FIGURE 8-6 *Squeezing the handle actuates the metered-dose inhaler held within this device. The MDI-Ease adaptor is shaped to fit only certain metered-dose inhalers: ipratropium (Atrovent) and combination ipratropium plus albuterol (Combivent).*

enough force to depress the metal canister of the metered-dose inhaler in its plastic holder. A simple adaptive device was created by the manufacturers of Ventolin brand of albuterol and is called VentEase. It can be used with any metered-dose inhaler that is the same size as Ventolin.

The entire metered-dose inhaler device (metal canister and plastic holder) fits into the VentEase adaptor. With a simple hand-grip action (thumb force not required) applied to the VentEase, the top of the canister is forced downward by a plastic rocker and the metered-dose inhaler actuated. The manufacturers of ipratropium (Atrovent) have made a similar device for hand-grip actuation of the ipratropium (Atrovent) and combination ipratropium and albuterol (Combivent) inhalers, which are slightly shorter in length than albuterol inhalers. This latter assist device is called MDI-Ease (Fig. 8-6). The VentEase and MDI-Ease devices are not readily available in pharmacies; they are best obtained from GlaxoSmithKline and Boehringer-Ingelheim drug representatives, respectively.

KEY POINT   Although they may be difficult to locate, special devices (VentEase and MDI-Ease) are available to help patients with arthritic hands and poor thumb strength actuate metered-dose inhalers with a simple hand-grip movement.

Breath-actuated metered-dose inhaler

Another approach to improving patient coordination with metered-dose inhalers would be to build a device that releases its spray only when the patient begins to breathe in. If timing of actuation of the inhaler could be linked to the patient's inhalation, a major source of errors with metered-dose inhaler use could be eliminated—such as actuating the inhaler *after* inhaling and having the spray be blown back out into the room during exhalation. One manufacturer has successfully created such a device, a breath-actuated metered-dose inhaler, called the Autohaler. They (i.e., product developers at 3M) designed it for use with their quick-acting bronchodilator, pirbuterol (Maxair). Pirbuterol is very similar to albuterol in its onset of action, duration of action, and side-effects profile. Pirbuterol is now available only in the form of the Maxair Autohaler; and the Autohaler is designed to be used only with Maxair. Other metered-dose inhaler canisters will not fit into the Autohaler device.

The Autohaler retains the general shape of a metered-dose inhaler, but the metal canister is hidden within the plastic holder (Fig. 8-7). In preparation for use, the Autohaler is spring-loaded by raising a red lever on the top of the plastic holder into the vertical position. The device is now ready to release its medication when it "detects" inspiratory airflow at the mouthpiece. The detection system is a small plastic vane just inside the mouthpiece that is pulled upward (like a door swinging open) when one begins to inhale with lips tightly sealed at the mouthpiece. (Use of the Autohaler relies on the closed-mouth technique, described above.) When the vane swivels open, the device immediately "fires" automatically, releasing its spray. Actuation is accompanied by an audible click.

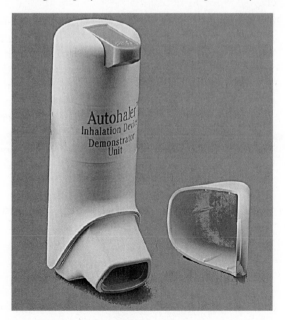

FIGURE 8-7   *The quick-acting inhaled beta-agonist bronchodilator, pirbuterol (Maxair), is made available in a breath-actuated inhaler, called the Autohaler. Photograph courtesy of Kenneth M. Bernstein.*

After each release of medication (or puff from the inhaler), the red lever at the top of the plastic holder needs to be returned to its starting position (parallel with the top of the device). When ready for a second puff, lift the lever to the vertical position, seal lips around the mouthpiece, and begin to inhale. Patients need to be reminded to continue a slow, steady breath in after the medicine has been released with its somewhat startling associated "click," and also—as usual—to hold one's breath at the end of an inhalation.

To trigger the device, inhalation must begin with sufficient force to pull open the plastic vane within the mouthpiece. Adequate force is generated by an inhalation with the speed of 30 L/min, an inspiratory flow that under most circumstances is readily achieved. However, a child or an elderly adult with too-tentative a breath in may not succeed in actuating the device each time. Actuation is also prevented if one accidentally blocks the airflow into the device by occluding the plastic grate at the base of the inhaler with one's thumb. At purchase the Maxair canister contains 400 doses of medication, twice the amount in an albuterol (Ventolin, Proventil) canister.

KEY POINT   The breath-actuated metered-dose inhaler, Maxair Autohaler, delivers the quick-acting, rescue bronchodilator, pirbuterol. The breath-actuated mechanism ensures that the spray of medication is released only after the patient begins to breathe in.

One other feature of the Maxair Autohaler is worth noting. It includes a way to release a spray of medication without using the breath-actuation method. At the base of the plastic holder, one can slide the white plastic grate forward (toward the mouthpiece opening), releasing a puff of medication. The purpose is to allow priming of a canister that has been unused for several days. It would also indicate an empty inhaler if one can see no medication being released.

In summary, the steps for using the Autohaler are as follows:

• Remove the mouthpiece cap and shake the inhaler
• Hold the Autohaler in an upright position
• Lift the red lever on top of the device
• Take care not to cover the vents at the bottom of the device with your fingers
• Put the lips and teeth over the mouthpiece
• Breathe in steadily and deeply
• A click is heard as the spray is released
• Hold the breath for several seconds
• Return the red lever back down to the horizontal position

HFA propellant-driven metered-dose inhalers

The propellant used to pressurize traditional metered-dose inhalers is a chloro-fluorocarbon (CFC), similar to the CFCs that for many years were used in our air conditioners, refrigeration units, and pressurized spray cans. Beginning in the 1980s, scientists came to realize that CFCs released into the atmosphere were the major cause of depletion of the ozone layer high in the stratosphere. The growing "ozone hole" threatened increased ultraviolet radiation exposure at ground level and had major potential implications for the health of marine animals and humans alike. Recognizing the serious health risks involved, representatives from nations around the world came together in 1987 to sign what came to be known as the Montreal protocol, banning all manufacture and use of CFCs—with a time-limited exception for medical devices. CFCs will also be banned from metered-dose inhalers "when suitable alternatives become available," with a target date of approximately 2008.

Alternatives have taken two forms. One consists of devices that do not rely on pressurized sprays at all, the dry-powder devices discussed subsequently. The other is development of an alternative propellant for metered-dose inhalers, one that does not chemically interact with ozone. This "ozone-friendly" propellant is presently available; it is called hydrofluoroalkane or HFA. More and more manufacturers are transitioning to HFA-driven metered-dose inhalers. Currently available are the following: the bronchodilators, albuterol (Proventil HFA, Ventolin HFA, and ProAir HFA) and ipratropium (Atrovent HFA); and the inhaled steroids, fluticasone (as Flovent HFA) and beclomethasone (as QVAR). (As this book goes to press, the fluticasone-salmeterol combination, Advair, is being readied for release as an Advair-HFA metered-dose inhaler.)

Teaching use of HFA-driven metered-dose inhalers is virtually identical to instruction for traditional CFC-driven metered-dose inhalers. They are all of the same so-called "press-and-breathe" design: a spray is released when the canister is depressed in its plastic holder. Actuation needs to be timed to initiation of inhalation, a slow and deep breath sustained, followed by a brief breath-hold prior to exhalation. HFA-driven metered-dose inhalers can likewise be used with spacers. Differences include the following. The spray released at the nozzle of the metered-dose inhaler has a different speed and shape to its plume (Fig. 8-8). The medication aerosol is released at a slower speed and warmer temperature. Patients will sense a different feel to the spray compared to traditional metered-dose inhalers, less of a "cold blast" delivered to the back of the throat. They may need to be reassured that effective medication delivery is achieved despite this change in sensation. Priming continues to be needed for HFA-driven metered-dose inhalers. Finally, the beclomethasone-HFA inhaler, QVAR, is unique among the HFA-metered-dose inhalers in that it contains medicine held in solution rather than a suspension. No creaming occurs with standing, and the rather small and uniform particle size (approx. 1 micron in diameter) is optimized for medication delivery to the airways, especially the small, peripheral bronchi. With this system, as much as 50% of the dose released from the device makes its way to the lungs when inhalational technique is optimal.

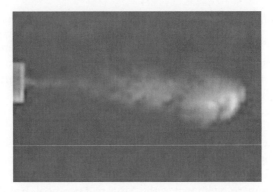

FIGURE 8-8   *Visualization of the plume released from a metered-dose inhaler. Reproduced from Hickey AJ, ed.,* Inhalation Aerosols (Lung Biology in Health and Disease *series), vol. 94, New York: Marcel Dekker, 1996 by permission of Routledge/Taylor & Francis Group, LLC. Copyright 1996.*

KEY POINT   Metered-dose inhalers with hydrofluoroalkane (HFA) propellant release a warmer, less forceful blast of medicine than traditional CFC-driven inhalers. However, the inhalational technique for the two types of metered-dose inhalers is identical.

Determining if a metered-dose inhaler is empty

Your patients will want to know when their metered-dose inhaler is empty. It is a surprisingly difficult question to answer. Even when it contains no more medication, the canister can feel partially full when shaken and release a spray when actuated. It will run out of medication before it empties of propellant and other contents. The biggest danger is that in an emergency your patient may seek relief from a device containing no medication. Less dangerous but quite frustrating is the need to discard a partially full inhaler because of the doubts about its status. At a cost of up to $0.50 per spray, the financial waste may be considerable.

At one time it was proposed that the fullness or emptiness of a canister could be judged by a "float test." Pull the metal canister from its plastic holder and float it in a small tub of water. If the canister sinks to the bottom of the tub, it is full, or nearly so. If it floats along the surface, nearly horizontal with the surface of the water, it is empty. Partially filled canisters bob "head down" at various angles from the surface depending on their weight (Fig. 8-9).

The float test has been abandoned for several reasons. First, at its best it is a qualitative assessment. It cannot distinguish "a few doses left" from completely empty. Second, empty canisters of different weight and construction will behave differently. This variable behavior appears to be particularly true with the metered-dose inhalers containing HFA propellant. Third, if water enters the dosing valve, it can interfere with medication delivery when the canister is placed back into the dosing well of its plastic holder. As a result of these shortcomings, we no longer recommend the float test.

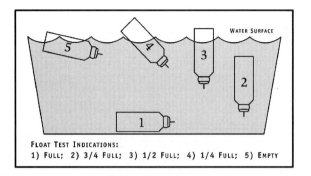

FLOAT TEST INDICATIONS:
1) FULL; 2) 3/4 FULL; 3) 1/2 FULL; 4) 1/4 FULL; 5) EMPTY

FIGURE 8-9   *The float test 1. Empty; 2. 1/4 full; 3. 1/2 full; 4. 3/4 full; 5. full.*

KEY POINT   The "float test" is no longer recommended for assessing when a metered-dose inhaler is empty because of its imprecision and the potential for interfering with medication release if water enters the nozzle of the canister.

In fact, a highly accurate device has been developed to keep track of the exact number of doses of medication used from an individual metered-dose inhaler (although its use has not caught on). Called a "Doser," this patented device (Fig. 8-10) is placed on top of the exposed end of the metal canister. Now, the metered-dose inhaler is actuated by pressing down on the Doser; and a computer chip in the Doser records each actuation. The Doser is programmed with the number of doses contained in a full canister and then *counts down* to zero

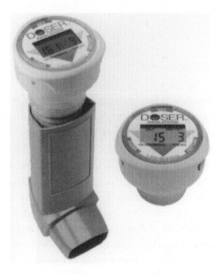

FIGURE 8-10   *A dose-counting device (Doser) that can be used with multiple different metered-dose inhalers. Reproduced with permission from www.doser.com.*

with each actuation. Shortcomings of the Doser device are that it can only be used on one inhaler at a time; it requires some initial programming set up; and it is costly—approximately $35 per device.

The number of doses of medication contained within each canister at the time of purchase—as indicated on the package insert—is highly reliable. For instance, an albuterol inhaler (200 doses/device) will reliably deliver 200 doses of medication, each dose containing nearly exactly 90 mcg of albuterol. If a patient uses his inhaler regularly and reliably—say, for example, two puffs morning and night for an inhaled steroid—one can readily calculate the number of days that a full inhaler will last. For instance, a fluticasone (Flovent) inhaler containing 120 doses/canister initially. If two sprays are used twice daily, it should be discarded after 30 days. Simply mark the metered-dose inhaler with the calculated finish date, and you will accurately know when it is empty. Unfortunately, labeling the inhaler with a completion date does not work for medications taken on an as-needed basis, such as quick-acting bronchodilators, or when one periodically *primes* an inhaler by squirting doses to the atmosphere.

As we will discuss below, some of the newer dry-powder devices have built-in dose counters indicating precisely the number of doses remaining. As this book is readied for release, the first metered-dose inhaler with built-in dose counter, Ventolin-HFA, is about to be launched.

Cleaning the inhaler

It is easy to wash a metered-dose inhaler that becomes soiled. One simply pulls the metal canister from its seat in the bottom of the plastic holder, then washes the plastic holder with soap and water and allows it to dry. When reassembling the unit, one should take care that the nozzle of the metal canister fits firmly back into the well at the bottom of the plastic holder and that no water remains in that well (that might interfere with proper release of medication from the inhaler nozzle).

DRY-POWDER INHALERS

Development of delivery systems for inhaled medication without use of CFC propellants took a second path, besides development of an alternative, ozone-safe propellant (hydrofluoroalkane or HFA). Other pharmaceutical firms have made their inhaled medications available in the form of an ultra-fine powder that is released not as a pressurized spray but as an aerosol created by the force of the patient's inhalation pulling the powder from the device.

You may remember an early dry-powder inhaler called the Intal Spinhaler, used to deliver the mast cell stabilizing medication, cromolyn. In the United States, the Spinhaler has been replaced by other, current cromolyn delivery systems, either the metered-dose inhaler or a solution for nebulization.

The Intal Spinhaler system made medication available in individual gelatin capsules. The capsules were placed into an appropriately-sized well atop a small, plastic propeller. After puncturing holes in the gelatin capsule, the patient put one end of the device between his or her lips and pulled a breath in. One could hear the propeller spin during inhalation, and a coarse white powder was emptied from the capsule. Those who remember the Spinhaler will remember that the powder was somewhat irritating. Some granules would remain to be cleared from one's mouth; and it was advised that one stop use of the medication during asthmatic attacks lest it precipitate worsened bronchospasm in the context of heightened airway hyperresponsiveness.

We mention this early dry-powder device not just for historical interest, but to emphasize that newer dry-powder inhalers have overcome some of these early drawbacks. The very fine powder in modern formulations is not irritating, leaves no visible residue in the pharynx, and need not be stopped during asthmatic attacks.

With each new release of an inhaled medication from a different pharmaceutical firm comes a new delivery device; each is a proprietary product that has been developed and approved for use with medications made by that company only. At present, five patented dry-powder devices are marketed, four with asthma medications and one with the long-acting anticholinergic bronchodilator used to treat COPD, called tiotropium (Spiriva). Although instructions for use are included with the package inserts, for most people a single demonstration is worth a thousand words of printed instructions. It is safe to say that a large percentage of physicians will be uncertain about how to instruct patients in proper use of these newer devices. You will need to become familiar with each of them, and remain open to learning about future devices as they are released onto the market. Your ability to teach patients the proper use of these devices is invaluable in achieving their potential effectiveness. The currently available dry-powder devices are listed here. The Diskhaler, once used to deliver fluticasone (Flovent), is no longer marketed. We include discussion of the Spiriva Handihaler because of suspicion that as an asthma educator you may also be asked to teach patients with COPD about use of this inhaler. (As this book goes to press, the Pulmicort Turbuhaler is being replaced with a slightly modified device, called the Flexhaler.)

Device	Medication (generic)	Medication (brand)
Diskus	Salmeterol; Salmeterol and fluticasone combination	Serevent; Advair
Turbuhaler	Budesonide	Pulmicort
Twisthaler	Mometasone	Asmanex
Aerolizer	Formoterol	Foradil
Handihaler	Tiotropium	Spiriva

In general, dry-powder inhalers are easier for patients to coordinate than are metered-dose inhalers. However, each device is unique and requires special instruction.

One feature that distinguishes some of these dry-powder devices from others is their single-dose versus multidose design. The single-dose model is similar to that developed for the Intal Spinhaler described above: each dose is contained within a gelatin capsule that is taken from its foil package and placed into the dry-powder device—one at a time. The multidose design contains multiple doses (enough for one month or more) within the inhaler and incorporates a mechanism to make the exact amount of medication available for each use. The Diskus, Turbuhaler, and Twisthaler utilize the multidose design.

Because medication is pulled from dry-powder inhalers with the force of an inhalation, unlike with metered-dose inhalers patients do not need to match timing of medication release with initiation of inhalation. There is no canister to press down or squeeze and no visible spray released into the air. Spacers cannot be used with dry-powder inhalers. Oropharyngeal deposition of medication remains high despite creation of miconized particles (<5 microns in diameter). Patients should be advised to rinse their mouth with water after each use of an inhaled steroid delivered by dry-powder inhaler (as for metered-dose inhalers).

A reasonable concern regarding dry-powder inhalers is whether young children or patients with severe airflow obstruction will have sufficient force of inhalation to create an aerosol from the medication reservoir. The minimal required inspiratory flow varies from one device to another, but in general it is quite little—on the order of 30–60 L/min. Although not widely used, a device is available to test the inspiratory flow that a person is capable of generating prior to prescribing a dry-powder inhaler. Called "In-Check Dial," it is a portable, hand-held device that can compare the strength of the patient's forceful inhalation with the flow required for different dry-powder devices. In general, children over the age of 4 years can generate adequate inspiratory flow to use dry-powder inhalers.

Currently there is no dry-powder system available in the United States to deliver a quick-relief beta-agonist bronchodilator such as albuterol. For a time the single-dose dry-powder inhaler called Rotahaler was marketed to deliver the Ventolin brand of albuterol, but this device has since been withdrawn from the market.

Diskus

You are likely already familiar with the Diskus device (Fig. 8-11). It is used to deliver the most widely prescribed controller medication, the salmeterol-fluticasone combination, Advair. It has three very favorable features: one is its built-in dose counter; two is its multidose design (each device should last at least 30 days); and three is dose adjustment such that it is always to be used as only one inhalation with each administration. The dose counter indicates the number of doses left.

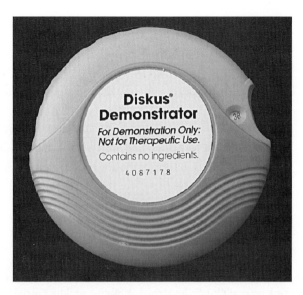

FIGURE 8-11   *Diskus dry-powder inhaler. Photograph courtesy of Kenneth M. Bernstein.*

It counts down from the initial number of 60 doses at purchase (28 doses contained within samples distributed by pharmaceutical representatives to doctors' offices). The counter advances to the next number when the lever used to prepare each dose for inhalation is moved into position. The numbers turn to red when five or fewer doses are left, presumably as a reminder that refill will soon be necessary.

The outer covering of the Diskus rotates open to expose the oval, fish mouth-like surface that is the mouthpiece. A thumb-grip indentation in the rim of the device is provided to facilitate this rotation. A lever is then exposed. In order to prepare the next dose of medication, one advances the lever about 1 inch, until it clicks into place at the other end of the space available. With movement of the lever, the white orifice from which the medication emerges can be seen in the center of the mouthpiece. The patient now places his or her lips onto the mouthpiece and forcefully pulls in a deep breath—followed by a brief breath-hold. Blowing into the orifice is to be avoided; it could disperse the medication into the air. The patient needs to breathe in, not out, once the device is put to the mouth. One breath in should empty all of the medication from its (concealed) packet. The internal workings of the device are such that each dose of medication is contained within a sealed foil packet along a coiled strip of such packets. Advancing the lever opens the next packet along that strip, while the remaining doses are kept protected from exposure to moisture.

After a dose of medication is inhaled, the device needs to be closed again. Using the thumb-grip indentation, one can pull the cover (and move the lever) back into place with one motion. No harm is done if one pulls the lever back to its starting position and *then* rotates the cover closed.

To summarize use of the Diskus dry-powder inhaler:

- Keeping the inhaler in a horizontal position, place thumb in thumb grip and pull cover fully open until a click is heard and the mouthpiece is exposed.
- With the mouthpiece toward you, slide the lever across as far as it will go until it also clicks into place.
- Bring the inhaler to the mouth and close lips tightly around the mouthpiece.
- Breathe in forcefully and steadily, followed by a brief breath-hold.
- Using the thumbgrip, close the cover (and with it, reposition the lever to its starting position).

Turbuhaler

The Turbuhaler was the first dry-powder inhaler introduced into the United States (in 1998). It too is a multidose device, each new Turbuhaler containing 200 doses of the medication, budesonide (Pulmicort). For patients who use only one or two "hits" per day, one device will last months. Its inner structure is illustrated in the accompanying diagram (Fig. 8-12).

The device is approximately the size of a large thumb. It has a plastic cover that serves to keep the mouthpiece clean and the medication port free of liquid or debris. The cover is removed by twisting it clockwise. A dose of medication is then made available by twisting the brown wheel at the bottom of the device as far as it will go to the right (clockwise) (approximately a $1/4$ turn), then twisting it back to the left (counterclockwise) to its original position. Upon return to its original position a soft click can be heard—and the medication is ready for inhalation. It is best to hold the device vertically while preparing the dose in this way. Before the very first dose from a new device, prime the system by rotating

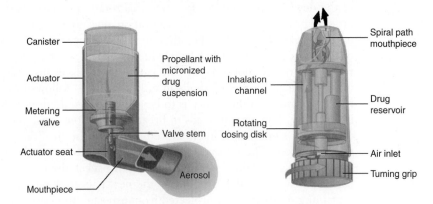

FIGURE 8-12   *Schematic diagram showing the inner workings of a traditional metered-dose inhaler (left) and the Turbuhaler dry-powder device (right). Reproduced with permission from Nelson HS. Beta-adrenergic bronchodilators. N Engl J Med 1995;333:499–506. Copyright 1995 Massachusetts Medical Society. All rights reserved.*

the brown wheel to the right, then left, without inhaling a dose. The Turbuhaler does not need any subsequent priming.

The patient then brings the Turbuhaler to his mouth, holding it horizontally. He seals his lips around the top of the device and pulls a deep, steady breath in, followed by a brief breath-hold. One deep breath in delivers the full 200 mcg of medication made available for each inhalation. If an additional amount is prescribed (for instance, "take two inhalations of medication twice daily"), the procedure is repeated: hold the device vertically, rotate the wheel to the right and then back to the left, hold it horizontally to one's mouth and lips, and pull another deep breath in. When done, place the plastic cover over the top of the inhaler and screw it back into position. As you know, budesonide (Pulmicort) is a steroid; patients should be reminded to rinse their mouth after each use.

Sometimes patients are encouraged to exhale gently before placing the device to the lips for a deep inhalation. Doing so maximizes the size of a breath available for inhalation, which is helpful for those with a small lung capacity. If teaching this step to patients, you need to advise them to exhale *away* from the orifice at the top of the Turbuhaler, so as not to blow medicine out of the inhaler or add moisture from the exhaled breath to the powder. In the same way, it is best to keep the Turbuhaler away from very moist areas, like an indoor pool or steamy bathroom.

The powder released from the Turbuhaler is difficult to feel: its very fine particle size is not felt in the mouth, and for most people it has no taste. Compared to the irritating powdered medications of yore, which left unpleasant residues in the mouth, these features can be viewed as pluses. However, some patients find it disconcerting that they cannot detect that medication is actually being delivered. "How do I know," they wonder, "that I am actually getting any medication?" Here's a simple solution to allay the doubts of such a skeptic. The patient should prepare the next dose for inhalation as one normally would. Then take a thin, colored-cloth (like a colored handkerchief or shirt edge) and tightly cover the top of the Turbuhaler. Place one's lips over the cloth and top of the inhaler, and pull in a breath *through the cloth*. Remove the cloth and on its inner surface (the surface touching the top of the Turbuhaler), one can see the white powder of the budesonide medication. *Voila!*

The Turbuhaler does not have a true dose counter, but it does have a qualitative dose indicator that warns when the device is nearly empty. Once the cover has been removed, one can see along the side wall of the inhaler (approximately 1 inch from the top), a small rectangular *window* made of clear plastic. When only 20 doses of medication are left, a plastic red indicator will fill half the window. When the device is empty, the plastic indicator fills the entire window. Take a moment to show your patient this dose indicator—because it is unlikely that anyone else will!

We summarize use of the Turbuhaler as follows:

- Unscrew and lift off the white cap.
- Holding the inhaler vertically, twist the brown wheel at the bottom to the right and then back to the left until a click is heard.

- With the inhaler now held horizontally, place the top end between the lips and breathe in forcefully and deeply, followed by a brief breath-hold. Do not blow out into the opening at the top.
- For a second puff of medicine, repeat the previous two steps.
- Screw the cover back onto its base.
- Rinse mouth thoroughly after use.
- Keep the inhaler away from damp environments, such a bath or pool area.

Twisthaler

The newest dry-powder inhaler, first made available in the summer of 2005, is the Twisthaler, developed to deliver the inhaled steroid preparation, mometasone (Asmanex). Its overall shape and size are similar to the Turbuhaler (Fig. 8-13), and it too is a multi-dose inhaler. However, it has several distinctive features. The first feature to note is that when one twists off the plastic cover, one feels some resistance. The act of twisting off the cover prepares the next dose of medication; there is no wheel at the bottom to be rotated. Once the cover has been removed, the medication is ready to be inhaled. One holds the inhaler horizontally to the lips, then pulls a strong, deep breath in, followed by a brief breath-hold. When done, the cover is screwed back into place until it closes with a click. If a second dose is prescribed, one again unscrews the cover, making another dose available for inhalation.

At the base of the inhaler is a dose counter with the precise number of doses remaining. It is visible even when the cover is in place. Twisting off the cover

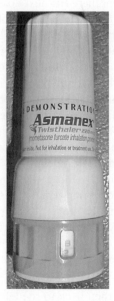

FIGURE 8-13 *Twisthaler dry-powder device.*

advances the dose counter to the next number. In prescribing the medication, practitioners need to indicate the number of doses within one inhaler: it is marketed with 30, 60, or 120 doses per device (for patients using one, two, or four doses per day). Another novel feature is that when the inhaler is empty, a locking mechanism is activated that prevents removal of the cover. In effect, the device becomes locked closed. Each inhalation (one puff) delivers 220 mcg of medication. Because mometasone is a corticosteroid, patients should rinse their mouth after use.

The following steps summarize use of the Twisthaler:

- Unscrew and remove the cover by twisting it counterclockwise.
- Holding the inhaler horizontally, place the top end to the lips and inhale forcefully and deeply, followed by a brief breath-hold.
- For a second puff, twist the cover on (it clicks into place) and then off again.
- Do not blow into the open inhaler.
- Rinse the mouth after use.
- When done, again screw the cover back over the top of the inhaler until it clicks into place.

Aerolizer

Because the Aerolizer is a single-dose dry-powder inhaler, no dose counter is needed. Each dose of the formoterol (Foradil) medication is contained within a gelatin capsule. The capsules come sealed within aluminum foil blister packs, six capsules per strip. The first step in using the Aerolizer is to remove the formoterol capsule from the blister pack. In fact, this step can require some fine motor manipulation. One is meant to tear off one compartment of medication along perforations, peel back covering white paper, and then push along the bubble side, forcing the capsule out through thin foil covering. Piercing the package along the edge of the blister pack with a pointed object, like a pen tip, works well to allow easy release of the capsule.

The Aerolizer has an easily removed blue cover (Fig. 8-14); one just pulls it straight off. Doing so reveals a long, hollow tube atop a white rectangular base. In the base is a well with a shape matching that of the capsule. To expose this well, rotate the tube portion away from the base. An arrow embossed on the plastic tube portion helps to indicate the direction in which to twist it open. It swings open 180°.

Now one is ready to place the capsule into the well within the base of the Aerolizer. The capsule does not go into the hollow tube above the base, and it definitely should not be swallowed! Return the tube portion back to its original position, covering the capsule and closing the device. Next is the step that patients must remember: pierce holes in the capsule (to allow the powder to escape) by squeezing together the blue wings on either side of the base. One hears a click as the capsule is pierced. Squeeze the piercing device only once for each capsule.

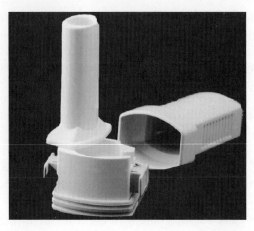

FIGURE 8-14   *Aerolizer dry-powder inhaler. Photograph courtesy of Kenneth M. Bernstein.*

The medicine is then ready for use. Hold the Aerolizer horizontally, seal one's lips around the end of the tube portion, and take a deep, strong breath in, followed by a brief breath-hold. As one inhales, one can hear the capsule rattling in its well (as it is supposed to do); and one may be able to appreciate a slight sweet taste to the medication.

Usually, one deep breath suffices to empty the capsule of its powder. Patients can check to see that in fact this is the case. They swing open the tube portion to expose the capsule in its well, shake out the capsule, and then open it by pulling apart its two halves. If powder remains in the capsule, they are not getting a full dose with just one inhalation. They may need two deep breaths to get all the medication from each capsule.

The single-dose system has advantages and disadvantages compared to multi-dose dry-powder inhalers. An advantage is the ability to examine individual capsules after use to ensure that all of the medication has been inhaled (as just described). A disadvantage is the extra work needed to prepare each dose. One needs to keep both the inhaler and the medication blister packs on hand and load the inhaler with a capsule each time one uses it. A widespread myth is that the formoterol (Foradil) capsules need to be refrigerated. They are kept refrigerated by the pharmacist before dispensing and may arrive by mail in a cold pack; but patients can safely keep the medicine at indoor room temperature (68–77°) for up to 3 months. A new Aerolizer device is provided with each month's supply of medication.

The following are steps recommended in the use of the Aerolizer:

- Pull off the blue cover.
- Rotate the long white tube (or neck) of the Aerolizer away from its base.
- Place the capsule of medication into the well in the base.
- Swing the tube back over the base until it closes with a click.
- Press together simultaneously the plastic buttons on either side of the base to pierce the capsule.

- Hold the inhaler horizontally, seal lips over the top of the tube, and inhale forcefully and deeply, followed by a brief breath-hold. One or two breaths will empty the capsule of medication.
- Rotate the tube back open to remove the empty capsule.
- Rotate the tube back to the closed position, and slide the blue cover back over the top.

Handihaler

The Handihaler is a single-dose dry-powder inhaler used to deliver the long-acting inhaled anticholinergic bronchodilator, tiotropium (Spiriva). We wish to emphasize again that tiotropium is not approved for use in asthma; it is recommended in the treatment of COPD. We include it here in our discussion of dry-powder inhalers because of our suspicion that you may at times be called upon to be a COPD educator as well as an asthma educator!

Use of the Handihaler is similar to the Aerolizer in that a capsule is removed from its foil packaging, placed in a well within the device, and then punctured to create holes through which medication can escape during inhalation. The Handihaler has an oval shape (Fig. 8-15). The cover is attached at one end; it is opened by bending it back at its hinge, but it cannot be removed from the device. Opening the cover reveals the mouthpiece. It too is hinged at one end and needs to be pulled open to expose the medication well. It rotates back in the same direction as the cover. A metal mesh on the underside of the mouthpiece

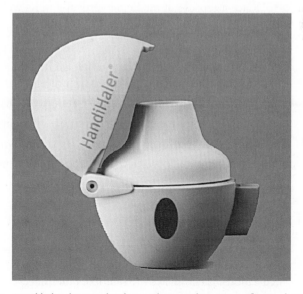

FIGURE 8-15   *Handihaler dry-powder device. Photograph courtesy of Kenneth M. Bernstein.*

covers the medication well during inhalation and prevents any particulate matter from being inhaled. The capsule is placed vertically into the well; it doesn't matter which end of the capsule faces up or down.

Once the capsule containing the tiotropium powder is placed into its well, the mouthpiece needs to be swung back into its closed position (while the cover remains open). It clicks back into place. As for the Aerolizer, the patient needs to remember to pierce the capsule prior to inhalation. This is done by compressing a blue piercing button on one side of the device. Only one compression is needed. Then the patient takes a strong, deep breath in, followed by a brief breath-hold. One can hear the capsule vibrate in its well during inhalation. It is recommended that two deep breaths be performed to empty fully the medication from the capsule. Do not breathe out into the mouthpiece.

After completing the two inhalations, the empty capsule can be removed. One again pulls open the mouthpiece and shakes the empty capsule from its well. The mouthpiece is swung closed, and then over it the cover (also called the dust cap). Both components snap into place.

Capsules come in packages of six, arranged as two parallel strips of three capsules. To remove the first capsule from one of the strips, the foil covering is pulled back over only that one capsule, to a line marked "stop" on the packaging. When the next dose is needed, that same foil is pulled back further—to the next "stop" line—allowing the second capsule in that strip to be removed. It is intended that the capsules be kept sealed in their foil packaging until immediately before use.

We summarize use of the Handihaler as follows:

- Swing open the hinged cover.
- Pull open the mouthpiece in the same direction.
- Place a capsule of medicine vertically in its well at the base of the inhaler.
- Swing the mouthpiece back closed over the base until it clicks into place.
- Pierce the capsule once using the blue button on the side of the device.
- Holding the inhaler horizontally, seal lips over the mouthpiece. Breathe in forcefully and deeply, followed by a brief breath-hold.
- Two breaths are recommended to empty the capsule fully.
- Open the mouthpiece again to remove the empty capsule.
- Swing the mouthpiece back until it clicks closed.
- Then swing the cover closed; it too will click into place.

NEBULIZERS

At first glance the use of nebulizers to transform medication in liquid form into an aerosol mist for inhalation would seem to be the ideal way to deliver inhaled medications. It eliminates the multiple potential errors in technique involved with dry-powder inhalers and, even more, metered-dose inhalers. The medication can be inhaled with slow, relaxed tidal breathing. All that is asked of the patient is that he or she breathe in and out comfortably while the mist is being created by the nebulizer system—and it is easy for the patient or caregiver to see when the mist is being generated. Patients do not need to remember when to inhale, when to exhale, when to hold the medicine to the mouth, and when not to breathe into the device. Many patients are asked to master the proper use of a metered-dose inhaler for their rescue medication, dry-powder inhaler for their controller medication, and peak flow meter to monitor disease severity. How uncomplicated nebulizer use seems: almost no teaching is needed other than to advise normal breathing while holding the mouthpiece between one's lips (Fig. 8-16) or an attached face mask to a young child's face.

There are other advantages as well. One nebulizer can be used to deliver a variety of different medications; and medications can be combined at one time in the nebulizer cup (e.g., the rescue medication, albuterol, can be mixed with the controller medication, budesonide [Pulmicort]). It is possible to vary the dose administered by varying the amount of the liquid that is placed into the nebulizer cup or by using only a portion of a nebulizer treatment. And then there is the matter of cost. Under the current system of health insurance, patients with Medicare will be reimbursed 80% of the cost of medicines available in liquid formulation for nebulization (but not if the same medicine is purchased as a dry-powder inhaler or metered-dose inhaler!).

Despite these advantageous features, nebulizer systems are far from ideal. For one thing, nebulization is time-consuming. The duration of a treatment depends on the particular nebulizer system and the volume of medicine to be nebulized, but on average it takes 5–10 minutes before the output begins to sputter, indicating near-completion of the treatment. Compared to less than a minute or two for metered-dose inhalers and dry-powder inhalers, this length of time can seem agonizingly long if one is trying to give medicine to a young, fussing

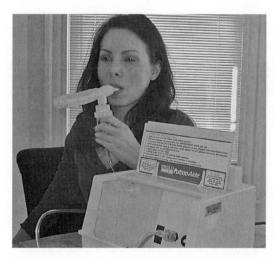

FIGURE 8-16 *Electric air compressor with attached hand-held nebulizer.*

child or to take medicine while getting ready for work in the morning or gym class in the afternoon. For another thing, medication delivery is highly inefficient with currently available nebulizers. Most of the dose of medicine put into the nebulizer cup settles on the inside of the equipment; some of it is lost into the air during exhalation. In most instances, only 10–15% of the initial dose is deposited onto the airways. Another drawback is lack of portability. Although small (palm-sized), battery-operated units are available, they tend to be costly. More widely used are electric, plug-in systems about the size of a toaster, obviously not suited for being carried in a purse or pocket.

KEY POINT Although some newer nebulizer systems are relatively compact and shorten the time needed for a medication treatment, in general nebulizers remain less portable and more time-consuming to use than metered-dose inhalers or dry-powder inhalers.

There are two types of nebulizer systems. One is called a jet (or wet) nebulizer. It is the type most likely to be familiar to you if you have had experience treating asthma in the hospital or urgent care setting. In the hospital, the flow of gas needed to convert a liquid into an aerosol comes typically from pressurized air or oxygen sources with wall outlets and attached flow meters. One can adjust the rate of gas flow using the regulating meters. For home use, the source of gas flow is an air compressor—the component that needs electricity to run. Different air compressors will generate different flow rates, making the outputs from nebulizer cups variable from one machine to another. The cost of a jet nebulizer system is approximately $80–$125 if purchased, although many insurance plans will pay for its rental as "durable medical equipment."

The other system is called an ultrasonic (or vibrating mesh) nebulizer. Aerosolization of the liquid medicine is generated by vibration of an electric crystal. No tubing is needed for conducting airflow to the nebulizer cup. Ultrasonic nebulizers generate larger particle sizes (smaller portion in the respirable range) and are less well suited for administration of a medication suspension, such as budesonide (Pulmicort). On the other hand, they significantly shorten the time needed for administration of a dose of medicine; they can be made small and lightweight; and they can run on batteries and be fitted with adaptors for automobile cigarette lighters. The cost of an ultrasonic nebulizer system ranges from approximately $250–$400. The cost may sometimes be covered by health insurance plans when use of a battery-operated, portable nebulizer is justified by a "letter of medical necessity" from the patient's healthcare provider.

Like valved holding chambers, nebulizers can be fitted with face masks in place of mouthpieces, thereby adapting them for use in children younger than 4–5 years of age. A swivel elbow on some models helps to keep the nebulizer cup upright while positioning the face mask to the reclining child's mouth and nose. A relatively tight seal is needed with the face mask to optimize medication delivery, and a tight-fitting face mask is commonly met with fussing and crying. Studies indicate that medication delivery to the airways becomes very poor when children are crying. Caregivers will sometimes adopt a compromise method to deliver nebulized bronchodilators to young children—the "blow-by" method. Medicine is blown from the mask or tubing in the direction of the child's nose and mouth. The child may stay happier, but the amount of medicine actually inhaled falls off dramatically. The blow-by technique is unacceptable for an inhaled steroid, such as budesonide (Pulmicort), because of increased delivery to the eyes and facial skin.

Because of their collection of moisture, nebulizer cups are a potential reservoir for contamination and bacterial overgrowth. Accumulation of dirt will also affect the aerosol output from the nebulizer. Consequently, they should be cleaned regularly with soap and water and periodically sterilized (e.g., soaked for 30 minutes in a solution that is one part white vinegar and three parts warm water). Many models are dishwasher safe. Do not wash the tubing. The average functional half-life of a nebulizer cup is approximately 3 months, although some models are guaranteed to have a stable output for at least 6 months (e.g., Pari Jet nebulizer).

To use a compressor and jet nebulizer, we advise the following steps:

- Connect one end of the plastic tubing to the compressor outflow port and the other end to the base of the nebulizer chamber.
- Keeping the nebulizer chamber in an upright position, unscrew its top, pour in the medication, and reseal the top.
- Turn on the power (on-off switch).
- Place mouthpiece in the mouth between the teeth (or mask over nose and mouth) and breathe normally until the output sputters and no more mist is created.
- Turn off the power.
- Disconnect the nebulizer chamber from the tubing, wash it, and allow it to dry prior to its next use.

Medications currently available for nebulization are the following:

Type of Medicine	Generic Name	Brand Name
Short-acting bronchodilator	Albuterol	Ventolin, Proventil, AccuNeb
	Metaproterenol	Alupent
	Levalbuterol	Xopenex
	Ipratropium*	Atrovent*
	Combination albuterol and ipratropium*	Duoneb*
Corticosteroid	Budesonide	Pulmicort Respule
Mast cell stabilizer	Cromolyn	Intal

*Used to treat chronic obstructive pulmonary disease and, on occassion, severe asthmatic attacks.

Of the medicines for nebulization listed above, only levalbuterol (Xopenex) is exclusively available as a liquid formulation—and it is likely that levalbuterol by metered-dose inhaler will be approved for sale by the time that this book is published. In other words, for all asthma medications one can choose to deliver them by metered-dose inhaler or dry-powder inhaler rather than by nebulization. (The budesonide dry-powder inhaler [Pulmicort Turbuhaler] cannot be adapted for very young children, but alternative inhaled steroid preparations can be given via metered-dose inhaler with attached valved holding chamber and face mask.)

Why then choose to use a nebulizer system? The answer is largely one of personal preference—a decision often made jointly by patient and provider. It is a matter of choosing which system seems—on balance—easier to use for a given person and given lifestyle, is least costly, and proves to be reliably effective. In our experience, nebulized quick-acting bronchodilators are often a desirable *back-up* for rescue therapy in severe asthmatic attacks, especially among patients who have required emergency room care on multiple occasions in the past. Nebulized medication may also be best suited to some caregivers of young children who together cannot manage metered-dose inhalers with spacers. Patients with Medicare as their primary health insurance may prefer nebulized delivery of their medication because of the cost saving. In the end, having multiple choices for delivery of inhaled medication is a good thing, without expectation that there will be one *right* method for all patients.

KEY POINT   Some patients may benefit from using a nebulizer system because of the specific medication to be delivered, its ease of use, its economic advantages, or its utility to deliver bronchodilator during severe asthmatic attacks.

Self-Assessment Questions

QUESTION 1

Advantages to the inhaled route of delivery for bronchodilators are rapid onset of action, potent bronchodilation, and few side effects. Disadvantages include which of the following?

1. Long-term irritation to the larynx
2. Long-term injury to the bronchial mucosa from aerosol propellants
3. Small fraction of medicine that actually reaches the airway walls
4. Variable amount of medication released in each puff
5. Unreliable number of doses per canister

QUESTION 2

Which of the following is not a key step in the use of metered-dose inhalers?

1. Shake inhaler before use.
2. Actuate inhaler at the very start of a breath in.
3. Inhale slowly and deeply after actuation of the inhaler.
4. Hold one's breath for approximately 5 seconds after deep inhalation.
5. Exhale rapidly and forcefully at the end of breath-hold.

QUESTION 3

Which of the following claims regarding the value of valved holding chambers (spacers) is not true?

1. They make possible administration of medication from metered-dose inhalers to very young children.
2. They reduce oropharyngeal deposition of inhaled steroids.
3. They should be used to delivery one puff of medication at a time, not loaded with multiple puffs prior to inhalation.
4. They can be readily adapted to use with dry-powder inhalers.
5. A built-in whistle in some models serves to signal too rapid an inhalation.

QUESTION 4

Currently, the only available breath-actuated metered-dose inhaler, called the Autohaler, is used to deliver the rapidly-acting beta-agonist bronchodilator, pirbuterol (Maxair). Which statement about the Maxair Autohaler is correct?

1. Only pirbuterol (Maxair) can be administered using the Autohaler device; no other medications can be substituted.
2. The Maxair Autohaler and albuterol (Ventolin, Proventil, ProAir) metered-dose inhalers contain 200 doses when full.

3. A counter indicates the number of remaining doses in the Maxair Autohaler.

4. One cannot *prime* the Autohaler because each puff requires an inhalation at the mouthpiece to trigger firing of the device.

5. A built-in whistle signals release of medication after the start of an effective inhalation.

QUESTION 5

Newer metered-dose inhalers use hydrofluoroalkanes (HFAs) in place of chlorofluoro-carbons (CFCs) as propellants. Which of the following statements about the HFA-driven metered-dose inhalers is true?

1. They are more sensitive to temperature extremes.

2. The spray released at the nozzle (i.e., the medication *plume*) is slower and warmer than that released from traditional metered-dose inhalers.

3. They do not require priming.

4. Oropharyngeal deposition of medication is increased because of the larger particle size in the medication aerosol.

5. Because of long-term safety concerns, the HFA-driven metered-dose inhalers are contraindicated below age 12 years.

QUESTION 6

A patient asks you, "How do I know when my fluticasone (Flovent-HFA) inhaler is empty?" The best strategy is:

1. Divide the number of puffs used per day into 120 (number of puffs in a full canister). The result is the number of days that you can use the inhaler; after that it is empty.

2. Float the inhaler in a tub of water. If it floats along the surface, it is empty.

3. You can use your inhaler until no more mist is released when you actuate it.

4. Shake the inhaler close to your ear. If you can hear contents moving within the canister, it is not empty.

5. Buy a new canister every month.

QUESTION 7

The parent of a 5-year-old asthmatic child has heard from another parent about "some-thing called InspirEase." She is not exactly sure what it is but wonders if it might be helpful for her child. You inform her that InspirEase is the brand name for:

1. A dry-powder inhaler device to deliver an inhaled steroid

2. An ultrasonic (vibrating mesh) nebulizer

3. A spacer system with an accordion-like reservoir bag

4. An adaptor for metered-dose inhalers used by patients with severely arthritic hands

5. A device to measure inspiratory flows in children being considered for use of dry-powder inhalers

QUESTION 8

As a general rule, it can be said about the dry-powder inhalers (compared to metered-dose inhalers) that they are:

1. Easier to clean

2. Easier to learn proper inhalational technique

3. More portable

4. Better suited for children under age 4–5 years old

5. Associated with fewer oropharyngeal side effects

QUESTION 9

Which of the following steps used to instruct a patient in the use of the dry-powder Diskus device (used to deliver salmeterol [Serevent] and combination fluticasone-salmeterol [Advair]) is incorrect?

1. Open the device with the thumbgrip until the cover clicks into place

2. Slide the lever to open the next packet of medication

3. Place lips on the exposed mouthpiece

4. First, blow out a gentle, comfortable breath into the device

5. Then, take in a strong, steady, full breath from the device

QUESTION 10

Instructions for the use of single-dose dry-powder inhalers, such as the formoterol (Foradil) Aerolizer and the tiotropium (Spiriva) Handihaler, include all of the following except:

1. Do not swallow the capsule.

2. Place capsule in receptacle well within the device.

3. Puncture hole in capsule with piercing button(s).

4. Pull in strong, steady breath at mouthpiece.

5. Rinse receptacle well and mouthpiece after each use.

QUESTION 11

A major advantage to medication delivery by nebulizer as opposed to metered-dose inhaler is:

1. No need for coordination of carefully timed breathing.

2. Improved particle size maximizes medication deposition on airways.

3. No risk of oral candidiasis when inhaled steroids are delivered by nebulizer.

4. A wider selection of medications is available for nebulization.

5. Allows administration of cromolyn (Intal) to young children.

QUESTION 12: TRUE OR FALSE

Patients N.P.O. for a surgical procedure can safely use nebulized bronchodilator preoperatively?

1. True

2. False

Answers to Self-Assessment Questions

ANSWER TO QUESTION 1 (DISADVANTAGE TO INHALED ROUTE OF BRON-CHODILATOR ADMINISTRATION)

The correct answer is #3; only 10–15% of the medication released at the nozzle of the metered-dose inhaler makes its way onto the bronchial tubes, even with optimal inhalational technique. Regular use of inhaled bronchodilators, even for many years, is not associated with laryngeal (answer #1) or bronchial mucosal (answer #2) injury. Metered-dose inhalers deliver a consistent amount of medication in each puff (answer #4). You get extra credit if you know that a reduced amount of medication may be released in the first puff if the metered-dose inhaler has been left standing for a long time, in which case *priming* with a wasted puff may be necessary. The number of doses of medication in each canister—when full—is highly reliable (answer #5).

ANSWER TO QUESTION 2 (TEACHING USE OF METERED-DOSE INHALERS)

The correct answer is #5. There is no reason to exhale rapidly and forcefully after taking a dose of medication from a metered-dose inhaler. One can simply relax and exhale naturally. The other steps are all appropriate aspects of metered-dose inhaler use: shake the device before use (answer #1); actuate the inhaler immediately before or at the very start of a breath in (answer #2); inhale slowly and deeply (answer #3); and hold one's breath at the end of the deep inhalation (answer #4).

ANSWER TO QUESTION 3 (VALUE OF VALVED HOLDING CHAMBERS [SPACERS])

The correct answer is #4; valved holding chambers cannot be used with dry-powder inhalers. They can be fitted with an attached face mask, making possible medication administration from metered-dose inhalers to very young children (answer #1). They reduce oropharyngeal deposition of inhaled steroids via metered-dose inhalers from more than 50% of the delivered dose to less than 10% (answer #2). Each puff of medication should be withdrawn from the spacer with a separate breath (answer #3); do not load the spacer with multiple puffs before inhaling. Some models contain a whistle that sounds when too rapid an inhalation is taken, encouraging a slow, steady breath in (answer #5).

ANSWER TO QUESTION 4 (USE OF THE BREATH-ACTUATED METERED-DOSE INHALER, THE AUTOHALER)

The correct answer is #1; there is no way to substitute any other canister for the pirbuterol (Maxair) canister in the Autohaler device. The Maxair Autohaler contains 400 doses when full (answer #2). There is no dose counter incorporated into the Maxair Autohaler (answer #3). A white plastic slide at the base of the Maxair Autohaler allows manual actuation of the inhaler without a breath in (answer #4). A "click" sounds when the Autohaler effectively releases a dose of medication, but there is no built-in whistle (answer #5).

ANSWER TO QUESTION 5 (FEATURES OF THE HYDROFLUOROALKANE- [HFA-] DRIVEN METERED-DOSE INHALERS)

The correct answer is #2. Users will notice that the *blast* of medication as it leaves the mouthpiece of the metered-dose inhaler is warmer and gentler with HFA-driven devices compared to traditional CFC-driven inhalers. It is not true that HFA-driven metered-dose inhalers are more sensitive to temperature extremes (answer #1) or that they do not require priming (answer #3). The array of particle sizes released from HFA-driven metered-dose inhalers is the same or smaller than conventional MDIs (answer #4). There are no known long-term safety concerns about inhalation of hydrofluoroalkanes (answer #5).

ANSWER TO QUESTION 6 (DETERMINING WHEN A METERED-DOSE INHALER IS EMPTY)

The correct answer is #1. If one uses a metered-dose inhaler daily (without wasted doses for priming), one can calculate the number of days that it will last based on the number of puffs taken each day and the number of doses contained within a full inhaler. It is sometimes useful to mark on a new inhaler the anticipated date that it will become empty, based on this calculation. The float test is no longer recommended because of its inaccuracy and the potential for water trapped in the nozzle to interfere with the proper functioning of the device (answer #2). The metered-dose inhaler may become empty of medication even when some mist is expelled from the mouthpiece on actuation (answer #3) and when a sound of internal contents is heard with shaking (answer #4). Depending on the number of doses used each day, an inhaler may become empty in less than one month (answer #5).

ANSWER TO QUESTION 7 (PROVIDING INFORMATION ABOUT INSPIREASE)

The correct answer is #3; InspirEase is a type of spacer system using a collapsible reservoir bag into which medication from a metered-dose inhaler is sprayed and from which the medication is then inhaled with repeated tidal breaths. InspirEase is not the name of a dry-powder inhaler device (answer #1) or an ultrasonic nebulizer (answer #2). Adaptors for metered-dose inhalers to be used by patients with severely arthritic hands are called VentEase and MDI-Ease (answer #4). The device used to measure inspiratory flow is called In-Check Dial (answer #5). It is a peak inspiratory flow meter used to assess whether a child can generate sufficient inspiratory flow to use dry-powder inhalers.

ANSWER TO QUESTION 8 (COMPARISON OF DRY-POWDER INHALERS WITH METERED-DOSE INHALERS)

The correct answer is #2; in general, it is easier to teach (and learn) proper use of dry-powder inhalers than metered-dose inhalers. Neither type of inhaler is difficult to clean (answer #1); and both are highly portable (answer #3). The dry-powder inhaler is not suitable for very young children (answer #4). Inhaled steroids released from dry-powder inhalers have the same oropharyngeal effects as when delivered by metered-dose inhalers (answer #5).

ANSWER TO QUESTION 9 (INSTRUCTION IN USE OF THE DISKUS DRY-POWDER DEVICE)

The correct answer is #4; do *not* blow into the Diskus after the packet of medication has been opened. The other steps represent proper procedure for use of the Diskus device: open the cover with the thumbgrip until it clicks into place (answer #1); slide the lever to open the next packet of medication (answer #2); place lips on the mouthpiece (answer #3); and then take in a strong, steady, full breath (answer #5).

ANSWER TO QUESTION 10 (INSTRUCTION IN USE OF SINGLE-DOSE DRY-POWDER INHALERS SUCH AS THE AEROLIZER OR HANDIHALER)

The correct answer is #5; it is not necessary to rinse the receptacle well and mouthpiece after each use of the device. Always good advice: remind patients not to swallow the capsule containing the medicine for inhalation (answer #1)! The other answers represent proper procedure: place the capsule in the receptacle well (answer #2); puncture the capsule with the piercing button(s) (answer #3) and then pull in a strong, steady breath (answer #4).

ANSWER TO QUESTION 11 (ADVANTAGES TO MEDICATION DELIVERY BY NEBULIZER)

The correct answer is #1. Medication is inhaled from the nebulizer system with routine, quiet (tidal) breathing; no carefully coordinated timing of inhalation is needed. The larger size of droplets in the nebulizer output (compared to the metered-dose inhaler spray) favors deposition of medicine in the nebulizer apparatus; less than 10% of the output reaches the bronchial tubes (answer #2). Inhaled steroids delivered by nebulizer (budesonide in the form of Pulmicort Respules) can cause oral candidiasis (answer #3). Several medications available for metered-dose inhaler (e.g., pirbuterol, fluticasone, beclomethasone, triamcinolone, and flunisolide) have no liquid formulation for nebulization (answer #4). Cromolyn can be administered to young children by metered-dose inhaler with valved holding chamber as well as by nebulizer (answer #5).

ANSWER TO QUESTION 12 (PREOPERATIVE ADMINISTRATION OF INHALED BRONCHODILATORS)

The correct answer is #1 (True). The main purpose of withholding food and drink prior to surgery is to ensure an *empty stomach* in order to reduce the risk for vomiting and aspiration. Medication inhaled onto the airways will not affect gastric contents or alter this risk.

9

MANAGING ASTHMATIC ATTACKS

C H A P T E R O U T L I N E

  I.   Epidemiology

 II.   Prevention

III.   Assessment
       a. Physical examination
       b. Peak flow measurement
       c. Oximetry and arterial blood gases
       d. Chest x-ray

IV.   Treatment
       a. General principles
       b. Bronchodilators
       c. Corticosteroids
       d. Other therapies
       e. Mechanically-assisted ventilation

 V.   Discharge planning

Much of our emphasis in routine asthma care—and asthma education—is devoted to maintaining healthy patients with normal or near normal lung function. We strive to minimize asthmatic symptoms and maximize exercise capacity. We are achieving our goals when our patients are free of cough, wheeze, or chest tightness; when they are exercising without limitation due to shortness of breath; and when their sleep is not disturbed by respiratory symptoms.

Another equally important goal is the prevention of asthmatic attacks. For people with asthma, acute asthmatic attacks are often the most frightening and frustrating part of living with asthma. For parents of asthmatic children, they can be a source of constant worry. One night spent watching your young child struggle to get air leaves an indelible mark on your memory. And then there are the days lost from work or the vacation plans canceled because of the visit to the urgent care center for your or your loved one's asthmatic exacerbation.

Perhaps you have experienced an episode of severe asthma yourself; you have likely heard patients talk about the experience:

- *It was like a 600-pound gorilla sitting on my chest and refusing to get off. Imagine running up a flight of stairs and then being forced to breathe through a tiny cocktail straw.*

- *Each breath was more and more difficult, and running through my mind was the thought that this one might be my last.*

Modern asthma care is highly effective in preventing asthmatic attacks. We can help our patients avoid the triggers that stimulate attacks. We can treat with medications that reduce bronchial hyperresponsiveness and lessen the frequency and severity of attacks. As we have previously discussed, routine use of anti-inflammatory therapy, especially inhaled steroids, has been shown to decrease the frequency of emergency room visits for asthma, hospitalizations for asthma, and fatal asthmatic attacks.

EPIDEMIOLOGY

And yet, despite our best efforts and the best efforts of our patients (or their parents), asthmatic attacks occur—frequently. In the United States, nearly 2 million times each year, people with asthma rush to their local emergency departments for treatment of asthmatic attacks. Approximately 500,000 hospitalizations for asthma occur annually in this country, and approximately 5000 times each year asthmatic attacks progress to the point of asphyxiation and death.

Asthmatic attacks are a common part of the experience of living with asthma. In the large nationwide telephone survey to which we have previously alluded, conducted in 1998 among randomly selected U.S. households and called Asthma in America, 21% of adults with asthma reported that they had experienced attacks requiring urgent care within the preceding 12 months. More recently, in the Children & Asthma in America telephone survey—in which the experiences of 801 asthmatic children between the ages of 4 and 18 years were assessed—19% of the children had an attack requiring emergency room care and 32% had an acute care visit to their doctor within the preceding year. Half the children missed school or day care in the past year as a result of their asthma; and one quarter of the parents missed work due to their children's asthma. Asthma is the number one *chronic* condition causing children to be absent from school.

From the perspective of health care economics, asthmatic attacks are costly. Of the 16 billion dollars spent on asthma care annually in the United States, more than half go to hospital-based care. Asthma ranks third as the most common cause of pediatric hospitalizations. In Boston, it is the most common nonobstetrical cause for hospitalization among women of child-bearing age.

Paradoxically, asthma is also recognized as one of the most *preventable* causes of hospitalization. Quality improvement initiatives throughout the nation are targeting reductions in rates of admission and readmission for asthma as a measure of improved quality of care.

KEY POINT Asthmatic attacks continue to cause frequent emergency department visits, hospitalizations, and work/school absences. It has been identified as one of the most *preventable* causes of hospitalization.

As we have previously mentioned, racial inequalities in asthma manifest themselves in the frequency with which persons of color are hospitalized with asthmatic attacks compared to whites. African-Americans and Hispanics are hospitalized at least three times more commonly than Caucasians, and this disparity has not narrowed over the last 2 decades.

In this chapter we will consider the assessment and treatment of severe asthmatic attacks that require care in an urgent care setting or hospital. In the next chapter we will explore what patients (or their parents) can do at home to deal with an asthmatic exacerbation, often successfully preventing it from progressing to a severe or life-endangering attack. As we will see, many of the intensive treatments administered in the acute care setting can also be readily given at home.

PREVENTION

A renowned pulmonary physician, Dr. Thomas Petty, is credited with having said, "Treatment of status asthmaticus is best started three days prior to the attack." Status asthmaticus is a now somewhat outdated term used to describe asthmatic attacks that respond little, if at all, to initial intensive asthma treatment. Although Dr. Petty's aphorism is not particularly useful for the treating care provider in the emergency department, it makes a crucial point. Most (although not all) severe asthmatic attacks evolve over a period of days, with many opportunities for early intervention. Consider the following case example:

> *A 35-year-old woman presents to the emergency department with wheezing and shortness of breath. She has had asthma since early childhood. At her baseline she is fully active, including regular aerobic workouts, without limitation due to her breathing. She takes an inhaled steroid preparation, fluticasone (Flovent) 44 mcg/puff two puffs twice daily and an albuterol inhaler as needed, usually less than once a week. One week ago she developed a fever to 101°F, sore throat, and cough productive of yellow phlegm. Her 3-year-old daughter and husband were also sick with respiratory*

illnesses. Her fever resolved and cold symptoms improved, but she continued with a cough productive of small amounts of whitish phlegm. Over the last 3 days, she found herself using her albuterol inhaler as many as 5–6 times a day for shortness of breath. Sleep was interrupted by paroxysms of coughing, and she began to sleep in a reclining chair to help with her breathing at night. Carrying laundry up stairs became a chore, and yesterday she stayed home from work (as an O.R. nurse) because of her chest symptoms. This morning she was breathless just showering and dressing, and so she asked her husband to drive her to the emergency room.

Over a period of 3 or more days, this otherwise healthy young woman went from doing vigorous aerobic workouts (including being able to jog 3 miles) to becoming short of breath with the light exertion of bathing and dressing. There were many clues to the worsening of her asthma: more frequent use of her quick-acting (rescue) bronchodilator; waking up at night with asthmatic symptoms; and shortness of breath with stair climbing. A respiratory tract infection probably triggered her exacerbation; viral infections remain one of the most common causes of severe asthmatic exacerbations in both children and adults. Dr. Petty's point is well-taken: had she recognized these symptoms of deteriorating asthma control and reacted with appropriate interventions early on—before the morning of her emergency room visit—she might have been able to reverse the course of the illness. In general, mild or moderate asthmatic attacks respond more readily to treatment than do severe ones.

KEY POINT   In general, an asthmatic attack identified and treated early (when airways have narrowed to only a limited degree) responds to treatment more readily than a severe asthmatic attack.

In the next chapter we will consider what actions she might have taken at home to interrupt the downward spiral of her asthmatic attack. At this point we wish simply to emphasize that teaching patients how to recognize and respond promptly to asthmatic deteriorations is an important function of asthma educators. And it is potentially life-saving. In detailed reviews of the circumstances surrounding deaths due to asthma, often neither the patient nor the patient's family recognized the severity of the asthmatic crisis and so failed to take appropriate action in time.

ASSESSMENT

Imagine that you see our asthmatic patient—the 35-year-old O.R. nurse—soon after she arrives at the emergency department and is brought into a room.

She is in acute respiratory distress. She sits at the edge of her stretcher, arms extended straight at the elbows, hands gripping the edge of the mattress. Her respiratory rate is 28 breaths per minute and labored. She has a very prolonged expiratory phase. She is using her neck muscles to aid in expanding her upper chest; you can see her stern-ocleidomastoid muscles contract with each inhalation. Her exhalations are forced and she tenses her abdominal muscles with each breath out. She is mildly diaphoretic, although her temperature is normal. Even with the unaided ear, you hear loud expiratory wheezing.

Her heart rate is 112 beats per minute and regular. Her blood pressure is 130/80 mm Hg. When measuring her blood pressure, as you slowly release the pressure from the cuff, you notice that starting at 130 mm Hg and continuing to 110 mm Hg, you can only hear the sounds of her pulse (the Korotkoff sounds) during her exhalations. When she breathes in, the sounds disappear; when she breathes out, you can hear them normally. Below 110 mm Hg, you hear the sounds of her pulse as you would normally, throughout the respiratory cycle. In sum, she has an exaggerated fall in her systolic blood pressure during the inspiratory phase of respiration, notable over the range of blood pressures from 130 to 110 mm Hg. She has 20 mm Hg of paradoxical pulse (or pulsus paradoxus).

On auscultation of her chest, she has loud, musical, inspiratory and expiratory wheezing heard in all lung fields. When you ask her to lie supine on the stretcher so that you can start an intravenous line, she tries to do so but quickly sits up again. She apologizes, saying that she is just too short of breath to lie down flat.

Physical examination

On her physical examination she has many features indicative of a severe asthmatic attack. She is tachycardic and tachypneic. She is using her accessory muscles of respiration. She has a paradoxical pulse (fall in systolic blood pressure during inspiration of more than 12 mm Hg), caused by the effect of the large negative pressures that she generates within her chest as she forcefully tries to pull air into her lungs. She is diaphoretic and unable to lie supine due to shortness of breath. In a young child we may also note flaring of the nostrils with each inspiration. The spaces between the ribs may pull inward on inspiration, and the space in front of the trachea just above the sternum may likewise be sucked inward with inspiration ("tracheal tug").

KEY POINT   Physical findings that point to a *severe* asthmatic attack include the following: rapid heart rate, rapid respiratory rate, use of neck muscles during inspiration, "paradoxical pulse," and, in young children, nasal flaring and intercostal retractions.

As a minor digression, it is interesting to note that many of these physical findings of severe asthma are a manifestation of the intense work of breathing during *inspiration*, even though the primary abnormality by which we recognize asthma is reduced airflow on *exhalation*. In part, the explanation has to do with the fact that during an asthmatic attack the airways are narrowed on inspiration as well as on expiration. However, the excess respiratory work during inspiration results primarily from another problem: overinflation of the lungs. The amount of air left within the lungs at the end of an exhalation is abnormally large during an asthmatic attack. It becomes so by the following process: a breath in, followed by a slow breath out—so slow that before all the air can be emptied out, the patient begins to pull in another breath (Fig. 9-1). Repeated inspiration with not enough time for complete exhalation leads to hyperinflation of the lungs; now breathing takes place at a very large lung volume. Try it and you will quickly see that it is hard work for the muscles of inspiration: take a breath in, don't let any air out, and now begin your breathing—in and out—with that extra air held in your lungs. It is particularly hard to expand the chest further at these large lung volumes (the lungs and ribs become stiffer), and the breathing muscles find themselves working less effectively at these volumes. Perhaps for these reasons a person with a severe asthmatic attack will often say to you that the problem is getting enough air *in*. It feels to him or her that the problem is pulling in an adequate breath, and rightly so.

The physical findings described above are useful in helping us to recognize a severe asthmatic attack, but they are not sensitive indicators. It is possible to have an asthmatic attack with severe airflow obstruction but not manifest tachycardia, tachypnea, paradoxical pulse, accessory muscle use, or diaphoresis. And we have already emphasized (in Chap. 6, "Pulmonary Function Testing and Peak Flow Monitoring") that the intensity of wheezing correlates poorly with

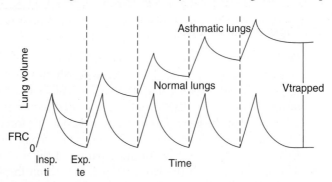

FIGURE 9-1   *In the presence of severe airways obstruction, exhalation is prolonged and the lungs may not empty fully before the next inhalation begins. The volume of gas held in the chest at the end of a routine exhalation (called the functional residual capacity or FRC) increases. This process of dynamic hyperinflation causes breathing to take place at a higher than normal lung volume (i.e, at an increased FRC). One consequence of this hyperinflation is increased work for the muscles of inspiration, such as the diaphragm. ti = inspiratory time; te = expiratory time; Vtrapped = volume of trapped gas. Reproduced from Levy BD, et al. Medical and ventilatory management of status asthmaticus. Intensive Care Medicine 1998;24:105–117. With kind permission of Springer Science and Business Media.*

the severity of asthma. If we rely on how loud or how intense the wheezes are to judge the severity of an asthma attack, we will often be wrong—and at risk for missing a dangerously severe attack.

KEY POINT Some patients with severe asthmatic attacks do not exhibit the typical physical findings. If you rely only on physical examination, you will misjudge the severity of some asthmatic attacks.

Peak flow measurement

Fortunately, we have at our disposal a simple and inexpensive test to measure the severity of an asthmatic attack: a peak flow measurement. It takes seconds to perform, and patients (over approximately 6 years of age) can do the test even in the midst of an asthmatic attack. If the patient appears to be in too much distress to give a quick, short, forceful exhalation, we will administer a bronchodilator treatment emergently and *then* measure peak flow. Trying to treat an asthmatic crisis without peak flow measurements is a bit like treating diabetes without checking blood sugar. It probably can be done, but it is certainly not desirable. Better to *quantify* the severity of the attack. It will help in triaging care, adjusting the intensity of therapy, monitoring the response to treatment, and providing medical documentation. And peak flow measurement will help protect you from underestimating the severity of a severe asthmatic attack even if characteristic physical findings are absent.

You may find that having the patient take a deep breath in and give a quick expiratory blast triggers a cough and a mild, transient increase in wheezing. No harm done. These symptoms tend to be mild and pass quickly (fewer than 5 minutes). The information gained is well worth the possible mild and brief discomfort.

Using peak flow results, we can categorize asthmatic attacks as mild, moderate, or severe. As already noted, you don't need a peak flow number to tell you that our patient, as described above, has severe asthma. One look at her struggling to breathe tells you as much. But other patients may report to you that they are having a hard time breathing and yet not appear in distress. They report difficulty walking up just one flight of stairs, but sitting there in the emergency department they seem quite comfortable. To clarify how severe their asthma attack is, you can walk with them up a flight of stairs (not recommended!) or check the peak flow. Diffuse expiratory wheezes on chest examination confirms the diagnosis of asthma, but it is the peak flow value of 120 L/min (normal for this hypothetical patient = 420 L/min) that indicates the severity of her airflow obstruction (and of her attack).

Perhaps you have a handy printed card or chart that lists normal peak flow values, based on people's age, gender, and height. If not, we offer the following as a *rough estimate* of normal values that you can remember for adults of average size and not at the extremes of age: 400 L/min for women, 500 L/min for men.

It is true that some people with asthma, even at their best, have abnormally reduced peak flow values. Their "personal best" peak flow is less than the average normal peak flow of someone of their age, sex, and height because of permanent changes to the bronchial walls, called "airway remodeling." The same would be true of a long-term cigarette smoker with chronic obstructive pulmonary disease (COPD); at his or her best, lung function is reduced. In this circumstance we need to rely on the patient's report of his or her best peak flow value or perhaps retrieve this information from the medical record, if available.

We can group asthmatic attacks into mild, moderate, and severe based on the extent of airflow obstruction. If the peak flow is greater than 70% of normal (or the patient's personal best peak flow), the attack is mild. Peak flow values between 50% and 70% indicate an attack of moderate severity. Values less than 50% of normal or personal best give evidence of a severe asthmatic attack. Because most adults will have a peak flow greater than 400 L/min when well, it is *generally* true that an initial peak flow measurement of 200 L/min or less points to a severe attack of asthma.

KEY POINT   A peak flow less than 50% of normal or of the patient's personal best peak flow value indicates a severe asthmatic attack. For most adults, a peak flow less than 200 L/min is evidence of a severe attack.

Oximetry and arterial blood gases

In assessing and treating asthma during an attack, another consideration becomes important besides airflow obstruction. It is the consideration of gas exchange: how well are the lungs able to put oxygen into the blood and remove carbon dioxide from the blood. These are generally not matters relevant to the routine outpatient management of asthma. Unlike in chronic bronchitis and emphysema (COPD), patients with asthma almost never develop significant *chronic* hypoxemia or hypercapnia. However, in an asthmatic attack, airways may become narrowed or closed to an extent that seriously impacts the exchange within the lungs of oxygen and carbon dioxide between the air and blood.

Most often, the hypoxemia associated with asthmatic attacks is mild. *On average*, the PO_2 during an asthmatic attack is in the range of 65–70 mm Hg (normal = 95–100 mm Hg), corresponding to an oxygen saturation reading of 93–95%. And the average blood carbon dioxide tension tends to be low, with a typical value being 33–35 mm Hg (normal = 36–44 mm Hg). What the low carbon dioxide values tell us is that most patients hyperventilate somewhat during an asthmatic attack. They do so not because of low blood oxygen (the hypoxemia is generally not severe enough to trigger hyperventilation) but for other reasons. Breathing more rapidly and deeply than usual is probably stimulated mostly by nerve endings within the airways and lungs and partly, at least in some instances, by a sense of panic over not getting enough air. It does not go away in response to administering extra oxygen. It resolves when the airway narrowing is alleviated.

Although mild hypoxemia and hypocapnia are the rule, if airway obstruction worsens still further, the consequences can be dire: severe hypoxemia and hypercapnia. Hypercapnia (arterial PCO_2 >44 mm Hg) occurs despite rapid breathing because the depth of breathing becomes less and less as the airways narrow more and more. The patient can no longer pull deep breaths, and with shallow breathing comes rising PCO_2. During very severe asthmatic attacks, first the PCO_2 rises to normal (approximately 40 mm Hg), and it may continue to rise to way above normal. As you know, low oxygen and high carbon dioxide levels (with associated acidosis) can be lethal. They can cause loss of consciousness, life-threatening cardiac arrhythmias, and death. As a result, we need to be attentive to the possibility of serious hypoxemia and hypercapnia during severe asthmatic attacks.

KEY POINT Hypoxemia and hypercapnia are potential complications of very severe asthmatic attacks.

As a safeguard against serious hypoxemia, in some emergency departments nurses and respiratory therapists routinely administer supplemental oxygen by nasal cannulae at 2 L/min flow to anyone presenting with an asthmatic attack. This is the standard approach for all children with asthmatic exacerbations. Another approach is to measure the patient's oxygen saturation with a pulse oximeter and administer supplemental oxygen only to patients whose SaO_2 is less than or equal to, say, 92%. (Not that an SaO_2 88–92% requires treatment with supplemental oxygen, but blood oxygen levels can fall transiently during bronchodilator therapy, and a "buffer zone" with some extra inhaled oxygen offers a margin of safety.) This latter approach has the virtue of not giving supplemental oxygen to those who do not need it.

It is worth noting that in general very low levels of supplemental oxygen correct the hypoxemia in asthma. You can expect the SaO_2 to return to normal (≥95%) with as little as 2 L/min flow. If a patient has profound hypoxemia during an asthmatic attack (SaO_2 ≤86%) or requires high levels of supplemental oxygen (>3 L/min), consider other causes. Among the possibilities are pulmonary complications (such as pneumonia, lobar collapse, or pneumothorax) or profound hypercapnia (because hypoventilation also contributes to hypoxemia).

KEY POINT In the absence of complications, the hypoxemia of asthma is usually mild and responds readily to low inspired concentrations of supplemental oxygen.

How can one determine if a patient has hypercapnia? At the present time, the only method is by analyzing arterial blood; it requires an arterial blood sample and arterial blood gas (ABG) analysis. It is safe to say that you and any patient you know would prefer not to undergo an arterial stick if it is not necessary. With some lidocaine infiltrated around the radial artery and a single pass of the needle, arterial sampling may not always be painful; but more often than not, it is. Does every patient with a severe asthmatic attack need to undergo an ABG?

Our answer to this question is "no." We would recommend performing an ABG in those patients who: (1) are in respiratory distress; (2) have a peak flow less than 25% of normal; and (3) are not improving with initial bronchodilator treatment. It turns out that hypercapnia develops only in those patients with very severe airflow obstruction: peak flow <25% of normal (Fig. 9-2). As a rough guide, these are patients whose peak flow is <150 L/min. If despite initial intensive bronchodilator therapy the patient continues to struggle to breathe with little sign of improvement—and the peak flow is less than 25% of normal—an arterial blood gas analysis is warranted. If the results indicate a PCO_2 of 40 mm Hg or above, particularly close monitoring is needed, perhaps in an intensive care unit. Repeat blood gas measurements will be required to determine if the trend in ventilation is towards improvement (decreasing PCO_2) or towards respiratory failure (increasing PCO_2). Other indications for checking arterial blood gases include unusually profound hypoxemia, loss of consciousness due to asthma, and somnolence that interferes with the ability to cooperate with therapy. In young children arterial blood gases are generally reserved for those who are being considered for intensive care unit admission.

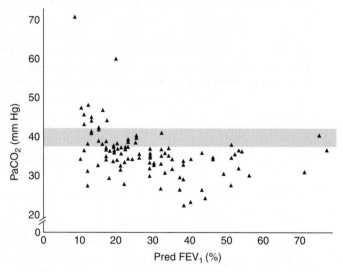

FIGURE 9-2 *Each point on this graph records the 1-second forced expiratory volume (FEV₁) and arterial carbon dioxide tension (PCO2) in a patient during an asthmatic attack. No episodes of hypercapnia (PCO2 greater than 44 mmHg) were observed when the FEV₁ was greater than 25% of the predicted normal value. Reproduced with permission from McFadden ER Jr Lyons HA. Arterial blood gas tension in asthma. N Engl J Med 1968;278:1027–32. Copyright 1968 Massachusetts Medical Society. All rights reserved.*

KEY POINT Measuring arterial blood gases is indicated in patients with respiratory distress, not improving with initial bronchodilator therapy, whose peak flow is less than 25% of normal.

Another potential cause of hypercapnia in asthmatic attacks is iatrogenic: inhibition of the drive to breathe by medications with centrally-acting respiratory depressant side effects. Years ago physicians were (mistakenly) inclined to treat the anxiety that frequently accompanies asthmatic attacks with anxiolytics, such as benzodiazepines (e.g., lorazepam [Ativan] or diazepam [Valium]). The consequence was a depressed drive to breathe and, in severe asthmatic attacks, the risk of worsening hypoventilation and resultant hypercapnia. This is a cautionary tale: use sedatives to treat the anxiety associated with asthmatic attacks only at your patient's risk!

Chest x-ray

One other test commonly performed in the assessment of asthmatic attacks is a chest x-ray. However, if one stops to ask what the value of a chest x-ray is in this setting, it proves difficult to find a justification. Most often (in fact, 98% of the time), the chest film will either be normal or simply show evidence of hyperinflation. Abnormal findings other than pulmonary hyperinflation—such as pneumonia, pneumothorax, pneumomediastinum, or areas of atelectasis—are rare, and they can usually be suspected on the basis of abnormal physical findings (such as fever, crackles on auscultation, unilateral wheezing, or subcutaneous emphysema) or excessive hypoxemia. For the routine asthmatic attack, it is safe to forego a chest radiograph. We reserve chest imaging for patients with one of the abnormal physical findings mentioned above, profound hypoxemia, doubt about the diagnosis of asthma or first-ever manifestation of asthma, or comorbid medical conditions (e.g., HIV/AIDS, recurrent pneumonias, history of aspiration, etc.).

KEY POINT During asthmatic attacks the chest x-ray is most often either normal or shows only nonspecific hyperinflation.

TREATMENT

Treatment of asthmatic attacks, particularly severe attacks, often begins in parallel with the assessment. It is appropriate to treat a patient with respiratory distress with the same sense of urgency as a middle-aged person with crushing anterior chest pain suspected of having a myocardial infarction. Every effort should be made to alleviate the patient's sense of breathlessness quickly.

General principles

The goal of therapy is rapid reversal of airway narrowing and, if necessary, correction of blood gas abnormalities (hypoxemia and hypercapnia). Just as during the day-to-day care of asthma, the causes of airway narrowing in asthmatic attacks are bronchial muscle contraction and airway wall inflammation with mucus hypersecretion. The fastest way to open airways is to stimulate the bronchial muscles to relax. In the emergency setting, bronchodilators are given immediately and repeatedly to achieve this goal. As we shall see, inhaled beta-agonists prove to be the most effective bronchodilators with the fewest side effects.

We have no immediate way to distinguish how much of a patient's airway narrowing is due to bronchoconstriction and how much is due to inflammatory changes in the airway wall. Patients can't tell based on how they feel, and health-care providers can't discriminate based on examination or testing. In those patients who do not improve dramatically and quickly in response to bronchodilators and in those patients with very severe asthmatic attacks, it is assumed that inflammation plays a major role. Treatment for inflammation involves corticosteroids; and in the setting of asthmatic attacks, this means systemically administered corticosteroids.

For the hypoxemic patient (as determined by pulse oximetry), we administer supplemental oxygen. That's simple. On the other hand, for the hypercapnic patient, complex decision making is needed. Therapeutic options include close monitoring for resolution of the hypercapnia in response to bronchodilator and corticosteroid treatment; noninvasive mechanical ventilation; and intubation and mechanically-assisted ventilation.

KEY POINT   The basic components for treating asthmatic attacks are bronchodilators (inhaled beta-agonists administered repeatedly), corticosteroids (administered systemically), and, when needed, supplemental oxygen.

Bronchodilators

Approximately 25 years ago, when subcutaneous epinephrine (adrenaline) was the standard emergency department treatment for asthmatic attacks, several clinical experiments were performed to compare how fast and how effectively different bronchodilator treatments reversed airway narrowing. Asthmatic patients were randomly assigned to receive one or another bronchodilator treatment for the first hour or more of their care, and no other medications were given during this time. The results of these experiments demonstrated the following: (1) inhaled beta-agonist bronchodilators, such as albuterol, given by hand-held (also called continuous flow, jet, or updraft) nebulizer, were equally effective as subcutaneous epinephrine (without the pain of injection); (2) this same conclusion proved true even in patients with very severe airways obstruction, when one might doubt that inhaled medications could reach their target, and (3) intravenous theophylline was a distant third (compared to inhaled beta agonists and subcutaneous epinephrine) in terms of bronchodilator potency, with considerably increased likelihood of side effects (Fig. 9-3).

In these experiments, the nebulized and subcutaneous bronchodilators were given every 20 minutes for the first hour of treatment. Although in the absence of an asthmatic attack, the duration of action of albuterol and epinephrine is approximately 4 hours, in an emergency circumstance the benefit appears to wear off more quickly. Repeated administration brings progressively greater bronchodilation with each dose. The downside is more frequent and more intense side effects with the cumulatively increasing dose. Common side effects from repeated doses of albuterol via hand-held nebulizer (2.5 mg/dose) are tremor, tachycardia (overall *average* increase in heart rate after three doses given in the first hour is 4–6 beats/min), and a racy, jittery feeling. Serum potassium decreases slightly. Average blood pressure remains the same or *falls* slightly. To reiterate, repeated doses of inhaled beta agonists generally do not cause hypertension.

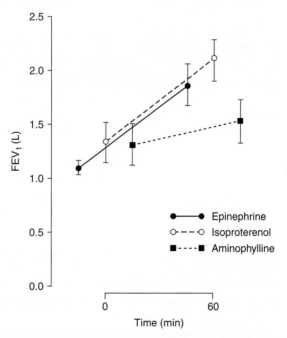

FIGURE 9-3   *In this study of the initial treatment of asthmatic attacks, patients were randomly assigned to receive an inhaled beta agonist (isoproterenol), subcutaneous epinephrine, or intravenous aminophylline during the first hour of their treatment in the emergency department. The results indicate comparable improvement in lung function (FEV$_1$) with inhaled beta-agonist bronchodilator compared with subcutaneous epinephrine. Intravenous aminophylline was a less potent bronchodilator. Reproduced with permission from Rossing TH, et al. Emergency therapy of asthma.* American Review of Respiratory Disease 1980;122:365–71. *Official journal of the American Thoracic Society. Copyright American Lung Association.*

Additional controlled clinical trials conducted in emergency departments have refined this basic message: that repeated doses of inhaled beta agonists are the preferred method to reverse bronchoconstriction in asthmatic attacks. They have tested whether adding intravenous aminophylline (or theophylline) to inhaled beta agonists provides additional bronchodilation during asthmatic attacks. It does not. They have likewise tested the combination of beta-agonist (albuterol) with anticholinergic bronchodilators (ipratropium). The combination seems to provide added bronchodilation only in those persons with *severe* airway obstruction. And they have explored whether the single isomer form of albuterol, levalbuterol (Xopenex), might be more effective with fewer side effects than the traditional albuterol preparation. The answer appears to be: marginally so, at best.

An innovative approach to patients with severe asthmatic attacks who exhibit only limited benefit from inhaled beta-agonist bronchodilators is the administration of intravenous magnesium sulfate. Magnesium sulfate acts as a bronchodilator, apparently by blocking the availability of calcium to contracting muscle tissue. At a dose of 2 g infused intravenously over 20 minutes, it provides some further bronchodilation in patients still severely obstructed after receiving inhaled beta agonists. A novel approach currently undergoing evaluation is the administration of magnesium by inhalation.

Another line of investigation has addressed how best to deliver inhaled bronchodilator medications. Comparisons have been made between albuterol by hand-held nebulizer versus albuterol by metered-dose inhaler with attached spacer device. Although the amount of albuterol released with each actuation of the metered-dose inhaler is only 90 mcg (compared to 2500 mcg in the aerosol solution placed in a nebulizer cup), other factors—such as particle size and loss of medication out of the expiratory port of the nebulizer system—favor delivery by metered-dose inhaler. Multiple experiments have demonstrated what many clinicians might have doubted: approximately four to six puffs delivered from a metered-dose inhaler provide identical bronchodilation compared to one treatment via nebulizer. The caveat is that the patient must carefully coordinate the actuation of the metered-dose inhaler with a slow, deep breath in from the attached spacer.

KEY POINT   Beta-agonist bronchodilators administered by metered-dose inhaler and spacer can provide identical improvement as the same beta-agonist medication delivered via hand-held nebulizer.

In many emergency departments and hospitals, nebulizers continue to be preferred for administration of beta agonists, in part because of their ease of use. Nebulizers require no special respiratory coordination, only quiet breathing in and out through the mouthpiece. In young children the nebulizer system can be attached to an appropriately sized face mask. In other emergency departments physicians have found that switching to metered-dose inhalers for beta agonist delivery works equally well and provides a significant cost savings. One protocol calls for albuterol by metered-dose inhaler, four puffs every 10 minutes, for up to several hours if necessary.

Patients often come to the emergency department reporting that they have used their albuterol inhaler at home, sometimes quite frequently, and they feel that now it seems to have "lost its effect" or "stopped working." You wonder how it is possible that albuterol by metered-dose inhaler can still prove effective in that circumstance? The answer likely has to do with two factors: the first relates to how well the medication is inhaled onto the airways; the other has to do with the dose. The proven efficacy of beta-agonist bronchodilators by metered-dose inhaler in emergency departments is dependent on careful coaching of patients in their proper use, aided by spacer devices. At home, under the stress or even panic of a severe asthmatic attack, all of the elements of proper metered-dose inhaler use—precise timing of medication release, a slow, steady breath in, and a subsequent short breath-hold—are hard to put into practice. Also, whether by metered-dose inhaler or nebulizer, the dose of beta agonist given in the emergency department is larger than most patients will comfortably self-administer at home. Four puffs of albuterol every 10 minutes provide 2.2 mg of albuterol in one hour (90 mcg released at the mouthpiece/puff); three nebulizer treatments (2.5 mg of albuterol per treatment) give 7.5 mg of albuterol over 1 hour. By comparison, a home regimen of two puffs of albuterol every 2–4 hours provides far less medicine (on average, approximately 0.05–0.1 mg per hour).

There is an important lesson that we can share with our patients based on these scientific observations. We can tell them: if you suffer an acute asthmatic crisis far from emergency medical care, at work, at school, on vacation, or at summer camp, you have at your disposal a powerful treatment every bit as effective as the nebulized bronchodilators given in many emergency departments. You can use your bronchodilator inhaler—your albuterol (Ventolin, Proventil), pirbuterol (Maxair), or metaproterenol (Alupent) metered-dose inhaler—to bring quick and powerful relief. In this circumstance, you can use not just the usual two puffs, but rather four puffs; and you can repeat the treatment as often as every 10–20 minutes. We would not suggest that this intervention replace seeking medical care, but it helps your breathing and "buys you time" while you get medical help.

Corticosteroids

While the majority of patients improve quickly and dramatically in response to intensive treatment with bronchodilators, some do not. Even after multiple doses of beta agonists—with or without ipratropium (Atrovent), theophylline, or magnesium—some patients continue with severe wheezing and shortness of breath. Their peak flows improve only a little, if at all. In them the bronchodilators really do seem to have stopped working.

In fact, in the vast majority of instances, failure to improve is not due to medication tolerance but to an alternative cause for the continued severe airflow obstruction, something more than bronchial smooth muscle constriction. Most often the persistent difficulty is due to swollen, mucus-filled bronchial tubes. No amount of bronchodilator, inhaled or intravenous, will reverse this inflammatory response. Improvement requires: (1) removal from the offending allergens or irritants, and (2) anti-inflammatory steroids. Over time, at rest in a clean hospital environment, patients tend to gradually experience improvement over a period of several hours to days. Corticosteroids accelerate the improvement (Fig. 9-4).

There was a time many years ago when steroids were withheld until late in the course of treating asthmatic attacks, used only as a "last resort." In recent years this approach has been reversed. Patients recognized as having a very severe asthmatic attack are begun on steroids immediately. Other patients are prescribed steroids after the first hour of bronchodilator treatment if at that point they continue with respiratory difficulty and a reduced peak flow (<40% of predicted). In addition, a course of corticosteroids given at the time of discharge home from the emergency department reduces the risk of a recurrent attack over the ensuing 2–3 weeks. Nowadays, only mild attacks or those occurring under special circumstances (e.g., patient ran out of his or her routine anti-asthmatic medications) do not prompt prescription of corticosteroids in the emergency department or at the time of emergency department discharge.

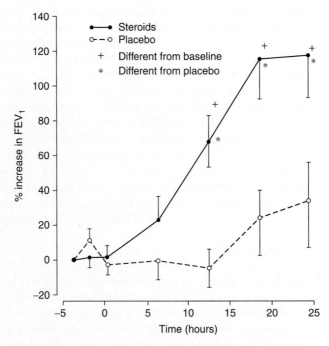

FIGURE 9-4 *Patients admitted to the hospital with severe asthma were randomly assigned to receive besides intensive treatment with bronchodilators either intravenous corticosteroids or placebo. The group given systemic corticosteroids achieved significantly more rapid improvement. Reproduced from Fanta CH, et al., Glucocorticoids in acute asthma: a critical controlled trial,* American Journal of Medicine 1983;74:845–851, *with permission from Elsevier.*

To treat an asthmatic attack, corticosteroids need to be given systemically (intravenously or as tablets or liquid for oral administration). Even highly potent *inhaled* steroids like fluticasone (Flovent) are not as effective as systemic steroids (which are brought to all layers of the airway wall via the bloodstream). On the other hand, it appears that orally and intravenously administered steroids are equivalent. Sixty milligrams of oral methylprednisolone (Medrol) is equally effective as 60 milligrams of intravenous methylprednisolone (Solu-Medrol). Oral steroids take approximately 1 hour to be absorbed from the stomach into the bloodstream. In most instances, this delay of 1 hour (compared to the instant blood levels achieved via an intravenous bolus) is not clinically important. After all, it takes several hours for systemic steroids to exert the chemical actions that dampen inflammation; a 1-hour delay is generally insignificant and undetectable.

KEY POINT   Treatment of severe asthmatic exacerbations requires systemic rather than just inhaled corticosteroids. Oral administration is as effective as intravenous administration when comparable doses are given.

These, then, are the evidence-based assertions upon which we can agree: corticosterioids speed the resolution of severe asthmatic attacks; they need to be given systemically in this setting to be fully effective; and when comparable doses are given, oral and intravenous steroids achieve the same outcomes. Where things get less certain are the following issues: how much steroids, for how long, and do we need to taper? Because very few scientific data are available to answer these questions, we are left with style, tradition ("because that's how we've always done it"), and individual experiences to guide our choices. As a result, you've seen used many different dosing schedules of steroids for severe asthma. We can share with you our experiences and biases, but we do not suggest that these are the only way or even the preferred way of doing things. It is only our way at the present time.

In the emergency department, we would give a single dose of prednisone 60 mg (it comes in 20 mg tablets) or methylprednisolone (Medrol) 64 mg (it comes in 16 mg tablets) to an adult of average size. In children, the recommended dose is 2 mg/kg/day, up to 60 mg. Liquid formulations are available, such as prednisolone (Pediapred or Prelone) and prednisone (both formulated as 5 or 15 mg per teaspoonful). Those who choose to give intravenous corticosteroids in the emergency department generally administer 60–125 mg of methylprednisolone (Solu-Medrol) as an intravenous bolus. Larger doses (e.g., 500 mg by intravenous bolus) have been shown to be no more effective.

Patients admitted to our hospital receive oral prednisone 60 mg every 8 hours for the first 24 hours of their hospitalization. The optimal dose of steroids in this setting is unknown. Our total daily dose is within the range (120–180 mg) recommended by the members of the Expert Panel of the National Asthma

Education and Prevention Program in their "Guidelines." To many clinicians, exposing the stomach to this large dose of orally-administered steroids seems heretical, but in fact there is no evidence to indicate that gastrointestinal side effects of orally-administered steroids are any greater than for intravenously-administered steroids. Our experience over the last 5–6 years bears out this prediction that oral administration of these large doses is well tolerated. Previously, when intravenous corticosteroids were the standard, we used to give intravenous methylprednisolone (Solu-Medrol) 60–125 mg every 6–8 hours.

After the first hospital day, we reduce the dose of systemic steroids: to prednisone 60 mg every 12 hours on Day 2 and to 60 mg once daily on Day 3. Patients are typically discharged home on a dose of 60 mg/day. A common schedule for steroid dose-reduction thereafter might be to reduce by 10 mg every second day (i.e., prednisone 50 mg/day for 2 days, then 40 mg/day for 2 days, then 30 mg/day for 2 days, etc.). This protocol gradually reduces the daily steroid dose to zero over 12 days. As you know, there are innumerable variations to this protocol, varying the speed and duration of the dose reduction. Are there any principles that can guide a rational approach to this hodge-podge of steroid tapers?

We would offer the following recommendations: (1) patients should be treated with oral steroids until their lung function has returned to normal (or to their personal best), or at least until very close to normal; (2) the number of days for complete or near-complete resolution of asthmatic attacks varies widely, but the vast majority of patients will have recovered within 10–14 days of treatment; (3) patients (and their care providers) can know when they have fully recovered by measuring their peak flows and comparing the results with their personal best values; and (4) once lung function has recovered back to baseline, oral steroids can be abruptly stopped or gradually tapered without any difference in effect on asthma.

The usual arguments in favor of a steroid dose *taper* are: sudden cessation of oral steroids can lead to adrenal insufficiency, and abrupt withdrawal can be followed by a rapid relapse of asthmatic symptoms. It is certainly true that after weeks and months of regular systemic steroid use, the medication cannot be stopped suddenly without dire consequences. However, a 2–3 week course of systemic steroids is not long enough to cause adrenal gland atrophy with its risk of adrenal insufficiency; and patients continued on inhaled steroids are generally protected from relapses when oral steroids are withdrawn. As a result, when prescribing a short steroid course many physicians have abandoned the traditional oral steroid taper. They recommend a 4–7 day course of relatively high doses (40–60 mg/day of prednisone), followed by discontinuation of oral steroids and continuation of inhaled steroids.

KEY POINT   Evidence does not support the need for a steroid taper. When the patient has recovered back to baseline, steroids can be stopped (as long as the patient is treated with inhaled steroids to prevent asthmatic relapse).

There are three other *fine points* about systemic steroids for severe asthmatic attacks that we wish to mention. First, oral steroids can be given as a single daily dose (our preference) or in multiple divided doses throughout the day. One popular, prepackaged medication pack, the Medrol Dose-Pak, has methylprednisolone tablets laid out for a 6-day taper, with three-times daily administration on the first 2 days, twice-daily dosing on the next 2 days, then once daily dosing.

Second, we encourage continuation of inhaled steroids throughout asthmatic exacerbations, even though they probably add little benefit to high doses of systemic steroids. The reason for our recommendation is that we wish to communicate to our patients the importance of inhaled steroids in their treatment regimen. Use your inhaled steroids everyday, whether you are well or sick; they are the key to preventive maintenance therapy for asthma. Another advantage to continuing inhaled steroids even during hospitalization for a severe asthmatic exacerbation is the opportunity for teaching. Care providers can review how patients use their inhaled steroid and can teach about the difference between controller medications and rescue medications while they are actually being used. Finally, the potential for confusion is great when patients are instructed, for instance, to restart their inhaled steroid when their dose of prednisone gets down to 20 mg per day. At that point, days after your last contact with the patient, the instructions are likely to be forgotten or misconstrued, and the inhaled steroids "lost to follow-up."

And third, intramuscular steroids can on occasion be substituted for a short course of oral steroids. For instance, lipid-based, repository forms of methylprednisolone (Depo-Medrol) and triamcinolone (Kenalog) are available. These formulations are meant to be slowly absorbed from the injection site into the blood over a period of several days. Their advantage: certainty regarding medication compliance. Their disadvantage: once given, the drug cannot be withdrawn or the dose modified. As an example, at discharge home from the emergency department, intramuscular triamcinolone 80–120 mg might be given instead of a schedule for taking oral steroids.

Other therapies

The mainstays of therapy for severe asthmatic attacks are nebulized bronchodilators, given frequently, and systemic corticosteroids, which can be given orally. It seems too simple! Is there something more that we should be doing, especially for the patient who has not yet shown signs of improvement, who continues to struggle to get enough air?

In most instances, the answer is "no." Continue the current course, and the patient will improve over the next few hours or days. (We will discuss the exception to this recommendation, the patient who is developing respiratory failure due to asthma, in a moment.) There are other therapies that you might wish to try—or have seen tried—but for the most part they lack scientific justification or proof of benefit. They may have worked in some patients some of the time, or they *seemed* to work, in that the patient improved at the same time that these treatments were being given. Their continued use is based on "anecdotal evidence," the observation that they appeared to help one or a few patients. In some cases this anecdotal evidence has been published in medical journals. Nonetheless, scientific justification for their use based on randomized, controlled clinical trials is lacking.

For example, one might wish to give treatments to help your patient clear thick secretions from her airways. She has repeated coughing and expectorates thick, clear mucus, like egg-white. Sometimes she can cough up small plugs of yellow phlegm that are the shape of small bronchial tubes. You are tempted to recommend hydration (oral or intravenous); a mist of humidified air to be breathed via face mask; mucolytics such as guaifenesin (or, in the past, drops of supersaturated potassium iodide—remember that?); or chest physical therapy. In desperate circumstances, physicians have performed lung lavage via the bronchoscope to wash secretions from the airways. None of these therapies can be recommended for routine use.

Hydration for an asthmatic attack has been a commonly uttered mantra for decades. It probably was born of the observation that very young children, those too young to report their thirst and ask for something to drink, can lose significant amounts of fluid via their labored respirations and become dehydrated. With dehydration come thickened airway secretions and worsened mucus plugging. Of course, very young children with dehydration should receive supplemental fluids. But most older children and adults can respond to fluid losses across the respiratory tract by sensing thirst and drinking liquids. Dehydration would be a highly uncommon presenting manifestation of a severe asthmatic attack among older children and adults. And forcing extra fluids in patients who are normally hydrated does no good, and for theoretical reasons might worsen lung function in asthma. Remember the golden rule of medical therapeutics, *Primum non nocere*—above all, do no harm! Pushing fluids because "we've always done it that way" is not sufficient justification.

KEY POINT   Hydration only helps with clearance of secretions in dehydrated patients. Most older children and adults with asthmatic attacks are not dehydrated.

In patients suffering acute exacerbations of COPD, antibiotics are routinely administered. The same is not true for asthmatic attacks. The major difference is that in COPD bacterial colonization of airways is common, and bacterial infections frequently trigger deterioration. In asthma the airways remain free of bacterial colonization, and viruses, not bacteria, are the usual infectious cause of exacerbations. Experiments comparing empiric antibiotics versus placebo during flares of COPD have documented the benefits of treating with antibiotics. Similar experiments in asthma are few, but those that have been performed showed no advantage to routine antibiotics during asthmatic flares. A short course of azithromycin does not treat viral respiratory tract infections! Even among patients admitted to the hospital with severe asthmatic attacks, we reserve antibiotics for treatment of a likely bacterial sinusitis or pneumonia.

KEY POINT   Unlike in COPD, antibiotics are not part of the routine treatment of asthmatic exacerbations.

Recent interest has focused on a respiratory therapy intervention for very severe asthmatic attacks: having the patient breathe a gas mixture of helium and oxygen rather than air. By replacing the nitrogen in air with helium, one can create a gas mixture that is 80% helium and 20% oxygen. Besides allowing you to sound like a cartoon character when you speak, this gas mixture has the property of being less dense than air, and it is possible that this less dense gas mixture might flow through narrowed bronchial tubes more easily than air. It has also been argued that bronchodilators nebulized with helium-oxygen mixture (rather than air or oxygen) have improved delivery to the airways and greater efficacy.

The helium-oxygen gas mixture is a well-proven therapy for upper airway narrowing, such as in epiglottitis or vocal cord dysfunction. Patients find it easier to breathe when this low density gas mixture passes through a single point of narrowing in the upper airway. Whether the same is true when the narrowing involves thousands of bronchial tubes throughout the lungs is less certain. For theoretical reasons having to do with different patterns of gas flow in the upper and lower airways (turbulent vs. laminar), a gas mixture of low density might not have much impact on the speed of exhalation in asthma. At this time, helium-oxygen gas mixtures for asthma remain experimental, both in its use to ease breathing and as a vehicle to deliver bronchodilators more effectively to obstructed bronchial tubes.

Mechanically-assisted ventilation

Asthmatic attacks cause *reversible* airways obstruction. With removal from the offending allergen or recovery from the triggering viral respiratory infection—and with the help of potent bronchodilators and anti-inflammatory steroids—the bronchial tubes are restored to their normal patency and breathing again becomes comfortable. The usual course of an asthmatic attack treated in the hospital is improvement over a matter of days.

The exceptions to this rule are the most frightening events. Some patients are brought to the emergency department only after they have stopped breathing; others are on the verge of respiratory arrest, with agonal gasps of breathing. Other patients with severe attacks remain in respiratory distress despite intensive initial therapy. As we have discussed, the onset of action of the anti-inflammatory steroids takes several hours from the time of administration. Patients remain at risk for further deterioration in those first few hours of care, despite very intensive bronchodilator therapy. After 12–24 hours of in-hospital care, most patients show improvement or at least a stable course. However, sometimes patients can worsen while in the hospital as a result of medical complications (e.g., pneumonia, pneumothorax, or lobar atelectasis) or of therapeutic *misadventures*, such as treatment with beta blockers, sedating medications, or aspirin or nonsteroidal anti-inflammatory drugs (NSAIDs) in the aspirin-sensitive asthmatic.

Common to these near-fatal asthmatic attacks is hypercapnia. As a result of very severe airways obstruction, ventilation of alveolar spaces decreases, and adequate removal of carbon dioxide from the lungs cannot be achieved. In one small series of 10 patients with 11 events of respiratory failure seen in an emergency department or on arrival to a respiratory intensive care unit, in whom arterial blood gases were drawn before initiation of treatment, the average arterial PCO_2 was 97 mm Hg. Important consequences of this severe degree of hypercapnia are: (1) low blood oxygen (hypoxemia); (2) low blood pH (acidemia); (3) sedation with further depression of respiratory drive (CO_2 narcosis); and (4) risk of cardiac arrhythmias, both bradycardias and atrial and ventricular tachycardias.

Recognizing impending respiratory failure due to asthma is an important task, so that appropriate interventions can be initiated before respiratory arrest occurs. We speak of the patient who appears to be *tiring*: one who has struggled with rapid, labored breathing for hours and now, despite persistent, severe wheezing, starts to have fewer, more shallow breaths. Other patients will manifest their worsening hypercapnia with a changed mental status and signs of confusion.

Another important clue is a patient's need for increasing amounts of supplemental oxygen to maintain adequate oxygen saturations (SaO_2) by pulse oximeter. In most uncomplicated asthmatic attacks, if supplemental oxygen is needed, flows of 1–3 litres by nasal cannulae suffice to maintain SaO_2 above 90%. Beware of the patient who requires larger amounts of supplemental oxygen. One is tempted simply to increase the flow of oxygen through the nasal cannulae. When you do so, the blood oxygen will rise and the pulse oximeter will finally stop alarming. But an explanation for this abnormally high oxygen requirement is needed. It may be pneumonia or other comorbid illness that accounts for this unusual degree of hypoxemia, but it may also be worsening hypercapnia and impending respiratory failure.

In the end the diagnosis of hypercapnia—and the assessment of its severity—requires arterial blood gas analysis. The patient with a severe asthmatic attack who appears to be tiring, the patient who has developed a change in mental status with confusion or sleepiness, and the patient who needs increasing amounts of supplemental oxygen all should have measurement of arterial blood gases (or, in the somewhat comical vernacular of the housestaff these days, they need to be *gassed*). The level of the arterial PCO_2 will guide triage (does this patient need observation in the intensive care unit?) and decision making regarding mechanically-assisted ventilation.

KEY POINT   A high or rising requirement for supplemental oxygen during a severe asthmatic attack may be a sign of hypercapnia and impending respiratory failure. Besides administering more oxygen, one should consider this is an indication to check the arterial blood gases.

Intubation and mechanical ventilation provide the means of correcting life-threatening hypercapnia and acidemia. This intervention "buys time" while one awaits resolution of the bronchoconstriction, airway swelling, and widespread mucus plugging that characterize very severe asthmatic attacks. On the other hand, it is also an invasive intervention, with attendant discomfort and risks of serious complications. The decision if and when to intervene with intubation and mechanical ventilation can be easy, for example in the patient with agonal breathing, the patient with hypersomnolence and confusion so that he or she can no longer cooperate with antiasthmatic treatments, or the patient with an arterial PCO_2 of 100 mm Hg and pH of 6.96. At other times, the decision can be very difficult, such as in the patient who is struggling to breathe but awake and conversant. Into the decision-making process go both evidence-based recommendations and a large measure of the "art of medicine." In general, we would offer the following advice: patients with a PCO_2 >55 mm Hg with an acute respiratory acidosis (pH <7.28) should be considered for mechanically-assisted ventilation, especially if the *trend* on serial ABGs is towards worsening hypercapnia despite maximal medical therapy.

An option that has been investigated more recently for patients with impending respiratory failure due to asthma is non-invasive face mask ventilation. It explores the possibility that positive-pressure ventilation can be delivered in some instances using a face mask, without the need for intubation. Continuous positive pressure ventilation (CPAP) and intermittent positive-pressure ventilation (e.g., bi-level positive airway pressure, Bi-PAP) can be delivered by a face mask in the cooperative patient. Their use requires physicians, nurses, and respiratory therapists skilled in their proper administration and an intensively monitored care setting (emergency department or intensive care unit). Noninvasive ventilation might be tried in that patient in "the gray zone," still awake and alert but in clear-cut respiratory distress with an elevated PCO_2, not improving despite intensive treatments. Sometimes the noninvasive ventilation brings symptomatic relief, improves arterial PCO_2, and gives the antiasthmatic medications time to work. Other times, hypercapnia worsens despite its use, and intubation becomes necessary.

Two final points about the use of mechanically-assisted ventilation in severe asthmatic exacerbations: First is the observation that mechanical ventilators do not help to improve exhalation. They provide mechanical assistance on inhalation, relieving fatiguing inspiratory muscles and giving bigger tidal breaths, but exhalation is passive. The lungs and bronchial tubes, and not the ventilator, determine the speed at which air empties from the lungs. Correcting this major problem in asthma—airway narrowing and expiratory airflow obstruction—will still require intensive medical treatments with bronchodilators and anti-inflammatory steroids.

The second point is that when adjusting the settings on mechanical ventilators, intensivists have discovered that they do not in all circumstances need to aim for normal arterial blood gases (PCO_2 of 40 mm Hg and pH of 7.40). Sometimes, to achieve these goals would require large and/or frequent breaths from the ventilator, with risk of major complications from excessive stretching of the lungs (high inflation pressures) or gas trapping within the lungs (high end-expiratory pressures or "auto-PEEP"). It turns out that all that need be asked of the ventilator is that it help prevent *life-endangering* rises in PCO_2 and falls in pH. This novel strategy for adjusting ventilator settings in severe obstructive lung disease is called "permissive hypercapnia." It means that maintaining the arterial PCO_2 elevated at 50–60 mm Hg or more is satisfactory until the asthmatic attack improves to the point that normal gas exchange can be achieved with safer ventilator settings. Whereas prolonged hypoxemia causes serious brain injury, prolonged hypercapnia almost never does.

KEY POINT Permissive hypercapnia refers to the strategy of ventilator management that accepts target arterial PCO_2 values higher than normal. The purpose is to avoid overdistention of the lungs due to dangerously high ventilator pressures used to force air into the lungs.

DISCHARGE PLANNING

An interesting consequence of modern therapeutic strategies for the hospitalized patient with asthma is that much of it can be given in the outpatient setting. Orally administered steroids and inhaled bronchodilators can be taken at home just as well as in the hospital. Gone are the days when physicians considered it necessary to admit patients to the hospital for the administration of intravenous aminophylline (1980s) or intravenous corticosteroids (1990s).

Nonetheless, there is still a good rationale for hospitalization of the acutely ill asthmatic patient. The reasons include removal from potential allergenic stimuli in the home or work environment; rest and limited need for physically demanding activities; certainty that medication is taken properly and on time; and close observation for the possibility of deterioration, with the ability to intervene should respiratory failure be imminent.

At the same time, as the patient recovers from an asthmatic attack and begins to feel better, there comes a point when he is able to continue recovery at home. The patient is considered to be well enough to care for himself at home. He can continue to self-administer the same medications that have been provided in the hospital, with the anticipation that he will continue the same course of improvement that was begun in the hospital.

Unfortunately, deciding when that point has been reached remains ill-defined, a decision made up of one part science and four parts "clinical judgment." A common approach is to wait until the patient's wheezing has completely or near-completely resolved and he can walk comfortably the distance of a few hundred feet. It makes sense that a measure of lung function should also inform this decision. However, there is no well-defined target value accepted as a safe discharge peak flow. In our opinion, once the peak flow has improved to 60–70%

of normal (or of the patient's "personal best" peak flow), the patient is safe for discharge with little risk of immediate deterioration (if the discharge treatment plan is followed).

In years past, discharge planning for asthmatics could be rather abrupt. The medical team would assess the patient's status on morning rounds and possibly declare the patient ready for discharge. Prescriptions were written for inhalers and an oral steroid course, and recommendation was made for a post-discharge medical follow-up visit in the near future. Some patients might have a compressor and nebulizer available at home to administer aerosolized bronchodilators; others were expected to make a sudden transition from nebulized aerosol to metered-dose or dry-powder inhaler.

You can imagine the potential for confusion on the part of the patients or patients' caregivers. They have just undergone a stressful and probably frightening experience in which their or their child's asthma was out of control. They now return home with inhalers to master, a varying schedule of medications to take (as the oral steroid dose is tapered or stopped), and possibly other equipment with which they need to become familiar (e.g., spacer or peak flow meter). They need to contact their physician and negotiate a follow-up appointment. In addition, for some patients, asthma is only one of a number of medical problems with which they need to contend, and asthma self-care is only one aspect of the demands of their complicated lives.

Predischarge planning and patient education are both a major challenge and a great opportunity for the asthma educator. This moment in the patients' medical lives can be viewed as a "teachable moment," a period during which they are particularly receptive to learning new information and skills related to their asthma. Just as you are eager to teach preventive strategies in asthma care, they too would like to know how best to avoid this unfortunate event—a severe exacerbation of asthma—from ever happening again.

KEY POINT Following an asthmatic attack, the asthma educator has an opportunity to teach the essentials of asthma knowledge and skills to the hospitalized patient. We should seize this "teachable moment."

We offer here an asthma education "checklist" of topics to be discussed with patients prior to discharge. It is not all-inclusive; you can add other items to the list that you may think equally important. We would view it as the "basics": teaching Asthma 101 to the patient while he or she is a captive audience in the hospital. Nor does this teaching need to await the day of discharge. In an ideal world, asthma education in the hospital begins as soon as the patient is no longer in acute respiratory distress.

- Teach the concepts of reversible airway narrowing and persistent bronchial hyperresponsiveness.

- Discuss the importance of reducing the patient's exposure to environmental stimuli for asthma (environmental control measures).
- Instruct the patient in the proper use of inhalers (inhaler technique).
- Instruct the patient in use of inhalational aids (spacers), if needed.
- Instruct the patient in the different purposes of his or her controller and rescue medications.
- Instruct the patient in measurement and recording of his or her peak expiratory flow rate (PEFR), including in selected pediatric patients.
- Discuss the importance of recognizing and responding appropriately to signs of an acute asthma attack (asthma "action plan," as discussed in the next chapter).
- Facilitate postdischarge medical follow-up.

Self-Assessment Questions

QUESTION 1

Preventing severe, potentially life-threatening asthmatic attacks is a key aspect of asthma co–management and a crucial goal of asthma education. It presumes that:

1. Patients will monitor their peak flow daily to detect subtle deterioration in lung function prior to the development of asthmatic symptoms.
2. Most asthmatic attacks typically develop gradually, over a period of many hours to days.
3. Asthmatic attacks are predictable based on knowledge of one's asthmatic triggers.
4. Viral respiratory tract infections, for which we have no specific treatment, infrequently cause asthmatic attacks.
5. Only patients with severe persistent asthma are at risk for severe, life-threatening attacks.

QUESTION 2

Which of the following physical findings would be highly atypical for a severe asthmatic attack?

1. Inward pull of the skin just above the sternum (tracheal tug)
2. Exaggerated fall of systolic blood pressure during inspiration (paradoxical pulse)
3. Visible contractions of the sternocleidomastoid muscles of the neck during inspiration (accessory muscle use)
4. Diaphoresis and refusal to lie supine due to shortness of breath
5. Stridor

QUESTION 3

An asthmatic patient with severe shortness of breath and wheezing is seen in the emergency department. She takes only her albuterol inhaler, which she has used 6–7 times already this morning. Arterial blood gases are obtained, with the following results: PO_2 68 mm Hg, SaO_2 94%, PCO_2 40 mm Hg, pH 7.42. Based on these blood gas results, you conclude that:

1. She has mild hypoxemia and should be given supplemental oxygen at 1–2 L/min flow via nasal cannulae.
2. She has normal arterial blood gases and can continue to receive nebulized bronchodilator without concern.
3. She has impending respiratory failure and should be triaged to receive especially close monitoring.

4. Her hypoxemia indicates that her nebulized bronchodilator treatments should be attached to oxygen rather than compressed air.

5. Her normal arterial PCO_2 indicates that her asthmatic attack is not as severe as was suggested by her wheezing and shortness of breath.

QUESTION 4

A chest x-ray obtained during an asthmatic attack is most likely:

1. To be normal or show hyperinflation (flattening of the diaphragms)
2. To show evidence for eosinophilic bronchitis
3. To show evidence for eosinophilic pneumonia
4. To show atelectasis (due to mucus plugging of bronchi with distal collapse of lung tissue)
5. To show small, bilateral pleural effusions

QUESTION 5

During an asthmatic attack, nebulized bronchodilator (e.g., albuterol) is frequently administered as often as every 20 minutes for the first hour of treatment. Common side effects observed with beta-agonist bronchodilator treatments given in rapid succession include all of the following except:

1. Tachycardia
2. Muscle tremor
3. Hypertension
4. Agitation
5. Heart pounding

QUESTION 6

Repeated administration of a beta-agonist bronchodilators such as albuterol is preferred for the initial treatment of asthmatic attacks over theophylline or inhaled anticholinergics such as ipratropium (Atrovent) because:

1. They are less expensive.
2. They are more likely to be a part of the patient's usual medical regimen.
3. They have fewer side effects.
4. They are more effective bronchodilators.
5. They have a longer duration of action.

QUESTION 7

Corticosteroids for severe asthmatic exacerbations:

1. Should be given systemically only to patients already receiving inhaled steroids for their asthma

2. Should be given only to patients who have failed bronchodilator therapy administered for the first 24 hours

3. Are contraindicated in patients over age 65 years

4. Are equally effective given by inhalation as when given orally in tablet form

5. Are equally effective given orally in tablet form as when given intravenously

QUESTION 8

Many different steroid regimens are prescribed in the outpatient setting for treatment of acute asthmatic exacerbations. They differ in dose, duration, and frequency of daily administration. These variations in style reflect uncertainties as to the optimal strategy and variability among different patients and in the same patient during different asthmatic attacks. Which of the following statements about an oral steroid course for an asthmatic exacerbation is supported by scientific evidence?

1. Twice-daily administration is more effective than a single daily dose.

2. An oral steroid course should be followed by use of inhaled steroids to prevent a recurrent flare of asthma.

3. A gradual steroid taper is needed to prevent a recurrent flare of asthma.

4. A gradual steroid taper is needed to prevent adrenal insufficiency, even if the steroid course is 4–7 days in duration.

5. Intramuscular steroids have more side effects and less benefit than a short course of oral steroids, even in patients with a history of poor medical compliance.

QUESTION 9

A 28-year-old teacher calls in January with symptoms of an asthmatic exacerbation. Her symptoms began with sore throat, rhinitis, low-grade fever, and malaise. Her cold quickly "settled into her chest": she developed a nonproductive cough, chest tightness, and shortness of breath. Her nose is "running like a faucet" with a discharge that looks like egg-white. Her peak flow, usually 400 L/min, was 250 L/min this morning before she took her inhalers (combination fluticasone-salmeterol [Advair] and albuterol). She reports that many of her students have been sick this winter, and she requests an antibiotic for what she suspects is a "bad bronchitis and maybe sinusitis." You recommend that she speak with her physician about:

1. Further treatment of her asthma and withholding antibiotics for now

2. Azithromycin

3. Guaifenesin and azithromycin

4. A chest x-ray

5. A sinus CT scan

QUESTION 10

A 14-year-old boy presents to the emergency department in severe respiratory distress. He is too short of breath to speak more than one or two words at a time. After a treatment with nebulized bronchodilator, he looks no better. He feels desperately short of breath, breathing at a rate of 30 breaths/min. Which of the following arterial blood gas results (obtained with the patient breathing air) would convince you of the need for immediate intubation and mechanical ventilation?

1. PO_2 = 60 mm Hg, SaO_2 91%, PCO_2 33 mm Hg, pH 7.47
2. PO_2 = 45 mm Hg, SaO_2 75%, PCO_2 43 mm Hg, pH 7.39
3. PO_2 = 45 mm Hg, SaO_2 75%, PCO_2 33 mm Hg, pH 7.33
4. PO_2 = 45 mm Hg, SaO_2 75%, PCO_2 75 mm Hg, pH 7.20
5. PO_2 = 81 mm Hg, SaO_2 97%, PCO_2 21 mm Hg, pH 7.56

QUESTION 11

Hospitalization for treatment of a severe asthmatic attack can reasonably be justified by all of the following hospital-specific advantages except:

1. Intravenous administration of corticosteroids
2. Removal from an environment with continued allergenic exposures
3. Close medical observation for the possibility of deterioration to the point of respiratory failure
4. Limitation of physical exertion
5. Assurance of medical compliance with needed treatments

QUESTION 12

A 21-year-old college student is being discharged home following hospitalization for an asthmatic exacerbation. She should receive all of the following except:

1. A follow-up appointment with her healthcare provider
2. A Visiting Nurse Association (VNA) referral
3. Instruction on the proper use of her inhalers with demonstration in return of their correct use
4. A home peak flow meter and instruction in its use
5. Review of potential asthmatic stimuli in her home environment

Answers to Self-Assessment Questions

ANSWER TO QUESTION 1 (PREVENTING SEVERE, POTENTIALLY LIFE-THREATENING ASTHMATIC ATTACKS)

The correct answer is #2. Prevention of severe, potentially life-threatening asthmatic attacks presumes that—in most instances—attacks develop gradually, with adequate time to intervene before dangerous airflow obstruction develops. Daily peak flow monitoring (answer #1) is not necessary to prevent severe attacks. Even with complete understanding of one's asthmatic triggers (answer #3), it may not be possible to predict (and prevent) all asthmatic exacerbations. Viral respiratory tract infections are a common cause of asthmatic exacerbations in both children and adults (answer #4). It is important to remember that even patients with mild asthma can develop asthmatic attacks, including severe, life-threatening ones (answer #5).

ANSWER TO QUESTION 2 (TYPICAL PHYSICAL FINDINGS IN SEVERE ASTHMATIC ATTACKS)

The correct answer is #5 (stridor). Stridor (a loud upper airway sound having a single note or tone, most often heard during inspiration) is a sign of upper airway obstruction (e.g., epiglottitis) and not of asthma. On the other hand, during a severe asthmatic attack, one may find a "tracheal tug" (answer #1), paradoxical pulse (answer #2), accessory muscle use (answer #3), and diaphoresis and a patient's refusal to lie supine because it makes him or her too short of breath (answer #4). Remember that the absence of these physical findings does not exclude the presence of severe airways obstruction (FEV_1 <1 liter) during an asthmatic attack.

ANSWER TO QUESTION 3 (ARTERIAL BLOOD GASES DURING AN ASTHMATIC ATTACK)

The correct answer is #3. Remember that most often during asthmatic attacks, patients hyperventilate, causing an abnormally low PCO_2 (on the order of 33–35 mm Hg). Although normal for a healthy person at rest, a PCO_2 of 40 mm Hg, as in this example, is distinctly abnormal for a patient with respiratory distress during an asthmatic attack. It gives evidence of severe obstruction and the inability to *blow off* carbon dioxide to the usual extent. As suggested in answer #3, such a patient "has impending respiratory failure and should be triaged to receive especially close monitoring." She has only mild hypoxemia and at present does not need supplemental oxygen (typically reserved for SaO_2 ≤90%) (answer #1). Her blood gases are not normal (mild hypoxemia), and her normal PCO_2 is worrisome, as discussed above (answer #2). As noted, her hypoxemia is mild and does not require supplemental oxygen, including during nebulizer treatments (answer #4). As above, her normal PCO_2 at a time when she continues with shortness of breath and wheezing indicates a very severe asthmatic attack (answer #5).

ANSWER TO QUESTION 4 (CHEST X-RAY FINDINGS DURING ASTHMATIC ATTACKS)

The correct answer is #1. Chest x-rays obtained during asthmatic attacks most often are normal or simply show evidence for pulmonary hyperinflation. Bronchial inflammation (whether eosinophilic bronchitis or an infectious bronchitis) is poorly visualized on chest x-ray; the chest x-ray appears normal despite its presence (answer #2). Eosinophilic pneumonia (answer #3) and atelectasis (answer #4) are infrequent complications of asthmatic attacks and not the usual findings. Small, bilateral pleural effusions would make one consider another diagnosis, perhaps congestive heart failure (answer #5).

ANSWER TO QUESTION 5 (SIDE EFFECTS OF REPEATEDLY ADMINISTERED BETA-AGONIST BRONCHODILATORS)

The correct answer is #3. The usual response to beta-agonist stimulation is a slight *fall* in blood pressure, not hypertension. Tachycardia (answer #1), muscle tremor (answer #2), agitation (answer #4), and heart pounding (due to forceful heart contractions) (answer #5) are all common side effects observed during intensive beta-agonist bronchodilator administration for asthmatic attacks.

ANSWER TO QUESTION 6 (PREFERENCE FOR BETA AGONISTS OVER OTHER BRONCHODILATORS IN THE TREATMENT OF ASTHMATIC ATTACKS)

The correct answer is #4. Beta agonists are more potent in stimulating bronchodilation (they stimulate a greater increase in expiratory flow) compared to theophylline or anticholinergics. Neither theophylline nor an anticholinergic such as ipratropium (Atrovent) is expensive (answer #1). It is not important that patients have previous experience with the bronchodilator treatment administered for asthmatic attacks (answer #2). Repeated administration of albuterol may have fewer side effects than theophylline but not than ipratropium (answer #3). The duration of action of beta agonist bronchodilators is said to be 4–6 hours (comparable to ipratropium and probably shorter than theophylline) (answer #5), although in acute asthmatic attacks more frequent administration is warranted.

ANSWER TO QUESTION 7 (ROLE OF CORTICOSTEROIDS IN THE TREATMENT OF SEVERE ASTHMATIC EXACERBATIONS)

The correct answer is #5. Several studies have demonstrated that when given in identical (or similar) doses, oral steroids in tablet form are equally effective as intravenously administered corticosteroids. Prior use of inhaled steroids is not a requirement for receiving systemic steroids (answer #1). Systemic steroids are often administered within the first hour of treatment for severe asthmatic attacks, especially those responding poorly to inhaled bronchodilators (answer #2). There is no age limit for administration of corticosteroids in asthmatic attacks (answer #3). Clinical trials have found that inhaled steroids are not as effective as systemic steroids in the treatment of asthmatic attacks (answer #4).

ANSWER TO QUESTION 8 (USE OF A COURSE OF ORAL STEROIDS IN THE AMBULATORY SETTING)

The correct answer is #2. Treatment with inhaled steroids following a course of oral steroids for an asthmatic exacerbation reduces the rate of recurrent attacks, both in the short term (2 weeks) and long term (2 years). Prescription of systemic steroids one, two, or more times daily seems to be a matter of style and personal preference, without demonstrated benefit of one regimen over another (answer #1).

Despite the time-honored approach of a steroid taper, there is no evidence that abrupt cessation of oral steroids for an asthmatic attack leads to a greater rate of recurrence, assuming use of inhaled steroids after oral steroids are stopped (answer #3). Adrenal insufficiency may complicate *long-term* use of oral steroids, meaning at least 2–3 weeks of use (answer #4). Intramuscular steroids represent a reasonable option to replace a short course of oral steroids in a patient with suspected poor medical compliance. Intramuscular administration is not associated with more side effects or less benefit (answer #5).

ANSWER TO QUESTION 9 (MANAGEMENT OF AN ASTHMATIC ATTACK TRIGGERED BY A RESPIRATORY TRACT INFECTION)

The correct answer is #1. The clinical history strongly suggests a viral respiratory tract infection. She has no history to suggest bacterial bronchitis or pneumonia (fever, purulent sputum production, chest pain, etc.) or bacterial sinusitis (fever, purulent nasal drainage, localized headache, teeth aching, etc.). Antibiotics are not indicated (answers #2 and #3). A chest x-ray would be appropriate—to exclude alternative diagnoses—if she does not improve with treatment of her asthmatic exacerbation (answer #4). A sinus CT scan is not indicated for an acute respiratory infection of this sort (answer #5).

ANSWER TO QUESTION 10 (INDICATIONS FOR INTUBATION AND MECHANICAL VENTILATION IN SEVERE ASTHMATIC ATTACKS)

The correct answer is #4. The usual indication for intubation and mechanical ventilation for a very severe asthmatic attack is hypercapnic respiratory failure. No longer is the patient able to breathe enough to remove carbon dioxide from the blood, and arterial PCO_2 rises. As the arterial PCO_2 climbs, the blood pH falls (acidosis). The set of blood gases in answer #4 is the only choice with hypercapnic respiratory acidosis. The first example (answer #1) has mild-to-moderate hypoxemia with respiratory alkalosis, typical of most asthmatic attacks. The second set of blood gases (answer #2) shows profound hypoxemia and a PCO_2 that has risen to normal. This patient requires supplemental oxygen and close monitoring for the development of hypercapnia. As discussed previously (Question 3 above), a normal PCO_2 of 43 mm Hg is a very worrisome finding in this setting. The third set of blood gases (answer #3) is complex. There is profound hypoxemia that requires supplemental oxygen. Despite a low PCO_2 typical of the hyperventilation seen during an asthmatic attack, the pH is low (not alkalemic, as expected [see answer #1]). This low pH indicates the presence of an (unexpected) metabolic acidosis. The cause is not clear in this patient with an asthmatic attack. Nonetheless, this finding is not an indication for intubation and mechanical ventilation. Rather, it dictates a work-up to find the cause of the metabolic acidosis. The fifth set of blood gases (answer #5) indicates a marked respiratory alkalosis. The patient has dramatic hyperventilation (PCO_2 down to 21 mm Hg) with a consequent rise in pH (to 7.56). There is no immediate danger to the patient from this hyperventilation, and treatment with intubation and mechanical ventilation would not help to correct the problem.

ANSWER TO QUESTION 11 (INDICATIONS FOR HOSPITALIZATION TO TREAT A SEVERE ASTHMATIC ATTACK)

The correct answer is #1. There is no evidence that intravenous corticosteroids speed the resolution of asthmatic attacks more than orally-administered corticosteroids, when given in comparable doses. On the other hand, hospitalization offers a patient: removal from an environment where there may be continued allergenic or irritant exposures (answer #2); close medical observation for deterioration, with available interventions if needed, including intubation and mechanical ventilation (answer #3); rest and limitation in physical exertion (answer #4); and assurance of medical compliance (compared with outpatient treatment) (answer #5).

ANSWER TO QUESTION 12 (DISCHARGE PLANNING FOLLOWING HOSPITAL-BASED TREATMENT FOR AN ASTHMATIC ATTACK)

The correct answer is #2. Rarely are patients home-bound following treatment of asthmatic attacks. A VNA referral is unnecessary. Good medical practice should include the following elements in discharge planning after an asthmatic attack: follow-up medical appointment (answer #1); instruction in proper inhaler use (answer #3); instruction in peak flow meter use (answer #4); and counseling about allergen and irritant avoidance in the home (and, if appropriate, in the work and school environments) (answer #5).

10

DEVELOPING AN ASTHMA ACTION PLAN

C H A P T E R   O U T L I N E

I.   Role of the Asthma Action Plan
    a. Rationale for asthma action plans
    b. Scientific evidence for the value of asthma action plans
    c. Getting started: key elements to an asthma action plan
    d. Put it in writing

II. Asthma Action Plan Templates
    a. Three-zone (traffic-light) model
    b. Sensitivity to cultural, linguistic, age, and literacy differences

III. Common Action Plan Recommendations
    a. Inhaled beta agonists
    b. Inhaled corticosteroids
    c. Oral steroids
    d. Interventions of no value

IV. Overview of Asthma Action Plans
    a. Mild intermittent asthma
    b. Mild persistent asthma
    c. Moderate persistent asthma
    d. Severe persistent asthma

V.   Case examples
    a. The college student
    b. The dental hygienist
    c. The 12-year-old boy
    d. The lawyer
    e. The toddler

ROLE OF THE ASTHMA ACTION PLAN

"My child can't breathe; what should I do?" As the parent of a child with asthma—or as an individual with asthma—this is probably the most terrifying moment of asthma care: dealing with an asthmatic attack. Some attacks are mild and require only a fine-tuning of the usual medical treatment. Other attacks are severe; one has to overcome one's sense of distress or, as a parent, one's anxiety and apprehension, to intervene quickly. In all instances, one is called upon to make decisions. Before the call can be made to the physician, before treatments can be begun in the emergency room, decisions need to be made in the home. "Is this attack serious?" "What medicine should I take (or give to my child)?" "Should I try to reach my doctor at this late hour?" "Should I call an ambulance?"

Of course, responses to any crisis will vary tremendously. Faced with the same problem, some people will overreact, others will deny its true severity, and still others will make appropriate decisions. The premise on which this book is based—and a fundamental belief underlying your studies as an asthma educator—is that the more a patient (or parent) knows about asthma and its treatments, the better he or she will able to cope at the time of an attack. Our common purpose is to equip patients with the knowledge, skills, and attitudes that will enable them to respond effectively to an emerging or full-blown asthmatic attack.

Rationale for asthma action plans

Preparing for asthmatic attacks is a special part of asthma education. Consider pilots learning to fly airplanes. They must learn the ins and outs of the operation of their airplane, and they become proficient in its operation: taxi, take-off, in-flight maneuvering, and landing. But all of this expertise is not sufficient. We also expect them to be capable of dealing with whatever unexpected event may suddenly arise. A major portion of their training focuses on preparing them to respond to emergencies: what to do if one engine loses power, what to do if the landing gear doesn't deploy, and so forth. We expect pilots to be ready to respond quickly and effectively to events that we hope they will rarely if ever actually need to face. And we assume that—in order for them to be ready—they have studied, anticipated, and practiced for these potential eventualities.

As asthma educators, we are the flight instructors. We need to put this same sort of expectation on our patients. Not only do we want them to understand the functioning of the respiratory system, not only should they be capable of managing their asthma during the day-to-day routine of their lives, but they need also to be prepared to deal with crises: asthmatic attacks. And we are not asking our patients to prepare for rare events. In any 12-month period as many as 40% of people with asthma will need urgent care at least once for an asthma flare.

When our pilot is confronted with the unexpected—a mechanical failure or in-flight turbulence—we want him or her to have a well thought-out plan of action. This is not the time to be looking in procedure manuals or exploring untried solutions. So too for our asthmatic patient: we want him or her to have a plan of how to respond to increased asthmatic symptoms. We want our patient (or the parent of an asthmatic child) to know *in advance* the steps to take to feel better again; what response to expect from these actions; and what to do if one doesn't get the anticipated response. In short, we want our patient to have an asthma action plan.

KEY POINT Asthma education needs to focus not only on day-to-day asthma management but also on the knowledge and skills that prepare a patient (or caregiver) to begin to deal with an asthmatic attack. We want our patients to be armed with a plan.

An asthma action plan provides not only greater safety for our patients; it also offers some measure of peace of mind. You know from your own experiences that facing a difficult challenge without any idea of how to manage it is an awful feeling. One can easily feel lost, helpless, in a state of panic and fear. And panic in a person who is breathless simply adds fuel to the fire. But if you are given the tools that you need to confront the challenge and a plan of attack, you become capable of a different response. You are ready to tackle the challenge, contribute as you can, and mobilize others to help if need be. You become a *doer*, rather than a helpless victim. This is the *empowerment* that asthma education hopes to confer. We wish to teach the skills to deal with an asthmatic attack and, along with them, the attitude: "I can manage this; I have a plan."

In a sense, teaching about asthma action plans is the culmination of asthma education. It incorporates understanding the components of airflow obstruction, assessing asthma severity, allergen avoidance, and knowing the role of asthma medications—their proper use, their anticipated effects, and their potential side effects. All of the information throughout this book comes together in teaching patients how to begin to treat themselves during an asthma attack. And it has the potential to save lives.

Scientific evidence for the value of asthma action plans

When the Expert Panel of the National Asthma Education and Prevention Program revised the *Guidelines for the Diagnosis and Management of Asthma* in 2002, they reviewed the scientific evidence regarding the role of asthma action plans in asthma management. They turned to randomized controlled trials of medical management alone versus medical management with the use of written asthma action plans to determine the scientific justification for recommending development of asthma action plans with our patients. They found seven published studies, many with limitations in their design and methodology. They concluded that "data are insufficient to support or refute the benefits of using written asthma action plans compared to medical management alone."

However, the Expert Panel report (www.nhlbi.nih.gov/guidelines/asthma/asthmafullrpt.pdf) went on to cite additional medical literature on this topic.

They noted that a systematic review of the literature provided by a Cochrane Collaboration review found that asthma self-management interventions using written asthma action plans compared to self-management interventions without action plans provided better outcomes. Patients receiving self-management interventions with action plans had fewer emergency room visits, fewer hospitalizations, and better lung function compared with patients who adjusted their medications only at the time of their regular medical visits to the doctor.

In addition, one study—using a case-control design—compared 51 patients who died of asthma with 202 patients who presented to the hospital with severe asthmatic attacks. These authors found that among patients with severe persistent asthma, having a written asthma action plan reduced the risk of dying from asthma by 70%.

Based on their review of the evidence, members of the Expert Panel came to the following recommendation:

"It is the opinion of the Expert Panel that use of written action plans as part of an overall effort to educate patients in self-management is recommended, especially for patients with moderate or severe persistent asthma and patients with a history of severe exacerbation."

KEY POINT Although evidence is not yet available to prove their benefit, the Expert Panel of the National Asthma Education and Prevention Program recommends the use of written asthma action plans as part of a comprehensive program in asthma self-management.

Getting started: key elements to an asthma action plan

The crucial step in developing an asthma action plan is getting started. It takes time. As asthma educators we need to find the time—or create the time—to begin the discussion: "Have you thought about what you would do if you have (or your child has) an asthma attack? Do you have a plan?" Once a diagnosis of asthma has been made, it is never too soon to raise the subject. Because even patients with mild asthma can suffer severe asthmatic attacks, it is a topic appropriate for all patients. Treatment of asthmatic attacks can and should begin at home (or wherever one is experiencing the attack). "As a person with asthma (or caregiver of someone with asthma), you will have to make decisions about what to do when your asthma flares. Let's come up with a plan of action together."

In some circumstances it may be most appropriate simply to urge your patient to discuss an asthma action plan with his or her physician. Alternatively, the patient's medical provider may have already created an action plan for your patient. It is always appropriate to review the plan and to make sure that the patient fully understands it. As the patient's medications change and his or her experience with asthma evolves, the action plan will need updating. "Let's take a look together at your asthma action plan," you might say. "Can you explain each step to me?"

There are four key elements to home management of asthmatic attacks: (1) recognizing an attack; (2) assessing its severity: (3) initiating treatment; and (4) knowing when and how to get help.

Step 1. The first step—recognizing an asthma attack—may seem pitifully obvious. A patient who is coughing, gasping, and struggling to get air needs no help in identifying an asthma attack. But asthma attacks need not be so severe to merit attention; and not all severe attacks manifest with such obvious symptoms. The biggest risk to our patients is that a serious attack of asthma goes unnoticed and ignored. It is not hard to imagine how this might happen. Imagine that a patient with asthma suffers a viral respiratory tract infection. He feels poorly with cough and low-grade fever. His chest aches and feels congested. He finds himself winded climbing the stairs up to the bedroom. "A bad cold," he concludes, ignoring the fact that it is distinctly abnormal for him to be short of breath with as little activity as climbing one flight of stairs. For whatever reason, he does not think of the possibility that his asthma has flared; or if he does consider that possibility, he downplays its importance. "I'll take my albuterol inhaler tonight, and check with the doctor tomorrow." Many people react to their illness with denial. "Even though I have used my albuterol four times already this evening, I'm sure I'll be better by morning."

Other patients are considered to be "poor perceivers" of asthmatic attacks. Persistent airway narrowing may make them less aware of further deterioration; lack of wheezing and associated chest vibrations may send fewer sensory signals to the brain. Or the brain may be set with a different sensitivity to the usual distress signals, including low oxygen or high carbon dioxide blood levels.

The same Expert Panel that considered the scientific evidence about the utility of asthma action plans examined the data in support of regular peak flow monitoring to detect asthmatic exacerbations. They found only four published studies testing whether written asthma action plans based on peak flow monitoring were superior to symptom-based action plans in terms of health care utilization, symptoms, or lung function. They concluded that "the evidence neither supports nor refutes" an advantage to regular peak flow monitoring. They recommended that "peak flow monitoring should be considered for patients with moderate or severe persistent asthma because it may enhance clinician-patient communication and may increase patient and caregiver awareness of the disease status and control." In particular, they noted that patients with an "inability to recognize or report signs and symptoms of worsening asthma" (poor perceivers) should consider regular peak flow monitoring of their asthma.

The alternative to regular peak flow monitoring is attentiveness to asthma signs and symptoms. We need to help our patients watch for indicators that their asthma may be out of control. A lingering cough in the absence of a cold, more shortness of breath with activities, a child's rapid respiratory rate or refusal to eat normally, and audible wheezing are all clues. They should not be dismissed as "normal for an asthmatic."

Step 2. Step two is assessing the severity of the attack. It's one thing to acknowledge that you are having a flare-up of your asthma; it's another, though related, step to recognize that this is a severe exacerbation. Patients with severe asthmatic attacks are at risk for respiratory failure and death. Their air passageways are compromised and unstable. Further narrowing of the airways can lead to large jumps in the work of breathing. The ability to deliver sufficient ventilation to the alveoli to rid the body of carbon dioxide may become jeopardized. A severe asthmatic attack is a medical emergency that deserves prompt attention, just like a blood sugar of 400 mg/dL.

When retrospective, in-depth analyses of deaths due to asthma are conducted, one often encounters the same sad report from family or friends: "he didn't look that bad; no one suspected that he was that ill." Often the patient— and sometimes the caregiver as well—underestimated the severity of the attack. If he stays relatively stationary, the patient may not notice how little activity it takes to make him short of breath. If he gets some relief, though transient, from his quick-acting bronchodilator, he may think that he is getting better. Our job as asthma educators is to help patients not to overlook the warning signs of a severe asthmatic attack.

Warning signs include the following: labored breathing with light exertion; speech that is interrupted in order to catch one's breath; the need to sit upright to be able to breathe comfortably; and in a child, nasal flaring and skin retractions between the ribs with each breath in.

Here is where a peak flow measurement can be invaluable. An asthmatic attack is severe when the peak flow is less than half the patient's normal value (less than half of his or her "personal best"). It is that simple and direct. Try as hard as one can, even after using the quick-acting bronchodilator, and if the indicator on the peak flow meter still registers less than half of one's best value, there need be no further discussion: this is a severe attack of asthma. In the words of the Expert Panel members in their 2002 review of the *Guidelines*, "peak flow monitoring during exacerbations of asthma is recommended [for patients with moderate or severe persistent asthma] to: determine severity of the exacerbation and guide therapeutic decisions." We have added the brackets, believing that checking one's peak flow during a flare of asthmatic symptoms is appropriate for all patients, regardless of the severity of their chronic asthma.

KEY POINT   Like the Expert Panel of the National Asthma Education and Prevention Program, we recommend use of peak flow meters during asthmatic exacerbations to assess the severity of the exacerbation and to guide treatment.

We recognize that a caveat is needed when making decisions based on home peak flow measurements. In some cases, bad data can be worse than no data at all. Peak flow recordings made at home are subject to the capabilities of those performing the test, and without question the results are highly effort-dependent. A shallow breath in, a weak exhalation, and lips not tightly sealed at the mouthpiece can all give falsely low readings. A decision to recommend oral steroids based on an erroneous report of a low peak flow number can do more harm than good. It is important to interpret peak flow data in the context of other signs and symptoms of asthma. If the whole picture does not fit, have the patient come to be seen in a medical office. Fortunately, peak flow meters will rarely give a falsely elevated value. They continue to be a valuable safety net so that severe asthmatic attacks are not overlooked.

Step 3. Having recognized the presence of an asthmatic attack, it is time to take action. If your patient knows what is triggering this exacerbation, it may be possible for him to remove himself from further exposure. He should get up and leave the smoky barroom or leave the house with the pet cat to which he is allergic. Continuing to breathe in allergens or irritants can lead to worsening lung function even when appropriate medications are taken. Our advice is to get out of the burning building, even if one is carrying a fire extinguisher!

The other appropriate response is to take medication that will begin to alleviate the exacerbation. The asthma action plan gives patients permission to take extra doses of medication without first discussing the matter with their medical provider. For the patient with mild intermittent asthma whose only available medication is an albuterol inhaler, it is not difficult to choose which medicine. Still, there are plenty of questions to be answered: how many puffs can I take at once; how frequently can I repeat a dose; how quickly should I expect to see a response; and how long should I wait before seeking additional treatment? For the patient whose medicine cabinet is full of antiasthmatic and antiallergic medications—albuterol, budesonide (Pulmicort), fluticasone-salmeterol combination (Advair), theophylline, montelukast (Singulair), loratadine (Claritin), and pseudoephedrine (Sudafed), with a nebulizer and compressor in the closet—choosing the right medication can be daunting. Unless, of course, the patient has an asthma action plan to which to refer!

As you develop an asthma action plan with your patient, your recommendations—preferably made in collaboration with the patient's physician—will vary according to several different factors. In part, they will be influenced by what medications and delivery devices the patient has available at home. The patient's past experiences with asthmatic attacks will also shape your recommendations. For instance, has he ever taken prednisone before and what was his response; has nebulized bronchodilator proven particularly effective? Other considerations include how accessible medical care is in an emergency, either through the doctor's office or local urgent care center. Is the doctor willing to prescribe prednisone for the patient to have available at home, to be begun during an asthmatic crisis?

Step 4. An effective asthma action plan also provides advice as to when and how a patient should seek medical help for treating an asthmatic attack. It is the intent of asthma education to help patients *begin* treatment in the home and, if the response is favorable, to continue treatment. The goal is not, however, to transfer the care of severe asthma from medical professionals to parents or patients themselves. It is not desirable to have patients running a mini-emergency room in their home. Continuing treatment for severe asthma at home even though symptoms and peak flow are not improving is a bad idea. It is dangerous.

This is an important point. Asthma education emphasizes the value of *co-management* approaches to asthma care. Collaborative management involves both patient (or caregiver) and clinician, and it frees the patient to make decisions and take actions appropriate to the moment, without needing physician approval at that instant. Although we sometimes refer to asthma *self-management*—again emphasizing how the informed patient can take charge of his or her care—the intent is never to ask the patient to assume the responsibilities of doctor and nurse too. To some extent we are asking our patients to tread a fine line. Begin treatment to prevent an asthma flare from worsening, we tell them; but don't wait too long to call for help. An important part of the equation is this safety net: there is professional help available, and your patient should use it if he or she is not improving with initiation of his or her action plan at home.

KEY POINT   Equally important as teaching the ability to recognize and treat asthmatic exacerbations is helping patients to know when they need medical help, whether telephone contact with their provider or urgent care in a medical office or emergency room.

Some physicians recommend that if the patient has taken two treatments of the quick-acting bronchodilator one after the other without improvement, he or she should call. Others insist that if their patient begins oral steroid tablets, he or she should contact them. Once again, a peak flow meter gives useful guidance. If your patient follows his or her asthma action plan and finds the peak flow decreasing or, in severe attacks, failing to increase, it is time to get help. Circumstances will dictate what form that help might take: call your doctor for an urgent appointment; call the after-hours covering physician for advice; go to the local emergency room or urgent care center; or call 911 for emergency medical technicians and an ambulance. You can help your patient by discussing these emergency options *in advance* and by writing down emergency phone numbers on his or her asthma action plan form.

Put it in writing

Imagine that you have just had a comprehensive and detailed discussion with a mother about her child's asthma action plan. You have reviewed medications to be used in an asthma attack, distinguished controller medications from quick-reliever medications, emphasized proper methods for medication delivery, and outlined guidelines for when to call the medical provider for further advice. You now go on to your next patient, and the patient prepares to leave the office—when a research assistant approaches this mother and asks for permission to ask her a few questions. An asthma researcher is conducting a study about medical communication, and the assistant wants to review with the mother exactly what it is that she heard you tell her just moments ago. "Can you show me," she asks, "which medicine is your controller medication and which the quick reliever?" "Which one are you supposed to give your child in an asthma attack?" "How many puffs should you give?" "How soon can you give it again?"

Despite the clarity of your explanation and your use of the technique of listener feedback—you asked the mother to repeat to you what you had taught her about the child's medicines—there is still room for error. In one study of patients and providers interviewed after their medical appointment, 20% of the time patients and providers disagreed about whether an asthma controller medication had been prescribed. Misunderstandings are common. When asked to identify their controller medication, 30% of patients in one study indicated their rescue inhaler.

Imagine now that the research assistant described above does not interview your patient immediately after your teaching session but 1 week later, or 1 month later. With the passage of time, and the vagaries of memory, the possibility of confusion multiplies. Finally, add the stress and distraction of a sick child, when the mother's asthmatic child is wheezing and struggling to breathe 6 months after your discussion of an asthma action plan, and you can imagine how difficult it will be for this mother—or anybody—to recall accurately the details of your conversation.

Two approaches can help to overcome these obstacles to implementing an effective asthma action plan. One is repetition. If you and the mother have a chance to review the action plan at multiple visits over the course of many months, it will become increasingly familiar and routine for her. It will be there in her memory even under times of high anxiety. The other—and most important—is developing a *written* asthma action plan. Even if she can't recall what you told her, she can look in her purse or on the refrigerator door to find the written plan of attack that you had discussed many months ago. There, for her to refer to, are the medications, the doses, the frequency of administration that she needs to know, as well as the emergency phone numbers if her child does not quickly improve. The written asthma action plan makes it possible for the mother to share the information accurately with other members of her family and other childcare providers in the home. It also makes this information available outside of the home—at sleepovers, daycare, school, or camp. You help your patient the most if you develop an asthma action plan and write it down. We will review various templates provided for creating an asthma action plan, or you may already have your favorite or decide to create one of your own. Most important is that you pick one that seems to work for you and your patient—and use it.

KEY POINT   To make an asthma action plan work, put it in writing and review it frequently.

ASTHMA ACTION PLAN TEMPLATES

Three-zone (traffic-light) model

Probably the most widely used style for asthma action plans utilizes the traffic-light model of green, yellow, and red zones. Green means "go," you're doing well. Yellow means slow down and be cautious; you are having a mild-to-moderate asthmatic attack, and you need to take action to get well again. Red means stop; this is a severe asthmatic attack and demands your urgent and full attention. Asthma action plans may utilize peak flow measurements, asthmatic symptoms, or a combination of both to indicate in which zone one finds oneself.

Using this format, patients are considered to be in their green zone if they have no symptoms and their peak flow is 80% or greater of their optimal or "personal best" peak flow. When they have cough, wheeze, chest tightness, shortness of breath with exertion, and nighttime awakenings due to their asthma—and when their peak flow falls to the range of 50–80% of their personal best—they are in their yellow zone. Red zone symptoms include severe shortness of breath—to the point of having difficulty walking or talking—or failure to respond to quick-relief medications. A child with nasal flaring, retractions of the skin between ribs during inspiration, or very rapid breathing is in the red zone. A peak flow of less than half of one's usual (<50% of one's personal best peak flow) puts one in the red zone as well.

A frightening asthma attack is probably not the best time for your patient to try to calculate percentages. The following quick reference chart can help you, the asthma educator, determine the green, yellow, and red zones for your patient (Table 10-1). When you develop an asthma action plan for your patient, make the calculations with him or her and indicate actual numbers (e.g., 250–400 L/min) rather than percentages (50–80%) on his or her written asthma action plan. Many peak flow meters are now sold with adjustable, color-coded green, yellow, and red indicators alongside the peak flow indicator (Fig. 10-1). You can calculate the ranges for the three zones with the patient and then help set the position of these zone indicators on their peak flow meter. Using these meters the patient can visualize directly in which zone his or her current peak flow value falls every time he or she makes a measurement.

TABLE 10-1

CALCULATING PERCENTAGES FOR PEAK FLOW ZONES

Personal Best PEFR	Green Zone PEFR	Yellow Zone PEFR	Red Zone PEFR
100	Greater than 80	80–50	Less than 50
125	Greater than 100	100–63	Less than 63
150	Greater than 120	120–75	Less than 75
175	Greater than 140	140–88	Less than 88
200	Greater than 160	160–100	Less than 100
225	Greater than 180	180–113	Less than 113
250	Greater than 200	200–125	Less than 125
275	Greater than 220	220–138	Less than 138
300	Greater than 240	240–150	Less than 150
325	Greater than 260	260–163	Less than 163
350	Greater than 280	280–175	Less than 175
375	Greater than 300	300–188	Less than 188
400	Greater than 320	320–200	Less than 200
425	Greater than 340	340–213	Less than 213
450	Greater than 360	360–225	Less than 225
475	Greater than 380	380–238	Less than 238
500	Greater than 400	400–250	Less than 250
525	Greater than 420	420–263	Less than 263
550	Greater than 440	440–275	Less than 275
575	Greater than 460	460–288	Less than 288
600	Greater than 480	480–300	Less than 300
625	Greater than 500	500–312	Less than 312
650	Greater than 520	520–325	Less than 325
675	Greater than 540	540–338	Less than 338
700	Greater than 560	560–350	Less than 350
725	Greater than 580	580–362	Less than 362
750	Greater than 600	600–375	Less than 375
775	Greater than 620	620–387	Less than 387
800	Greater than 640	640–400	Less than 400

KEY POINT One popular asthma action plan template uses the traffic-light model: the green zone indicates good asthma control; the yellow zone is a mild-to-moderate asthmatic exacerbation—take caution; and the red zone is a severe asthmatic attack—stop what you are doing and take immediate action.

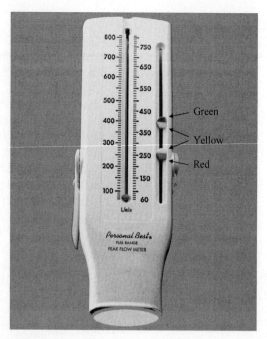

FIGURE 10-1 *Peak flow meter with color-coded peak flow zone indicators. Photograph courtesy of Kenneth M. Bernstein.*

As a reminder of our discussion in Chap. 6, "Pulmonary Function Testing and Peak Flow Monitoring," personal best peak flow is determined by having the patient make recordings using his or her home peak flow meter. The highest measurements made when feeling perfectly well or "as good as it gets" constitute the personal best value. If this information is not available, one can start with the predicted normal value for a person of a particular age, height, and gender (or just age in children), taken from a chart of normal values (see Tables 2-3 and 6-1). This number may need to be adjusted subsequently if it turns out that at best this particular patient has a peak flow that deviates from the average normal value. Individual variation, ethnic or racial differences, or airway remodeling with permanent decreases in lung function may account for this deviation. It is a good idea to ask your patient to re-establish her personal best peak flow whenever she obtains a new peak flow meter (even one made by the same manufacturer) and after the passage of time (to account for lung growth in children and age-related declines in lung function in adults).

In Massachusetts a consortium of groups interested in health care, including physicians, hospitals, health plans, purchasers of medical insurance, and government agencies, have come together to form Massachusetts Health Quality Partners. This group, together with other asthma advocacy groups, developed a pediatric asthma action plan for statewide use. It employs the green-yellow-red zone model and is suitable for peak flow or symptom-based asthma management. A sample of this full-page-sized model is included (Fig. 10-2).

Massachusetts Asthma Action Plan

Name:		Date:	
Birth Date:	Doctor/Nurse Name	Doctor/Nurse Phone #	
Patient Goal:		Parent/Guardian Name & Phone	
Important! Avoid things that make your asthma worse:			

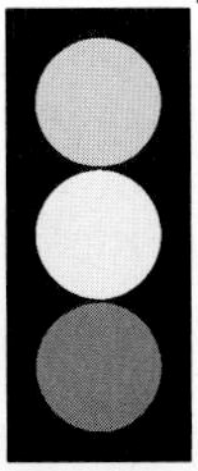

The colors of a traffic light will help You use your asthma medicine.

Green means **Go Zone!**
Use controller medicine.

Yellow means **Caution Zone!**
Add quick-relief medicine.

Red means **Danger Zone!**
Get help from a doctor.

Personal Best Peak Flow: _____

GO – You're Doing Well! ➡ Use these daily controller medicines:

You have **all** of these:
- Breathing is good
- No cough or wheeze
- Sleep through the night
- Can go to school and play

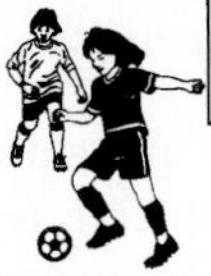

Peak flow from _____ to _____	MEDICINE/ROUTE	HOW MUCH	HOW OFTEN/ WHEN

CAUTION – Slow Down! ➡ Continue with green zone medicine and add:

You have **any** of these:
- First signs of a cold
- Cough
- Mild wheeze
- Tight Chest
- Coughing, wheezing, or trouble breathing at night

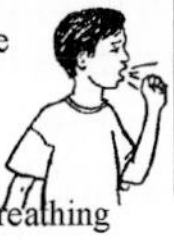

Peak flow from _____ to _____	MEDICINE/ROUTE	HOW MUCH	HOW OFTEN/ WHEN

CALL YOUR DOCTOR/ NURSE: _____

DANGER – Get Help! ➡ Take these medicines and call your doctor now.

Your asthma is getting **worse fast:**
- Medicine is not helping
- Breathing is hard and fast
- Nose opens wide
- Ribs show
- Can't talk well

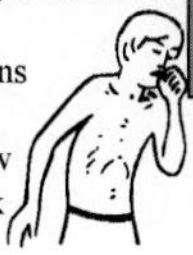

Peak flow from _____ to _____	MEDICINE/ROUTE	HOW MUCH	HOW OFTEN/ WHEN

GET HELP FROM A DOCTOR NOW! Do not be afraid of causing a fuss. Your doctor will want to see you right away. It's important! If you cannot contact your doctor, go directly to the emergency room and bring this form with you. DO NOT WAIT.
Make an appointment with your doctor / nurse within two days of an ER visit or hospitalization.

Doctor /NP/PA Signature: _____ Date:_____
I give permission to the school nurse, my child's doctor/NP/PA or _____ to share information about my child's asthma
Parent/Guardian Signature:_____ Date:_____

ADAPTED FROM NIH PUBLICATION (7/20/00)

FIGURE 10-2 *Pediatric asthma action plan developed by Massachusetts Health Quality Partners. From www.mhqp.org.*

Color copies can also be downloaded free of charge from the organization's website, www.mhqp.org or using the specific web address of www.mhqp.org/mhqp_attachments/asthmaActionPlan.pdf. This asthma action plan template is available in seven foreign languages: Chinese, Haitian Creole, Khmer, Portuguese, Russian, Spanish, and Vietnamese.

At Partners Asthma Center we have developed an asthma action plan card that folds to the size of a credit card, appropriate for carrying in a wallet. It emphasizes a two-step approach to asthmatic attacks: what you should do if you experience a mild-to-moderate attack, and what to do if you don't improve with these measures; and then another pair of recommendations for a severe attack. A sample is provided (Fig. 10-3) and can also be obtained (in English or in Spanish) from our website (www.asthma.partners.org).

Sensitivity to cultural, linguistic, age, and literacy differences

Generally good advice for developing the content of your patient's asthma action plan, as too for ambulatory asthma management in general, is "keep it simple." Avoid multiple options and varied branch points—too many "if this, then this" options. We encourage you to be as specific as possible for individual patients. Write "albuterol two puffs" rather than "use your beta-agonist bronchodilator"; "Flovent four puffs" rather than "use your inhaled steroid"; and "prednisone 40 mg" rather than "begin oral steroids." It is also appropriate to use terminology suited to your individual patient. If he or she refers to his or her Diskus device as the "purple donut," it is OK to use this expression on their asthma action plan. (Another version can be provided to the school nurse!)

KEY POINT   When writing the content of an asthma action plan, be as specific as possible and use terminology that you know the patient understands.

Asthma action plans are available for patients with low literacy skills. They employ pictures to depict asthma symptoms and medication actions at each level of care. Most people try to hide their limited literacy; it may take some probing to determine whether your patient can actually read the asthma action plan that you have created together.

Patient age is another determining factor in choosing the type of asthma action plan. Children under 5 years of age are usually unable to use peak flow meters effectively. For this age group asthma action plans must rely on levels of symptoms to categorize decreasing asthma control. For children over the age of 5, a low-range peak flow meter (peak flow values from 30–400 L/min) is available. For teenagers and adults the full-range peak flow meter (range = 40–800 L/min) is recommended.

Side One

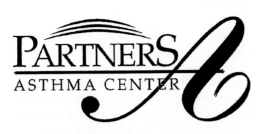

My Asthma Action Plan

Name: _____

My Physicians' Names:

Primary: Dr. _____

Asthma: Dr._____

My Asthma Medications:

_____

_____

My Other Medications:

_____

_____

_____

Medication Allergies: _____

Side Two

My Asthma Action Plan

Peak Flow Values

My BEST PEAK FLOW is:_____ liters/minute.
When my peak flow is less than:_____ liters/minute
(less than half of my best value), I am having a
severe attack.

A: In the event of a Mild or Moderate asthma
attack I would first:

_____

_____

If there is no improvement, my next step would be
to:

_____

_____

B: In the event of a SEVERE asthma attack, I would
first:

_____

_____

If there is no improvement, my next step would be
to:

_____

_____

If there is still no improvement,

Seek Emergency Help Immediately

EMERGENCY PHONE NUMBERS

My Asthma Doctor:_____

(ask to page your asthma doctor or the covering
fellow)

Ambulance:_____ or 911

FIGURE 10-3   *Partners Asthma Center's asthma action plan card.*

COMMON ACTION PLAN RECOMMENDATIONS

Just like asthma care in general, one size does not fit all when it comes to asthma action plans. It makes no sense to recommend nebulized bronchodilator use for the patient who does not have access to a compressor and nebulizer at home. "Begin an inhaled steroid" does not apply to the patient already taking daily inhaled steroids as a controller medication. Still, there are common principles that underlie our recommendations for all patients and some common strategies that are widely used to treat asthmatic flares. In addition, there are a number of popular but marginally effective or ineffective remedies that we would not encourage.

Inhaled beta agonists

From your reading of Chap. 9, "Managing Asthmatic Attacks," you know that asthmatic attacks may be characterized by bronchoconstriction, airway swelling and mucus accumulation, and—most often—both. You also know that the most rapid and potent means of reversing bronchial smooth muscle contraction is inhalation of rapidly-acting beta-agonist bronchodilators. Most widely used are albuterol (Ventolin, Proventil, ProAir), pirbuterol (Maxair), metaproterenol (Alupent), and levalbuterol (Xopenex). Virtually all patients with asthma will have access to a quick-acting inhaled bronchodilator; it is with this "rescue" bronchodilator that they need to begin to seek relief from their asthma exacerbation.

For some of our patients, using their bronchodilator to treat increased asthmatic symptoms is more like an "asthma reflex" than an object of asthma education. Nonetheless, other patients will confuse their controller inhaler with their quick-relief inhaler. For example, we have all had patients who mistakenly take their fluticasone (Flovent) inhaler two puffs as needed for relief of symptoms. So, as step one, make sure that your patient knows which inhaler to use for quick relief. Have them correctly identify their "rescue inhaler" for you.

We need to establish "ground rules" for rescue inhaler use in an asthmatic attack. On the one hand, we need to give explicit permission to use the inhaler more than the usual "two puffs four times per day" as needed. Many patients have come to believe that using it more frequently than every 4–6 hours is dangerous. Our goal in achieving good asthma control *on a chronic basis* is to reduce rescue inhaler use to as infrequently as once or twice per week; and pharmacists may refuse to refill prescriptions for beta-agonist bronchodilators if insufficient time has elapsed since the last refill. The reason for these cautions has mostly to do with emphasis on alternative treatments to bring asthma under good control. Excessive beta-agonist use is dangerous when it indicates poor asthma control and inadequate use of other (controller) therapies. It rarely causes harmful side effects itself. The therapeutic-to-toxic ratio for inhaled beta agonists is very broad. Toxic effects—for example, cardiac tachyarrhythmias—are rare. It is very hard to overdose on beta agonists administered by metered-dose inhaler.

A low risk of toxic effects does not preclude common and unpleasant side effects from repeated use of the quick-acting bronchodilators. Even the selective beta-2 agonist bronchodilators will cause some jitteriness, tremor, and heart racing and pounding if used in sufficiently high doses. However, when the alternative is desperate breathlessness and a choking cough, these side effects are considered an acceptable price for rapid-onset symptom relief.

In an asthmatic crisis, patients can take (and parents can administer) four puffs of a quick-acting beta agonist as often as every 20–30 minutes. They certainly do not need to wait 4–6 hours to readminister the bronchodilator if they remain symptomatic from their asthma. It is worthwhile reminding patients that four puffs means one inhalation at a time, each one carefully administered to maximize effect. In adults proper delivery involves a slow, deep breath followed by a brief breathhold prior to exhalation. If readily available, a spacer is helpful to optimize medication delivery to the airways. Optimal medication delivery to a child in distress is more difficult; strategies based on a child's age and motor skills are discussed in Chap. 8, "Inhalers and Inhalational Aids in Asthma Treatment."

KEY POINT The therapeutic-to-toxic ratio for inhaled beta agonists is very broad. Patients can take extra puffs from their quick-relief bronchodilator and multiple doses over a short period of time with little risk of serious adverse effects.

On the other side of our ground rules for rescue inhaler use are cautions about reliance on beta agonists as the sole treatment for an asthmatic attack. Tragic stories abound regarding fatal asthmatic attacks in which the victims were found clutching their bronchodilator inhaler. Evidence strongly suggests that the beta-agonist bronchodilators did not cause a fatal reaction in these patients. Rather, they died from asphyxiation despite the temporary—and in the end, nonexistent—relief provided by their inhaler. Many patients come to the emergency room for treatment of their asthmatic attacks complaining that their bronchodilator inhaler *stopped working*. You know that their problem is inflammatory swelling and blockage of their bronchial tubes, asthmatic reactions not expected to improve with a bronchial smooth muscle relaxer. They are in urgent need of medications to reduce this asthmatic inflammation. They need your teaching to avoid the dangerous pitfall of relying on bronchodilators until their airway obstruction becomes life-threatening.

How much bronchodilator use is too much? Given the broad safety of the beta-2 selective adrenergic-agonist bronchodilators, this is a difficult endpoint to define. We think that a better question is: when is it ill-advised to continue frequent beta-agonist administration at home? We would advise our patients that if after two to three doses within the first hour there is no definite improvement, seek help. If after two to three doses within the first hour you find yourself still within the red zone, seek help. If there is clear-cut improvement, it is safe to continue to administer four puffs of the rescue inhaler as often as every hour while waiting for other, anti-inflammatory medications to begin to act. As previously noted, some practitioners ask that they receive a call after two doses of bronchodilator have been administered in rapid succession to treat an asthmatic attack.

Patients who have ever experienced a life-threatening asthmatic attack should have a compressor and nebulizer available at home to administer inhaled bronchodilators during a severe asthmatic attack. Other good candidates for a compressor and nebulizer system are patients who have required emergency department visits for their asthma, where they improved quickly with administration of a nebulized bronchodilator; and young children and the elderly, if they have difficulty coordinating use of the metered-dose inhaler with spacer (with or without face mask). Bronchodilator medication, such as albuterol (Ventolin, Proventil, AccuNeb), metaproterenol (Alupent), or levalbuterol (Xopenex), is sold in premixed, unit-dose plastic vials. Just twist off the top, pour the medication into the nebulizer cup, press the "on" switch of the compressor, and breathe in and out quietly through the mouthpiece or face mask. Its ease of use, even during a severe asthmatic attack, makes this an appealing medication delivery method.

KEY POINT   We would recommend home compressor and nebulizer systems for the following groups of patients: those with prior life-threatening asthmatic attacks; those who have had rapid relief of asthmatic attacks in the emergency department when treated with nebulized bronchodilator; and young children or the elderly if they have difficulty coordinating use of the metered-dose inhaler.

The same precautions about overreliance on bronchodilators via metered-dose inhaler pertain to nebulized bronchodilators—and perhaps even more so, because the latter provide such potent bronchodilation. It is an easy mistake for your patients to make—repeatedly using their nebulized bronchodilator without attending to the inflammatory component of their asthma. The risk is that nebulized bronchodilators stop providing any benefit for swollen, mucus-filled bronchi. In the absence of definite and sustained improvement after the first two doses or over the first hour of treatment, your patient should get urgent help.

Inhaled corticosteroids

If oral steroids such as prednisone and methylprednisolone (Medrol) had no serious side effects, the next step in treating an asthmatic attack that persisted after inhaled bronchodilator treatment would be initiation of oral corticosteroids. They offer the most effective means of reducing airway inflammation and mucus hypersecretion during an asthmatic exacerbation. Systemic corticosteroids and frequently administered bronchodilators are the backbone of in-hospital care for asthmatic attacks.

But oral steroids, even when taken for short periods, have the potential for myriad side effects; and repeated courses over time have inevitable, cumulative harmful consequences. It is for this reason that one seeks an alternative, "kinder and gentler" option for treating milder asthmatic flare-ups. Enter inhaled corticosteroids.

A strategy for treating mild-to-moderate asthmatic attacks (yellow zone) that has emerged over the last decade or so is to begin or increase the dose of inhaled corticosteroids. Patients using only a quick-relief bronchodilator with or without a leukotriene blocker should begin an inhaled steroid during a mild or moderate asthmatic attack. Patients already taking an inhaled steroid as their controller medication should increase the dose, typically doubling it. For example, if your patient is routinely taking fluticasone (Flovent) 44 mcg/puff, two puffs twice daily (as in the case example in Chap. 9, "Managing Asthmatic Attacks"), he or she is advised to increase the dose to four puffs twice daily (or use Flovent 110 mcg/puff, two puffs twice daily). If your patient uses budesonide (Pulmicort Turbuhaler) two inhalations once daily, he or she should begin two inhalations twice daily—or even four inhalations twice daily—during a mild-to-moderate asthmatic attack.

Although this is a recommendation that we routinely make, it is, in truth, a curious one. We have often told our patients that it may take 1 or 2 weeks after beginning inhaled steroids before they notice the benefit. The anti-inflammatory effects may take some time to manifest. Yet in the context of a mild-to-moderate asthmatic attack, we hope for a quicker onset of action. We hope that the effect of *stepping up* anti-inflammatory therapy will be evident in a day or so, that symptoms will abate and peak flow values increase back into the green zone, and that after several more days the steroid dose can again be *stepped down* to the baseline dose. Because the asthmatic exacerbation is relatively mild, the slower tempo of improvement (compared to oral steroids) seems acceptable, given the minimal side effects associated with even high-dose inhaled steroids in the short term.

Randomized clinical trials have put this management strategy to the test—with variable results. Some studies showed benefit, others not. In the absence of better options, it remains the standard of care, with the following cautions given to our patients: if there is no improvement after 1–2 days, contact your healthcare provider; and if despite increasing your inhaled steroid dose, your lung function worsens, get medical help. In most instances, the medical provider—and perhaps the red-zone guidelines of the asthma action plan—will recommend a course of oral steroids at this point.

KEY POINT   Doubling the dose of inhaled steroids for a mild-to-moderate asthmatic attack is a reasonable strategy, although evidence demonstrating its value is limited.

Oral steroids

Oral corticosteroids are the "big guns" in the battle against an asthmatic attack. In a severe attack, they can be life-saving. When a patient with asthma struggles with labored breathing, repetitive coughing, and uncomfortable wheezing in the chest, persistent despite use of a rescue bronchodilator, oral steroids can bring relief. The beneficial effect may take up to 6–12 hours to manifest. As discussed in Chap. 9, "Managing Asthmatic Attacks," the fundamental strategy in treating severe asthmatic attacks involves frequent administration of inhaled bronchodilators to sustain breathing until—with the help of systemic corticosteroids—asthmatic inflammation begins to subside.

The usual recommended starting dose of prednisone, methylprednisolone (Medrol), or prednisolone (Prelone, Pediapred) is 1–2 mg/kg in children and 40–60 mg/day in adults. We prescribe oral steroids to be taken as a single daily dose ("take your first dose now, as soon as you obtain the medication; then begin taking the medication once a day in the morning, beginning tomorrow morning"). An alternative schedule is provided by a prepackaged formulation of methylprednisolone (Medrol Dose Pack) in which the first day (of a 5 day taper) is prescribed as two 4-mg tablets taken three times over the course of the day.

We have discussed the variety of dosing strategies used for a *short course* of oral steroids in the previous chapter, including some employing a tapering schedule, others not. For an asthma action plan, it is sufficient to have the patient begin treatment, then consult with the care provider. The most difficult decision for the patient (and oftentimes, for the provider as well) is "do I need (or do I prescribe) oral steroids now?" The details of the steroid course can be worked out later, as the asthmatic attack is improving.

Oral steroids are recommended for a severe asthmatic attack (red zone) that fails to improve after initial treatment (e.g., the first two to three doses) of inhaled bronchodilator. How this initiation of oral steroids takes place will vary widely depending on the patient, his or her relationship with the prescribing physician or nurse practitioner, and his or her prior experience with oral steroids. Some providers (including us) will entrust some of their patients, especially those who have taken oral steroids in the past, with a prescription for this medication to have on hand at home. In many instances, we encourage our patients to begin the medication in an asthmatic crisis, then call to notify us. Other providers will request that their patients not begin oral steroids without first contacting their office. Still others will insist that their patients call for a prescription of oral steroids when needed, uncomfortable relying on the judgment of their patients (or certain of their patients) to self-medicate appropriately. The asthma action plan can reflect this variability in practice patterns. The advice may be to "call your healthcare provider" (for a prescription of oral steroids) or "begin prednisone" (or "increase your dose of prednisone," for those few patients on chronic oral steroids).

It is important to acknowledge that the idea of taking oral steroids may be highly emotionally charged for your patient. If they have taken oral steroids in the past and experienced adverse reactions, they may dread the thought of resuming use. Other patients may have heard stories about oral steroids—from family, friends, or neighbors—and be filled with *fear and loathing* regarding steroids, as well as lots of misinformation. The part of the asthma action plan that indicates "take two to four puffs of your albuterol inhaler" is an easy sell. The part that suggests that your patient might take 40 mg of prednisone is a huge step. It requires lots of time on your part spent discussing its rationale, the importance of restoring breathing in an asthmatic crisis, and the likely consequence of worsening asthma in the absence of oral steroids (i.e., a trip to the hospital, where patients typically receive large doses of oral steroids, possibly prescribed for a relatively long course).

Lest you think that this sort of intensive asthma co-management strategy is fine only for a well-educated, highly-literate patient population, we wish to point out the success of this same sort of intervention applied in the inner city. In 1990 Dr. Paul Mayo and colleagues at Bellevue Hospital in New York City published the results of an intensive outpatient treatment program among 104 adult asthmatic patient identified because of their frequent need for hospitalizations with asthmatic attacks. Patients in the intervention group received outpatient care at a special chest clinic and received an optimized medical regimen. They also received an intensive educational program. "Emphasis was placed on teaching patients aggressive self-management strategies in case of marked asthma exacerbation," including self-initiation of oral steroids. Compared to the control group—and compared to their own experiences prior to the treatment intervention—these inner-city patients achieved a threefold reduction in the rate of hospital readmissions for asthma and a two- to threefold reduction in the number of in-hospital days. And as they say of achieving success in New York, "if you can make it here, you can make it anywhere"!

KEY POINT Asthma action plans that include instructions on self-initiation of oral steroids for severe attacks can reduce the need for emergency room visits and hospitalizations, even among inner-city residents of low socioeconomic status and low literacy.

Interventions of no value

There is a good chance that your patient has had prior experience dealing at home with at least one asthma flare-up and possibly many. He or she may have settled on some *home remedies* that seemed to help treat asthma attacks in the past. Or perhaps a neighbor, friend, or helpful great aunt has offered tips about treatments that worked for her. It is worthwhile asking openly about what ideas your patient (or patient's caregiver) may have for treating asthma attacks at home—including "complementary and alternative" remedies. Although we don't want to discount therapies born of experience, we also don't want to endorse folkloric treatments in place of proven, evidence-based care.

For instance, we cannot recommend drinking lots of fluids to treat an asthmatic attack. Preventing a very young child or a frail, elderly person from becoming dehydrated from lack of access to liquids is of course important, but trying to make inflamed, constricted bronchial tubes better by ingesting liters of extra fluids is futile. Breathing the mist generated by a hot shower may feel good during an asthmatic attack (or maybe not!), but it is not likely to increase your peak expiratory flow. As for breathing into a brown, paper bag: bad idea. If your patient is breathing fast and feeling anxious during an asthmatic attack, the likely cause relates to diffusely narrowed airways, not *hyperventilation* from primary anxiety. Rebreathing exhaled carbon dioxide in a paper bag will tend to drive up the blood carbon dioxide tension and further increase an already heightened drive to breathe.

With a medicine cabinet full of choices, your patient may try to feel better by taking an antihistamine, decongestant, cough suppressant, expectorant, mucolytic, acetaminophen (Tylenol), or some combination thereof—as provided in numerous over-the-counter cold remedies. These nostrums may help to treat nasal symptoms in the context of allergies or a viral upper respiratory tract infection, but they do not treat asthma. Nowadays many patients may also find an antibiotic available in their medicine cabinet. Remember, though, that viral infections, not bacteria, are the usual triggers of asthmatic exacerbations. A course of amoxicillin (Amoxil) or clarithromycin (Biaxin) in the absence of an escalation of antiasthmatic therapy simply delays effective treatment for an asthmatic exacerbation.

Finally, it is true that caffeine—like its close chemical relative, theophylline—is a bronchodilator. Three cups of caffeinated coffee will improve lung function. But it will do so at the cost of a sleepless night, and less effectively than one inhalation of a beta-agonist bronchodilator. We don't have a space for "drink black coffee" on our asthma action plans!

OVERVIEW OF ASTHMA ACTION PLANS

In this section we offer some sample strategies for completing the content of asthma action plans. These are meant as very broad guidelines, not specific examples to give to specific patients. As a result, we refer here to medication groups and do not use specific medication names. The latter would be appropriate for the actual action plan sheets or cards given to individual patients.

The examples use the three-zone model discussed above, and they are stratified according to the severity of the patient's asthma *at baseline*. It is worth emphasizing, however, that patients with all degrees of asthma severity, including mild asthma, are susceptible to very severe asthmatic attacks. Preparation for all eventualities is the key. We give particular emphasis here to options to treat young children.

KEY POINT   Even patients with mild asthma can suffer severe asthmatic attacks. Best to prepare for all eventualities.

Mild intermittent asthma

Green zone (feeling well; peak flow >80% of personal best):
- Inhaled bronchodilator 10–15 minutes prior to exercise.

Yellow zone (cough, chest tightness, wheeze, or limitation of exercise capacity; peak flow 50–80% of personal best):
- Inhaled corticosteroid via metered-dose inhaler and valved holding chamber (spacer) or via nebulizer. Rinse or wash out the mouth with water after use of the inhaled corticosteroid to prevent oral candidiasis.
- Inhaled bronchodilator every 4 hours as needed delivered via metered-dose inhaler and spacer, metered-dose inhaler with spacer and appropriately-sized face mask, or nebulizer (with or without a face mask).
- Contact your asthma care provider.

Red zone (more severe symptoms of asthma, including accessory muscle use, speaking in short, interrupted sentences, upright body positioning, and obvious respiratory distress; PEFR <50% of personal best):
- Contact your asthma care provider or, in an acute crisis, seek immediate emergency medical care.
- Quick-acting beta-2 agonist as often as every 20–30 minutes for at least two doses. Up to four puffs are permitted with each dose. If available, use a spacer to improve medication delivery. "Back-to-back" nebulized bronchodilator treatments can be given while awaiting medical contact.
- In this context a *burst* or short course of oral corticosteroids may be needed, such as prednisolone syrup in the example of a toddler.
- If there is not improvement after the first hour or two of treatment, seek urgent medical care.

Mild persistent asthma

Green zone:
- Low-dose inhaled corticosteroid or a leukotriene blocker
- Inhaled bronchodilator 10–15 minutes prior to exercise

Yellow zone:
- Inhaled corticosteroid via metered-dose inhaler and valved holding chamber (spacer) or via nebulizer. If already on an inhaled steroid, double your usual dose. Rinse or wash out the mouth with water after use of the inhaled corticosteroid to prevent oral candidiasis.
- Inhaled bronchodilator every 4 hours as needed delivered via metered-dose inhaler and spacer, metered-dose inhaler with spacer and appropriately-sized face mask, or nebulizer (with or without a face mask).
- Contact your asthma care provider.

Red zone:

- Contact your asthma care provider or, in an acute crisis, seek immediate emergency medical care.

- Quick-acting beta-2 agonist as often as every 20–30 minutes for at least two doses. Up to four puffs are permitted with each dose. If available, use a spacer to improve medication delivery. "Back-to-back" nebulized bronchodilator treatments can be given while awaiting medical contact.

- A short course of oral corticosteroids may be needed.

- If there is not improvement after the first hour or two of treatment, seek urgent medical care.

Moderate persistent asthma

Green zone:

- Low-dose inhaled corticosteroid and a long-acting inhaled beta-agonist bronchodilator; or low-dose inhaled corticosteroid and a leukotriene blocker; or medium-dose inhaled corticosteroid

- Inhaled bronchodilator 10–15 minutes prior to exercise

Yellow zone:

- Increase the dose of inhaled corticosteroids. In patients taking the fixed combination of fluticasone and salmeterol (Advair), this increase is best achieved either by using a higher steroid-dose preparation (e.g., Advair 500/50 while in the yellow zone) or by adding an inhaled steroid (e.g., Flovent 220 two puffs twice daily) to the same strength of Advair. Rinse or wash out the mouth with water after use of the inhaled corticosteroid to prevent oral candidiasis.

- Inhaled bronchodilator every 4 hours as needed delivered via metered-dose inhaler and spacer, metered-dose inhaler with spacer and appropriately-sized face mask, or nebulizer (with or without a face mask).

- Contact your asthma care provider.

Red zone:

- Contact your asthma care provider or, in an acute crisis, seek immediate emergency medical care. In an acute crisis, epinephrine pre-filled syringe with auto-injector (EpiPen), followed by call for emergency help (911).

- Quick-acting beta-2 agonist as often as every 20–30 minutes for at least two doses. Up to four puffs are permitted with each dose. If available, use a spacer to improve medication delivery. "Back-to-back" nebulized bronchodilator treatments can be given while awaiting medical contact.

- A short course of oral corticosteroids may be needed.

- If there is not improvement after the first hour or two of treatment, seek urgent medical care.

Severe persistent asthma

Green zone:

- High-dose inhaled corticosteroid plus long-acting inhaled beta-agonist bronchodilator with or without a leukotriene blocker. Daily or alternate-day oral steroids in some patients.

- Inhaled bronchodilator 10–15 minutes prior to exercise.

Yellow zone:

- Begin (or increase the dose) of oral steroids. A small dose (or dose increase) (e.g., prednisone 20 mg/day) may suffice.

- Continue other controller medications.

- Inhaled bronchodilator every 4 hours as needed delivered via metered-dose inhaler and spacer, metered-dose inhaler with spacer and appropriately-sized face mask, or nebulizer (with or without a face mask).

- Contact your asthma care provider.

Red zone:

- Contact your asthma care provider or, in an acute crisis, seek immediate emergency medical care. In an acute crisis, epinephrine prefilled syringe with auto-injector (EpiPen), followed by call for emergency help (911).

- Quick-acting beta-2 agonist as often as every 20–30 minutes for at least two doses. Up to four puffs are permitted with each dose. If available, use a spacer to improve medication delivery. "Back-to-back" nebulized bronchodilator treatments can be given while awaiting medical contact.

- Oral steroids (e.g., prednisone or prednisolone 1 mg/kg/day in children; 40–60 mg/day in adults).

- If there is not improvement after the first hour or two of treatment, seek urgent medical care.

Asthma attacks do not need to be managed in isolation. We encourage our patients and their caregivers to call us to ask questions about asthma management and to report changes in condition or medication use. Not only can we help with managing the asthmatic attack, we can also begin discussion about stepping down therapy after the exacerbation has resolved. It is especially important to make contact with the asthma care provider after an emergency department visit or hospitalization for asthma. An asthma attack of this severity should prompt review of the patient's medical regimen, assessment of risk factors for asthmatic attacks, and possible adjustment of the asthma action plan.

CASE EXAMPLES

Are you ready to help prepare an action plan for an asthmatic patient? We invite you to practice on five fictional patient scenarios. These are brief clinical vignettes; in real life you would likely obtain far more clinical history. For each case, we have prepared a sample asthma action plan, based on the Massachusetts pediatric action plan form (developed by Massachusetts Health Quality Partners), or our Partners Asthma Center action plan cards. (Massachusetts Health Quality Partners is in the process of creating an adult asthma action plan form.) We hope that you will create your own action plan for each patient, using a blank form, then compare your recommendations with ours (Figures 10-4 through 10-8). Feel free to improve on our versions!

▶▶▶ CASE 1

The college student

A 20-year-old college student is seen at the University Health Services. He uses albuterol as needed. His last asthmatic attack occurred when he was a freshman in high school.

Even a person with mild intermittent asthma and infrequent need of his rescue bronchodilator medication deserves an asthma action plan. As you discuss an asthma action plan with this student, you might check to see that he has an albuterol inhaler that has not expired, that he has good inhalational technique using a metered-dose inhaler, and that he knows that he can use his *rescue* inhaler preventively prior to exercise or exposure to other known triggers of his asthma. This would also be a good time to make sure that he has a peak flow meter for use at home and that he knows how to use it.

▶▶▶ CASE 2

The dental hygienist

A 42-year-old dental hygienist takes budesonide (Pulmicort Turbuhaler), two inhalations each morning, for her mild persistent asthma. She has a pirbuterol (Maxair) inhaler that she uses infrequently (approximately once every week or two). She has never been treated with oral steroids.

Our comments for Case 1 apply here as well. In a patient who has never taken oral steroids, we would be reluctant to have her self-initiate her first course at home some weeks or months after this encounter; we would likely not provide her with a prescription for prednisone or methylprednisolone (Medrol) to have at home. Still, at the time that we develop an asthma action plan with her, we might speak of oral steroids, their role, and their potential side effects. We would ask her to contact us at a time when she might first need them prescribed.

▶▶▶ CASE 3

The 12-year-old boy

A 12-year-old boy takes combination fluticasone and salmeterol (Advair 100/50) one inhalation twice daily. He has had a number of severe attacks of asthma, including one intensive care unit stay (no intubation).

This child is being treated for moderate persistent asthma. His history of multiple severe asthmatic attacks, including one of sufficient severity to necessitate treatment in the pediatric intensive care unit, puts him at high risk for severe, potentially life-threatening attacks. We would encourage having a compressor and nebulizer system at home and possibly a prefilled epinephrine-containing needle and syringe (Epi-Pen or Twinject) for emergency use. In addition, his caregivers should have oral steroids on hand for initial treatment of a severe attack.

▶ ▶ ▶ CASE 4

The lawyer

A 50-year-old lawyer has severe persistent asthma with associated aspirin sensitivity. Her medicines include fluticasone-salmeterol combination (Advair) 250/50, montelukast (Singulair), theophylline, and albuterol by MDI and nebulizer.

This patient takes three different controller medications (fluticasone-salmeterol combination, montelukast, and theophylline), none of which is suitable for a dose increase during a mild-to-moderate asthmatic attack. It is particularly important that she not increase her theophylline to treat an exacerbation, because of the risk of theophylline toxicity when the starting blood theophylline concentration is unknown. During discussion of her asthma action plan, you might remind her of the importance of avoiding not only aspirin but also all nonsteroidal anti-inflammatory drugs, many of which are contained in over-the-counter pain and cold remedies. She might consider wearing a medical alert bracelet containing the information that she has asthma and aspirin sensitivity.

▶ ▶ ▶ CASE 5

The toddler

A 2-year-old girl has recently been diagnosed with asthma after her third episode of cough and wheezing. She has been started on montelukast (Singulair Chewtabs) and has albuterol available by metered-dose inhaler with spacer and attached face mask.

Review of medication delivery with this child's caregiver is crucial. Medication delivery using a compressor-nebulizer system and attached face mask is an option (both for bronchodilator and corticosteroid delivery) if the caregiver and child cannot master the combination of metered-dose inhaler with spacer and face mask. If the asthma action plan is to include an inhaled corticosteroid, you will need to spend time with the child's caregiver explaining in detail its anticipated action, potential side effects, and techniques to avoid side effects—emphasizing its safety and considerable value in treating asthmatic attacks.

GO – You're Doing Well! ➡ **Use these daily controller medicines:**

You have **all** of these:
- Breathing is good
- No cough or wheeze
- Sleep through the night
- Can go to school and play

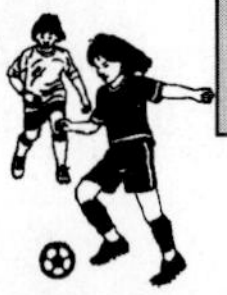

Peak flow from **500** to **400**

MEDICINE/ROUTE	HOW MUCH	HOW OFTEN/ WHEN
Albuterol inhaler	2 puffs	As needed, including before exercise

CAUTION – Slow Down! ➡ **Continue with green zone medicine and add:**

You have **any** of these:
- First signs of a cold
- Cough
- Mild wheeze
- Tight Chest
- Coughing, wheezing, or trouble breathing at night

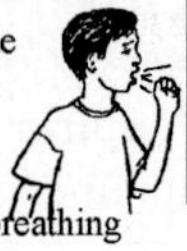

Peak flow from **400** to **250**

MEDICINE/ROUTE	HOW MUCH	HOW OFTEN/ WHEN
Albuterol inhaler	2 puffs	Four times daily until better
Call your doctor if there is no improvement in a few hours.		

CALL YOUR DOCTOR/NURSE: _____

DANGER – Get Help! ➡ **Take these medicines and call your doctor now.**

Your asthma is getting worse fast:
- Medicine is not helping
- Breathing is hard and fast
- Nose opens wide
- Ribs show
- Can't talk well

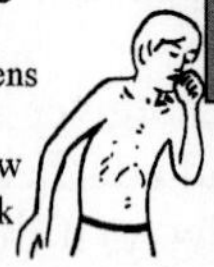

Peak flow from **250** to _____

MEDICINE/ROUTE	HOW MUCH	HOW OFTEN/ WHEN
Albuterol inhaler	4 puffs	Every 20-30 min for up to 2 hours
Call your doctor immediately or go to your nearest emergency room.		

GET HELP FROM A DOCTOR NOW! Do not be afraid of causing a fuss. Your doctor will want to see you right away. It's important! If you cannot contact your doctor, go directly to the emergency room and bring this form with you. DO NOT WAIT.
Make an appointment with your doctor / nurse within two days of an ER visit or hospitalization.

FIGURE 10-4 *Asthma action plan for Case 1, the college student.*

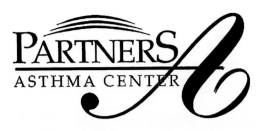

My Asthma Action Plan

Name: __The Dental Hygienist__

My Physicians' Names:

Primary: Dr. _____

Asthma: Dr. _____

My Asthma Medications:

__Pulmicort 2 inhalations once daily__

__Maxair inhaler as needed up to 4__
__times daily__

_____

_____

My Other Medications:
__Calcium with vitamin D__

__Omega 3__

_____

Medication Allergies: ___Sulfa___

My Asthma Action Plan

Peak Flow Values

My BEST PEAK FLOW is:___350___ liters/minute.
When my peak flow is less than:___175___ liters/minute
(less than half of my best value), I am having a
severe attack.

A: In the event of a *Mild or Moderate* asthma
attack I would first:
__Increase my Pulmicort to 4 inh. twice daily__
__Use my Maxair inhaler as often as every 3-4__
hours as needed until better
If there is no improvement, my next step would be
to:
__Call my doctor; may need oral steroids__

_____

B: In the event of a SEVERE asthma attack, I would
first: Use my Maxair inhaler as often as every
__20-30 minutes for up to 1-2 hours as needed__
__Call my doctor; may need oral steroids__

If there is no improvement, my next step would be
to:
__Seek emergency care immediately.__

_____

If there is still no improvement,

Seek Emergency Help Immediately

EMERGENCY PHONE NUMBERS

My Asthma Doctor:_____

*(ask to page your asthma doctor or the covering
fellow)*

Ambulance:_____ or 911

FIGURE 10-5   *Asthma action plan for Case 2, the dental hygienist.*

GO – You're Doing Well! ➡ Use these daily controller medicines:

You have _all_ of these:
- Breathing is good
- No cough or wheeze
- Sleep through the night
- Can go to school and play

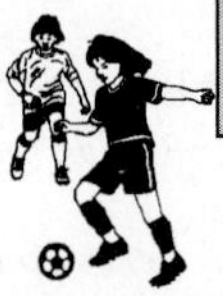

Peak flow from __250__ to __200__

MEDICINE/ROUTE	HOW MUCH	HOW OFTEN/WHEN
Advair 100/50	1 inhalation	Twice daily
Albuterol inhaler	2 puffs	As needed, up to 4 times a day

CAUTION – Slow Down! ➡ Continue with green zone medicine and add:

You have _any_ of these:
- First signs of a cold
- Cough
- Mild wheeze
- Tight Chest
- Coughing, wheezing, or trouble breathing at night

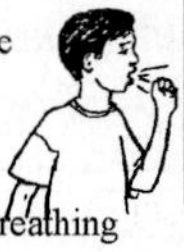

Peak flow from __200__ to __125__

MEDICINE/ROUTE	HOW MUCH	HOW OFTEN/WHEN
Advair 500/50	1 inhalation	Twice daily
Albuterol inhaler	4 puffs	Four times daily until better

CALL YOUR DOCTOR/ NURSE: _____

DANGER – Get Help! ➡ Take these medicines and call your doctor now.

Your asthma is getting worse fast:
- Medicine is not helping
- Breathing is hard and fast
- Nose opens wide
- Ribs show
- Can't talk well

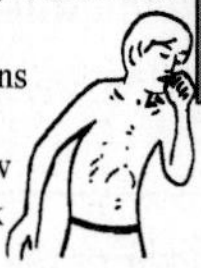

Peak flow from __125__ to _____

MEDICINE/ROUTE	HOW MUCH	HOW OFTEN/WHEN
Advair 500/50	1 inhalation	Twice daily
Albuterol by nebulizer	1 vial (2.5 mg)	Up to every 30 min
Prednisone	30 mg	Now, and call our office immediately

GET HELP FROM A DOCTOR NOW! Do not be afraid of causing a fuss. Your doctor will want to see you right away. It's important! If you cannot contact your doctor, go directly to the emergency room and bring this form with you. DO NOT WAIT.
Make an appointment with your doctor /nurse within two days of an ER visit or hospitalization.

FIGURE 10-6 *Asthma action plan for Case 3, the 12-year-old boy.*

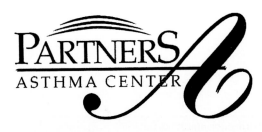

My Asthma Action Plan

Name: __The Lawyer__

My Physicians' Names:

Primary: Dr. _____

Asthma: Dr._____

My Asthma Medications:

Advair 250/50 1 inh. twice daily

Uniphyl 300 mg twice daily

Singulair 10 mg once daily

Ventolin 2 puffs as needed

My Other Medications:
Lisinopril 5 mg daily

Lipitor 20 mg daily

Medication Allergies: __Aspirin and all NSAIDs__

My Asthma Action Plan

Peak Flow Values

My BEST PEAK FLOW is:__320__ liters/minute.
When my peak flow is less than:__160__ liters/minute
(less than half of my best value), I am having a
severe attack.

A: In the event of a Mild or Moderate asthma
attack I would first:
Take my Ventolin every 4 hours until better
Add Flovent 220 2 puffs twice daily to my
Advair, Uniphyl, and Singulair
*If there is no improvement, my next step would be
to:*
Call my doctor; may need oral steroids

B: In the event of a SEVERE asthma attack, I would
first: Use my nebulizer with albuterol every 20-30
min as needed for up to 2 hours

Call my doctor; may need oral steroids

*If there is no improvement, my next step would be
to:*
Seek emergency care immediately.

If there is still no improvement,

Seek Emergency Help Immediately

EMERGENCY PHONE NUMBERS

My Asthma Doctor:_____

*(ask to page your asthma doctor or the covering
fellow)*

Ambulance:_____ or 911

FIGURE 10-7 *Asthma action plan for Case 4, the lawyer.*

GO – You're Doing Well! ➡		Use these daily controller medicines:		

You have _all_ of these:
- Breathing is good
- No cough or wheeze
- Sleep through the night
- Can go to school and play

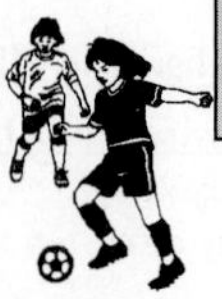

Peak flow from _____ to _____

MEDICINE/ROUTE	HOW MUCH	HOW OFTEN/WHEN
Singulair Chewtabs	4 mg	Once daily
Albuterol inhaler	2 puffs	As needed, up to 4 times a day

CAUTION – Slow Down! ➡		Continue with green zone medicine and add:		

You have _any_ of these:
- First signs of a cold
- Cough
- Mild wheeze
- Tight Chest
- Coughing, wheezing, or trouble breathing at night

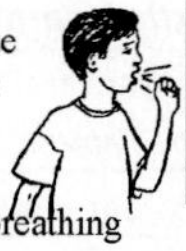

Peak flow from _____ to _____

MEDICINE/ROUTE	HOW MUCH	HOW OFTEN/WHEN
Pulmicort Respule by nebulizer	1 vial (250 mcg)	Twice daily
Albuterol by nebulizer	1 vial (1.25 mg)	Four times daily until better

CALL YOUR DOCTOR/ NURSE: _____

DANGER – Get Help! ➡		Take these medicines and call your doctor now.		

Your asthma is getting worse fast:
- Medicine is not helping
- Breathing is hard and fast
- Nose opens wide
- Ribs show
- Can't talk well

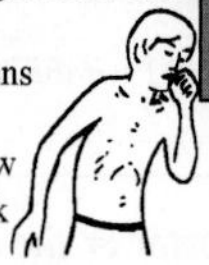

Peak flow from _____ to _____

MEDICINE/ROUTE	HOW MUCH	HOW OFTEN/WHEN
Pulmicort Respule by nebulizer	1 vial (250 mcg)	Twice daily
Albuterol by nebulizer	1 vial (1.25 mg)	Up to every 3-4 hours
Call office for oral steroids (Prelone)		

GET HELP FROM A DOCTOR NOW! Do not be afraid of causing a fuss. Your doctor will want to see you right away. It's important! If you cannot contact your doctor, go directly to the emergency room and bring this form with you. **DO NOT WAIT.**
Make an appointment with your doctor /nurse within two days of an ER visit or hospitalization.

FIGURE 10-8 *Asthma action plan for Case 5, the toddler.*

Self-Assessment Questions

QUESTION 1

Written asthma action plans are recommended by the National Asthma Education and Prevention Program based on:

1. Unequivocal scientific evidence from randomized, controlled clinical trials
2. Strong recommendations from asthma interest groups, such as Mothers of Asthmatics and the Asthma and Allergy Foundation of America
3. Review of the medical literature and consensus opinion of experts
4. Large-scale telephone survey data (*Asthma in America* and *Children & Asthma in America*)
5. Cost-savings analysis of emergency department and hospital utilization for asthmatic attacks

QUESTION 2

In discussing asthma management, the term "poor perceiver" is used to refer to patients who:

1. Have poor inhaler technique
2. Have low literacy skills
3. Are poorly aware of having a severe asthmatic attack
4. Respond poorly to instruction
5. Have difficulty with compliance due to low socioeconomic status

QUESTION 3

Which of the following is not a key element of initial self-management during an asthma flare?

1. Recognizing the presence of an asthmatic attack
2. Assessing the severity of an asthmatic attack
3. Intensifying antiasthmatic therapy
4. Knowing when and how to get medical help
5. Ready access to specialist referral

QUESTION 4

In the three-zone (traffic-light) model of an asthma action plan, the red zone indicates a severe asthmatic attack, when the peak flow is less than:

1. 70%
2. 60%

3. 50%

4. 40%

5. 30%

QUESTION 5

True or False: *Asthma action plans are best reserved for asthmatic patients over 5–6 years of age who can reliably use a peak flow meter.*

1. True

2. False

QUESTION 6

A pitfall of home peak flow monitoring is that improperly performed tests can give false values. The most common error is:

1. Overestimation of the severity of an attack (falsely low peak flow value)

2. Underestimation of the severity of an attack (falsely high peak flow value)

QUESTION 7

Which of the following recommendations about use of inhaled beta-agonist bronchodilators during an asthmatic attack is correct?

1. Do not use nebulized bronchodilator more than every 4 hours.

2. Do not use bronchodilator by metered-dose inhaler more than two puffs at a time.

3. Avoid use of valved holding chambers (spacers).

4. Do not rely on bronchodilator therapy alone if there is no improvement after 1 hour.

5. Avoid peak flow measurements immediately before or after use of bronchodilator.

QUESTION 8

True or False: *Self-initiation of oral steroids without first obtaining provider approval at the time of the attack should never be part of an asthma action plan.*

1. True

2. False

QUESTION 9

A complementary strategy that can reasonably be recommended along with a formal asthma action plan is:

1. Remain calm; breathe slowly and deeply.
2. Drink 6–8 glasses of water per day.
3. Mucolytics (e.g., guaifenesin) speed resolution of the attack.
4. If anxious, breathe into a small brown paper bag.
5. Drink caffeinated beverages during an attack.

QUESTION 10

A 27-year-old teacher with moderate persistent asthma takes combination fluticasone-salmeterol (Advair) 100/50 one inhalation twice daily along with inhaled albuterol as needed. During a mild-moderate asthmatic exacerbation (yellow zone), a reasonable strategy for initial self-management is:

1. Increase to two inhalations of combination fluticasone-salmeterol (Advair) twice daily.
2. Increase to combination fluticasone-salmeterol (Advair) 500/50 one inhalation twice daily.
3. Continue combination fluticasone-salmeterol (Advair) 100/50 one inhalation twice daily and increase albuterol use to two puffs four times a day.
4. Continue combination fluticasone-salmeterol (Advair) 100/50 one inhalation twice daily and add montelukast (Singulair) 10 mg once daily.
5. Discontinue combination fluticasone-salmeterol (Advair) and begin fluticasone alone (Flovent) 220 two puffs twice daily.

QUESTION 11

The parent of a 3-year-old child expresses concern about how best to prepare should her son experience an asthmatic attack. The child has mild persistent asthma and takes montelukast (Singulair Chewtab) 4 mg daily along with albuterol used as needed with a valved holding chamber and attached face mask. You suggest that a reasonable strategy for her to discuss with her physician would be to have available at home any of the following except:

1. Compressor and nebulizer for administration of albuterol
2. Compressor and nebulizer for administration of budesonide (Pulmicort Respules)
3. Fluticasone (Flovent) metered-dose inhaler 44 mcg/puff to be given via valved holding chamber and attached face mask
4. Combination fluticasone-salmeterol (Advair Diskus) 100/50 one inhalation twice daily
5. Prednisolone (Prelone) syrup

QUESTION 12

A 19-year-old college student has mild persistent asthma and uses mometasone (Asmanex) one inhalation once daily as his controller medication. Although he has never had a severe asthmatic attack, he has discussed strategies for dealing with flares of his asthma with his primary care physician, including more frequent use of his rescue bronchodilator, metaproterenol (Alupent), and doubling his dose of mometasone (Asmanex) to two inhalations each day. He asks your advice about what he should do in the event of a severe asthmatic attack that is not improving with these initial measures. You advise him that in that circumstance he should:

1. Stay home from class, rest, and drink plenty of fluids
2. Try an over-the-counter antihistamine-decongestant combination (such as Alka Seltzer Plus Cold and Sinus)
3. Increase his metaproterenol (Alupent) to four inhalations per each treatment
4. Increase his mometasone (Asmanex) further to two inhalations twice daily
5. Seek immediate medical attention by telephone or at an urgent care center

Answers to Self-Assessment Questions

ANSWER TO QUESTION 1 (SCIENTIFIC BASIS FOR USE OF WRITTEN ASTHMA ACTION PLANS)

The correct answer is #3. Members of the Expert Panel of the National Asthma Education and Prevention Program have recommended use of written asthma action plans based on their review of the medical literature and consensus among asthma care experts. The evidence from randomized, controlled clinical trials is divided about the value of asthma action plans (answer #1). Asthma interest groups did not dictate this recommendation from the National Asthma Education and Prevention Program (answer #2). The Asthma in America and Children & Asthma in America surveys did not address the issue of asthma action plans (answer #4). Cost-effectiveness analyses regarding the value of asthma action plans have not, to our knowledge, been performed (answer #5).

ANSWER TO QUESTION 2 (DEFINING THE CONCEPT OF "POOR PERCEIVER")

The correct answer is #3; poor perceivers fail to perceive the presence of a severe asthmatic attack. The term "poor perceiver" has not been used to describe those with poor inhaler technique (answer #1), low literacy skills (answer #2), poor response to instruction (answer #4), or difficulty with compliance due to low socioeconomic status (answer #5).

ANSWER TO QUESTION 3 (KEY ELEMENTS OF INITIAL ASTHMA SELF-MANAGEMENT DURING AN ASTHMA FLARE)

The correct answer is #5. Ready access to an asthma specialist may be helpful in managing severe asthma, but it is not a key element of initial self-management during an asthma flare. The other answers are the four key elements to an effective asthma action plan: recognizing the presence of an asthmatic attack (answer #1); assessing the severity of an asthmatic attack (answer #2); intensifying antiasthmatic therapy (answer # 3); and knowing when and how to get medical help (answer #4).

ANSWER TO QUESTION 4 (PEAK FLOW MEASUREMENT THAT INDICATES A SEVERE ASTHMATIC ATTACK [RED ZONE])

The correct answer is #3. The "red zone" is defined as 50% or less than one's personal best peak flow. The "green zone" is a peak flow greater than 80% of one's personal best. The "yellow zone" is defined as 50–80% of one's personal best.

ANSWER TO QUESTION 5 (ASTHMA ACTION PLANS WITHOUT PEAK FLOW MONITORING)

The correct answer is #2 (False). Asthma action plans are very much appropriate for the parents and other caregivers of children who are too young to perform peak flow measurements. In this circumstance the severity of the asthmatic attack must be gauged on the basis of asthmatic symptoms and physical findings. Similarly, asthma action plans can be developed for older children and adults who do not have or who do not wish to use peak flow meters.

ANSWER TO QUESTION 6 (DEALING WITH FALSE VALUES DERIVED FROM HOME PEAK FLOW MEASUREMENTS)

The correct answer is #1. It is far more common to generate a falsely low peak flow value than a falsely high number. A falsely low reading may result from an inadequate expiratory effort, poor coordination of a rapid exhalation, and an air leak at the mouthpiece.

ANSWER TO QUESTION 7 (USE OF BETA-AGONIST BRONCHODILATORS DURING AN ASTHMATIC ATTACK)

The correct answer is #4. Overreliance on beta-agonist bronchodilators during an asthmatic attack can result in dangerous airway obstruction due to untreated inflammation and mucus plugging. For initial treatment of an asthmatic attack, it is safe to use nebulized bronchodilator more than every 4 hours (answer #1) and to use bronchodilator by metered-dose inhaler more than two puffs at a time (answer #2). Valved holding chambers (spacers) can be helpful to optimize administration of bronchodilator from metered-dose inhalers (answer #3). Peak flow measurements made before and after administration of bronchodilators can help to assess whether or not the asthmatic attack is improving with therapy (answer #5).

ANSWER TO QUESTION 8 (SELF-INITIATION OF ORAL STEROIDS AT HOME)

The correct answer is #2 (False). We believe that it is appropriate in certain circumstances for a patient (or parent of a patient) to administer oral steroids as part of an asthma action plan, and then notify the healthcare provider after doing so. As an example, consider the patient who has had multiple severe asthmatic attacks, many courses of oral steroids in the past, and many emergency department visits for his asthmatic attacks. During a severe attack, when his usual physician is not readily available, he might take an initial dose of oral steroids at home as indicated on his asthma action plan, then subsequently inform his physician that he has done so.

ANSWER TO QUESTION 9 (COMPLEMENTARY STRATEGIES APPROPRIATE DURING AN ASTHMATIC ATTACK)

The correct answer is #1. Panic is never helpful during an asthmatic attack; it is good advice—not always easy to follow—to remain calm and take slow, deep breaths. We do not recommend forced hydration (answer #2), mucolytics (answer #3), breathing into a brown paper bag (answer #4), or caffeinated beverages (answer #5). Adding ineffective or potentially harmful recommendations to an asthma action plan distracts from the main message and threatens credibility.

ANSWER TO QUESTION 10 (INTENSIFYING THERAPY FOR A MILD-TO-MODERATE ASTHMATIC ATTACK IN A PATIENT TAKING AS HER CONTROLLER THERAPY THE FIXED COMBINATION OF FLUTICASONE AND SALMETEROL [ADVAIR])

The correct answer is #2. A commonly employed treatment for an asthmatic attack in the yellow zone is to increase the dose of inhaled steroids. In a patient using the fixed fluticasone-salmeterol combination (Advair), this strategy can be achieved by increasing the dose of Advair (to a higher fluticasone concentration per puff) such as in answer #2 or by adding more inhaled steroid to the same dose of Advair (e.g., adding fluticasone [Flovent] 220 two puffs twice daily to Advair 100/50 one inhalation twice daily). Increasing the number of inhalations of Advair 100/50 to two inhalations twice daily exposes the patient to twice the recommended dose of salmeterol (answer #1). Increasing the frequency of albuterol use to two puffs four times a day is an inadequate response to an attack in the yellow zone (answer #3). Adding a leukotriene blocker such as montelukast (Singulair) to a long-acting bronchodilator and inhaled steroid is an unproven strategy for managing mild-to-moderate asthmatic attacks (answer #4). Increasing the dose of inhaled steroid should not be accompanied by discontinuation of the long-acting beta-agonist bronchodilator during an asthmatic attack (answer #5).

ANSWER TO QUESTION 11 (STEPPING UP THERAPY IN A 3-YEAR-OLD CHILD RECEIVING A LEUKOTRIENE BLOCKER AS CONTROLLER THERAPY)

The correct answer is #4. A 3-year-old child would not be expected to be able to coordinate use of the Diskus dry-powder inhaler for administration of combination fluticasone-salmeterol (Advair). Potentially useful to have at home for managing asthmatic attacks would be albuterol administered via compressor and nebulizer (answer #1); an inhaled steroid administered via compressor and nebulizer (answer #2); an inhaled steroid administered by valved holding chamber and attached face mask (answer #3); and oral steroids (answer #5).

ANSWER TO QUESTION 12 (ASTHMA ACTION PLAN RECOMMENDATIONS FOR A SEVERE ASTHMATIC ATTACK)

The correct answer is #5. It is good to remember that asthma self-management at home has its limits. *Get help* is the correct advice when initial treatment strategies are not working. Staying at home for rest and hydration is dangerous when airway obstruction is worsening during an asthmatic attack (answer #1). Over-the-counter antihistamines and decongestants may help with cold symptoms, but they do not treat an asthmatic attack (answer #2). A further increase in bronchodilator dose will not address worsening airway inflammation (answer #3); and a further increase in the dose of inhaled steroids may not prove adequate (answer #4). It is best to get professional medical guidance when initial steps in one's asthma action plan are not working.

INDEX

Note: Page numbers followed by "*f*" denote figures; those followed by "*t*" denote tables.

A

Accolate. *See* Zafirlukast
Adrenaline. *See* Epinephrine
Advair. *See* Fluticasone
Aerobid. *See* Flunisolide
Aerolizer, 313–315, 314*f*,
   323, 326
Age, at asthma onset, 49–50, 50*f*
Air pollution, 275
Airway. *See* Bronchi
Airway narrowing. *See*
   Bronchoconstriction
Airway remodeling, 28–29,
   39, 43
Albuterol
   inhaled
      administration routes, 96*t*
      in asthmatic attacks,
         340–343
      in childhood asthma,
         178–179, 180
      mechanisms of action, 95,
         95*t*, 121, 125
   oral
      in childhood asthma, 179
      formulations, 102*t*
      vs. inhaled, 103, 122,
         126–127
Allergens. *See also* Allergies
   asthmatic reactions to, early
      vs. late, 11–13, 11*f*,
      12*f*, 38, 42. *See also*
      Bronchial
      inflammation
   avoidance
      approach to patient,
         275–276
      home visits, 279
      multidimensional
         intervention,
         277–279, 278*f*, 283,
         287

childhood asthma and,
   192–193
common
   cats, 267–268, 282, 286
   cockroaches, 263,
      269–271, 282, 286
   dogs, 268
   dust mites, 264–266, 264*f*,
      282, 285
   indoor mold, 268–269
   outdoor mold, 272–273,
      273*f*
   overview, 257*t*, 262–263
   pollens, 271–272, 272*f*,
      283, 286
   rats and mice, 271
   vs. irritants, 256–257
Allergic conjunctivitis,
   54, 253
Allergic rhinitis, 253
"Allergic salute," 54, 54*f*
"Allergic shiners," 54
Allergies. *See also* Allergens
   in asthma
      early vs. late reactions,
         11–13, 11*f*, 12*f*, 38, 42.
         See also Bronchial
         inflammation
      interventions
         approach to patient,
            275–276
         home visits, 279
         immunotherapy,
            141–143, 159, 163
         multidimensional,
            277–279, 278*f*, 283,
            287
         overview, 253–255, 254*f*,
            280, 284
      diagnosis
         blood tests, 261–262,
            281, 285

patient history, 256–257,
   280–281, 284
skin tests, 257–261, 259*f*,
   281, 285
Allergy-proof wraps,
   265–266
Alpha-adrenergic agonists, 94.
   See also Epinephrine
Alupent. *See* Metaproterenol
Alveoli, 5, 5*f*
Americans with Disabilities Act,
   192, 199, 203
Anabolic steroids, 106–107
Anaphylaxis
   in allergy testing, 261
   epinephrine for, 94
Angiotensin converting
   enzyme (ACE)
   inhibitors,
   18, 125
Anticholinergic
   bronchodilators,
   102*t*, 103–105. *See
   also specific drugs*
Anti-immunoglobulin
   E monoclonal
   antibody. *See*
   Omalizumab
Anti-inflammatory drugs
   corticosteroids. *See*
      Corticosteroids
   leukotriene blockers. *See*
      Leukotriene blockers
   mast cell stabilizers,
      112–113. *See also*
      Cromolyn
Anti-Parkinsonian
   medications, 104
Anxiety
   airway narrowing and,
      15–16
   in asthmatic attacks, 339

Arterial blood gases, in
        asthmatic attacks
    indications for measuring,
        350
    interpretation, 336–338,
        338*f*, 355–356, 359
Asmanex. *See* Mometasone
Aspergillosis, 140
Aspiration, foreign body,
        64, 180
Aspirin-sensitive asthma
    analgesic selection in, 124,
        128
    incidence, 114–115
    pathophysiology, 115–117,
        116*f*
Asthma
    action plans. *See* Asthma
        action plans
    allergies and, 253–255, 254*f*,
        280, 284. *See also*
        Allergens; Allergies
    aspirin-sensitive. *See*
        Aspirin-sensitive
        asthma
    attacks. *See* Asthmatic
        attacks
    in children. *See* Childhood
        asthma
    complementary and
        alternative therapies,
        148–150, 160,
        163–164
    definition, 29
    diagnosis
        diagnostic tests
            allergy testing, 63
            bronchoprovocative
                challenge, 61–62,
                82, 86
            exhaled nitric oxide
                concentration, 62
            imaging, 63
            peak flow. *See* Peak flow
            spirometry. *See*
                Spirometry
            therapeutic trial, 58
        excluding alternatives
            in adults, 65–67, 66*t*
            in children, 64

history
    age of onset, 49–50, 50*f*
    characteristic symptoms,
        48–49, 81,
        84, 85
    common associated
        illnesses, 50–51, 51*t*
    typical triggers, 49
    physical examination,
        52–55
difficult-to-control,
        140–141, 159, 163.
        See also Severe
        persistent asthma
epidemiology
    distribution, 33–34, 40, 44
    incidence, 31
    morbidity, 33*f*
    prevalence, 34–35
    by severity level, 79–80, 80*f*
etiology, 29–31
exacerbations. *See* Asthmatic
        attacks
exercise-induced. *See*
        Exercise-induced
        asthma
genetics, 30, 39, 43–44
goals of care, 36, 130
hygiene hypothesis, 35, 40,
        44–45
mild intermittent. *See* Mild
        intermittent asthma
mild persistent. *See* Mild
        persistent asthma
moderate persistent. *See*
        Moderate persistent
        asthma
mortality, 109, 109*f*
nonallergic
    characteristics, 255
    irritant exposures,
        274–275
nontriggers, 18, 37, 41
occupational. *See*
        Occupational asthma
outgrowing, 20
pharmacologic therapy. *See*
        also specific drugs
    bronchodilators. *See also*
        Bronchodilators

anticholinergic, 102*t*,
        103–105
beta–1 adrenergic,
        94–95, 95*t*
beta–2 adrenergic. *See*
        Beta–2 adrenergic
        agonists
compliance, 90
corticosteroids. *See*
        Corticosteroids
goals of care, 36, 130
historical perspective,
        91–92, 91*f*
leukotriene blockers. *See*
        Leukotriene blockers
mast cell stabilizers,
        112–113. *See also*
        Cromolyn
model for categorizing
        and teaching, 93, 120,
        124–125
step-care approach. *See*
        Step-care approach
stepping down, 143–144
pregnancy and. *See*
        Pregnancy
severe persistent. *See* Severe
        persistent asthma
severity staging system
    categories, 71–75, 71*t*,
        83, 87. *See also specific*
        categories
    criteria, 69–70, 82–83, 87
    development, 68–69
    limitations, 75–77
    purpose, 67–68
specialist referral for,
        139–140
triggers. *See* Triggers
Asthma action plans
    case examples, 388–399,
        390–394*f*
    communicating to patient
        or parent, 371–372,
        376
    evidence supporting,
        365–366, 395, 398
    getting started, 366–367
    for mild intermittent asthma,
        385, 388, 390–391*f*

for mild persistent asthma, 385–386
for moderate persistent asthma, 386, 388–389, 392f
rationale, 364–365
recommendations
inhaled beta agonists, 378–380, 396, 399
inhaled corticosteroids, 380–381, 397, 400
interventions of no value, 383–384
oral corticosteroids, 382–383, 396, 399–400
for severe persistent asthma, 387, 389, 393f, 397–398, 401
steps
access to medical help, 370, 397–398, 401
assessment of severity, 368–369, 395, 398
initiation of treatment, 369–370
recognition of attack, 367–368
three-zone model, 372–376, 373t, 374f, 375f, 377f, 395–396, 399
Asthma Control Test, 170
Asthmatic attacks
assessment
chest x-ray, 339
oximetry and arterial blood gases, 336–339, 338f, 355–356, 359
peak flow measurement, 335–336
physical examination, 333–335, 334f, 355, 359
in childhood asthma, 168–169, 169f, 172
discharge planning, 352–354, 358, 362
epidemiology, 330–331
mold exposure and, 273

preparation. See Asthma action plans
prevention, 331–332, 355, 358–359
respiratory infection as trigger, 357, 361
self-management. See Asthma action plans
treatment
antibiotics, 348–349
bronchodilators, 340–343, 341f, 378–380, 396, 399
corticosteroids
inhaled, 380–381, 397, 400
oral/intravenous, 343–347, 344f, 382–383, 396, 399–400
helium-oxygen gas mixture, 349
hospitalization indications, 352, 358, 362
interventions of no value, 348, 383–384
mechanical ventilation, 349–352, 357–358, 361
principles, 340
supplemental oxygen, 337, 340
Atopic diseases
associated with asthma, 50–51, 81, 85, 280, 284
definition, 252
by organ of involvement, 51t
physical findings, 53–55, 54f
types, 252–253
Atropine, 104
Atrovent. See Ipratropium
Autohaler, 301–302, 301f, 321–322, 325
Autonomic nervous system, 93–94
Azmacort. See Triamcinolone
Azmacort inhaler, 297–298, 297f

B
B-lymphocytes, 25
Beclomethasone
in childhood asthma, 184t, 185t
delivery system and doses, 110t
historical perspective, 92
in mild persistent asthma, 135
in moderate persistent asthma, 138
in severe persistent asthma, 139
Beta–1 adrenergic agonists, 94–95, 95t
Beta–2 adrenergic agonists. See also specific drugs
drug interactions, 104
inhaled
in asthmatic attacks, 340–343, 341f, 378–380, 396, 399
in childhood asthma, 180
delivery devices. See Inhalers and inhalational aids
long-acting, 98–99
mechanisms of action, 93–94
in moderate persistent asthma, 138
safety, 99–101, 100t, 121–122, 126
in severe persistent asthma, 139
short-acting, 94–98, 95t, 96t
in step-care approach, 131t
oral, 102t, 103
Beta-adrenergic antagonists (blockers), 16, 37, 41, 94, 120–121, 125
Bi-level positive airway pressure (Bi-PAP), 351
Breathing
anatomy and physiology, 5–9, 5f, 8f
in asthmatic attacks, 333–335, 334f

Brethine. *See* Terbutaline
Bronchi, 5–6, 5*f*, 6*f*
Bronchial hyperresponsiveness
  challenge test for. *See*
      Bronchoprovocative
      challenge test
  definition, 19
  inflammation as cause of.
      See Bronchial
      inflammation
  outgrowing, 20–21
Bronchial inflammation
  characteristics, 21–23
  definition, 19
  hyperresponsiveness and,
      23–24
  pathophysiology
    airway remodeling, 28–29,
      39, 43
    chemical mediators,
      26–27, 38–39, 43
    eosinophils, 27–28
    immunoglobulin E, 26,
      38, 42–43
    lymphocytes, 25
    mast cells, 26, 27*f*
Bronchitis
  chronic, 65. *See also* Chronic
      obstructive pulmonary
      disease
  recurrent, 65
Bronchoconstriction
  allergen challenge and,
      11–13, 11*f*, 12*f*
  characteristics, 7*f*
  clinical symptoms, 9
  exercise-induced. *See*
      Exercise-induced
      asthma
  mechanisms, 9–10
  triggers. *See* Triggers
Bronchodilators. *See also*
      Inhalers and
      inhalational aids;
      specific drugs
  anticholinergic, 102*t*,
      103–105
  in asthmatic attacks,
      340–343, 341*f*, 356,
      360, 378–380

beta-adrenergic agonists. *See*
      Beta–1 adrenergic
      agonists; Beta–2
      adrenergic agonists
  in childhood asthma, 180,
      198–199, 202
  in exercise-induced asthma,
      133–134
  in mild intermittent asthma,
      130, 132–133,
      157, 161
  in mild persistent asthma,
      135
  spirometry results before
      and after, 228, 229*f*,
      230
  in step-care approach, 131*t*
  theophylline. *See*
      Theophylline
  therapeutic trial, in asthma
      diagnosis, 58
Bronchoprovocative challenge
    test
  in asthma diagnosis, 20,
      61–62, 82, 86
  in children, 174
Bronchospasm, 10
Budesonide
  in childhood asthma, 184*t*,
      185*t*
  delivery systems, 110*t*, 111
  doses, 110*t*, 111
  in mild persistent asthma,
      135–137
  in pregnancy, 111, 137, 156
  in severe persistent asthma,
      139
  Turbuhaler, 310–312, 310*f*

C

Candidiasis, 107
Cat allergy, 267–268,
    282, 286
Challenge test, bronchial. *See*
      Bronchoprovocative
      challenge test
Chest radiograph
  in asthma diagnosis, 63
  in asthmatic attacks, 339,
      356, 359–360

Childhood asthma
  allergic sensitivities in,
      253–254
  asthmatic attacks in,
      168–169, 169*f*, 172,
      197, 200. *See also*
      Asthma action plans
  costs, 167
  diagnosis
    alternative considerations,
      173, 173*t*, 194–196
    case example, 170–171
    history and physical
      examination,
      171–172, 197, 201
    testing, 172–175,
      197, 201
  in inner-city residents,
      multidimensional
      intervention,
      277–279, 278*f*,
      283, 287
  interference with activities,
      167–168
  mortality, 166–167
  nocturnal symptoms,
      168
  pharmacotherapy
    controllers
      bronchodilators, 180,
      198–199, 202
      cromolyn, 180–181
      inhaled corticosteroids,
      181–185, 184*t*, 185*f*,
      198, 202
      leukotriene blockers,
      185–186, 199,
      202–203
    delivery devices
      age-related
      considerations, 198,
      202
      compressor and
      nebulizer, 175–176
      dry-powder inhaler,
      177–178
      metered-dose inhalers,
      176–177, 294–295,
      294*f*
  follow-up, 188–189

initial failure
  alternative diagnoses,
    193, 193t, 194–196,
    199–200, 203
  concomitant illnesses
    and, 192–193
  review of expectations
    and administration
    technique, 189
  specialist referral
    indications, 190,
    190t, 200, 203
  unidentified triggers
    and, 191–192, 191t
  preventive maintenance,
    187–188
  quick relievers, 178–180
  stepwise approach, 183t
prevalence, 166
risk factors, 171–172, 172t,
    197, 200–201
rules of two, 169–170
school absenteeism and,
    167–168
Chlorofluorocarbon (CFC), 303
Chronic obstructive pulmonary
    disease (COPD)
  anticholinergics for,
    104–105
  vs. asthma, 65t
  diagnosis, 65–67
  spirometry results in, 66,
    228, 229f
  wheezing characteristics, 53
Churg-Strauss syndrome,
    118–119
Cocaine, inhaled, 274–275
Cockroaches
  characteristics, 269–270,
    270f
  childhood asthma and, 263
  controlling exposure to,
    270–271, 282, 286
Complementary and
    alternative therapies,
    148–150, 160,
    163–164
Compressors, for nebulization.
    See Nebulizer
    systems

Confidence intervals,
    in spirometry results,
    218
Congestive heart failure, 67
Conjunctivitis, allergic,
    54, 253
Continuous positive airway
    pressure ventilation
    (CPAP), 351
Controllers, 129–130
Corticosteroids
  vs. anabolic steroids,
    106–107
  inhaled
    advantages vs. oral, 106
    in asthmatic attacks, 347,
      381, 396–397, 400
    benefits, 108–109, 109f,
      122, 127, 182
    in childhood asthma,
      181–185, 183t, 184t,
      185f, 198, 202
    doses, 110t, 111–112
    historical perspective, 92
    long-term effects, 136,
      158, 162, 182, 184
    in mild persistent asthma,
      135–137
    in moderate persistent
      asthma, 138
    patient questions,
      136–137
    in pregnancy, 137
    preparations, 110t
    selection, 111
    in severe persistent
      asthma, 139
    side effects, 107–108, 123,
      127, 136
    in step-care approach,
      131t
  intramuscular, 347
  oral/intravenous
    in asthmatic attacks,
      343–347, 344f,
      356–357, 360,
      382–383, 396,
      399–400
    in childhood asthma,
      187

side effects, 105–106,
    122, 127
  tapering, 346
Cough
  habit, 195
  pathophysiology, 9
CPAP (continuous positive
    airway pressure
    ventilation), 351
Cromolyn
  in childhood asthma,
    180–181
  delivery system, 113
  mechanisms of action,
    112–113
  preventive use, 113, 123,
    127, 133
Cyclooxygenase inhibitors,
    in aspirin-sensitive
    asthma, 116
Cystic fibrosis
  clinical presentation,
    195–196
  diagnosis, 54, 64, 196
Cytokines, 25

D
Dehumidifiers, 269
Diaphragm, in breathing, 8, 8f
Diskus device, 308–310, 308f,
    323, 326
Dog allergy, 268
Doser, 305–306, 305f
Dry-powder inhalers
  Aerolizer, 313–315, 314f,
    323, 326
  for children, 177–178
  Diskus, 308–310, 308f, 323,
    326
  Handihaler, 315–316, 315f,
    323, 326
  history of development,
    306–307
  inspiratory flow strength
    and, 308
  vs. metered-dose inhalers,
    308, 310f, 323, 326
  Turbuhaler, 310–312, 310f
  Twisthaler, 312–313,
    312f

Dust mites
    allergy to, 264–265
    characteristics, 264f, 265,
        282, 285
    controlling exposure to,
        265–267
Dysphonia, with inhaled
    corticosteroids,
    107–108

E
Eczema
    childhood asthma and, 171
    physical findings, 54
Electrostatic precipitators,
    279
Emphysema. *See also* Chronic
        obstructive pulmonary
        disease
    diagnosis, 65–66
    pathophysiology, 65
    wheezing characteristics, 53
End-expiratory wheeze, 53
Environmental tobacco smoke,
        childhood asthma
        and, 274, 283,
        286–287
Eosinophils, 27–28
Epinephrine
    in asthmatic attacks,
        340–341, 341f
    mechanisms of action, 94,
        95t, 125
    side effects, 94
Exacerbations. *See* Asthmatic
        attacks
Exercise-induced asthma
    management, 133–134,
        157–158, 161–162
    pathophysiology, 14–15

F
FET (forced expiratory time),
    215
FEV$_{25-75}$, 215–216
FEV$_1$ (forced expiratory
        volume in 1 second)
    before and after
        bronchodilator use,
        228, 229f, 230

definition, 214, 241, 247
normal ranges, 211,
    216–218
obstructive pattern,
    222–224, 226
restrictive pattern, 232
FEV$_1$/FVC
    definition, 214–215, 241,
        247
    normal ranges, 216–218
    obstructive pattern,
        222–224, 226
    restrictive pattern, 232–233
Flare, 259, 260f
Float test, 304, 305f
Flovent. *See* Fluticasone
Flow-volume curve
    in inadequate test, 220f
    normal, 218–219, 219f
    obstructive pattern,
        224–225, 225f, 226,
        227f, 242, 247–248
    restrictive pattern, 233, 234f
Flow-volume loop
    normal, 220, 221f
    obstructive pattern, 225f,
        227f
    restrictive pattern, 233, 234f
Flunisolide
    in childhood asthma,
        184t, 185t
    delivery system and doses,
        110t
    in mild persistent asthma,
        135–136
    in severe persistent asthma,
        139
Fluticasone
    in childhood asthma, 184t,
        185t
    delivery system and doses,
        110t
    in mild persistent asthma,
        135–136
    in moderate persistent
        asthma, 138
    potency, 111
    with salmeterol. *See*
        Salmeterol-fluticasone
        combination

in severe persistent asthma,
    139
Focal wheeze, 53
Food allergy, 193
Foradil. *See* Formoterol
Forced expiratory time (FET),
    215
Forced vital capacity. *See* FVC
Foreign body, aspirated, 64,
    180
Formoterol
    Aerolizer, 313–315, 314f
    duration of action, 98–99
    in exercise-induced
        asthma, 134
    in moderate persistent
        asthma, 138
    safety, 99–101
FVC (forced vital capacity)
    causes of reduced, 242,
        244–245, 246–247,
        249
    definition, 214, 241, 247
    normal ranges, 216–218
    obstructive pattern,
        222–224, 226
    restrictive pattern, 232

G
Gastroesophageal reflux
        disease (GERD), 193

H
Habit cough, 195
Handihaler, 315–316, 315f,
    323, 326
Helper T lymphocytes, 25
HEPA filters
    dust mite allergy and, 266,
        282, 285
    in multidimensional
        allergen intervention,
        277
Hives, 54
Home visits, 279
Hospitalization, in asthmatic
        attacks, 358, 362
House dust mites. *See* Dust
        mites
Humidifiers, 266

Hydrofluoroalkane (HFA), 303, 322, 325
Hygiene hypothesis, 35, 40, 44–45
Hypercapnia
  in asthmatic attacks, 337–339, 350
  permissive, in mechanical ventilation, 351–352
Hyperresponsiveness, bronchial. *See* Bronchial hyperresponsiveness
Hypoxemia, 336–337

I

Immunoglobulin E (IgE antibody)
  blood tests, 261–262, 281, 285
  in bronchial inflammation, 26, 38, 42–43, 145
  monoclonal antibody for. *See* Omalizumab
Immunotherapy, 141–143, 159, 163
In-Check Dial, 308
Inhalers and inhalational aids
  advantages, 289, 324, 327
  disadvantages, 321, 324
  dry-powder. *See* Dry-powder inhalers
  history of development, 290–291
  metered-dose. *See* Metered-dose inhalers
  nebulizer systems. *See* Nebulizer systems
InspirEase holding chamber, 298–299, 299f, 322–323, 325–326
Intal. *See* Cromolyn
Intal Spinhaler, 306–307
Interleukins, 25
Intermittent Positive Pressure Breathing (IPPB) device, 91
Intermittent positive pressure ventilation, 351
Intradermal skin test, 258

Ipratropium
  in asthmatic attacks, 342
  disadvantages, 104
  formulations, 102t
  indications, 104
Isoproterenol
  adrenergic effects, 95t
  in asthmatic attacks, 340–341, 341f
  side effects, 95

J

Jet nebulizer, 318. *See also* Nebulizer systems

L

Leukotriene(s)
  actions, 26–27, 39, 43, 114, 123, 128
  in aspirin-sensitive asthma, 115–117, 116f
  formation, 115, 116f
Leukotriene blockers
  in childhood asthma, 185–186
  efficacy, 118
  formulations and dosage, 117t
  indications, 118
  mechanisms of action, 114, 117–118
  in mild persistent asthma, 136–137
  in moderate persistent asthma, 138
  side effects, 118–119
Levalbuterol
  vs. albuterol, 96–98, 97f, 121, 126
  in childhood asthma, 179, 180
  route of administration, 96t
Lung volume, 231–232
Lymphocytes, 25

M

Magnesium sulfate, 342
Marijuana, 274
Mast cell stabilizers, 112–113. *See also* Cromolyn

Mast cells, 26, 27f
Maxair. *See* Pirbuterol
Maxair Autohaler, 301–302, 301f, 321–322, 325
MDI-Ease, 300, 300f
Mechanical ventilation, 349–352, 357–358, 361
Metaproterenol
  inhaled, 96t, 103
  oral, 102t, 103
Metered-dose inhalers
  adapters for hand weakness, 299–300, 300f
  in asthmatic attacks, 343
  breath-actuated, 301–302, 301f, 321–322, 325
  characteristics, 290–291, 291f
  for children, 176–177
  cleaning, 306
  creaming, 293
  determining doses remaining, 304–306, 305f, 322, 325
  vs. dry-powder inhalers, 308, 310f, 323, 326
  HFA propellant-driven, 303, 322, 325
  history of development, 290–291
  plume shape, 304f
  priming, 293
  spacers for. *See* Spacers
  tail-off, 294
  technique for use, 292–293, 321, 324
Methacholine challenge test, 61–62, 82, 86. *See also* Bronchoprovocative challenge test
Methylprednisolone, 345–346, 382. *See also* Corticosteroids
Methylxanthines. *See* Theophylline
Mice allergy, 271
Mild intermittent asthma
  asthma action plans, 385, 388, 390–391f

Mild intermittent asthma (*Cont.*):
  case examples, 77–78, 83,
    87
  clinical characteristics,
    71–72, 71*t*
  incidence, 79–80, 80*f*
  step-care approach,
    130–133, 131*t*,
    150–151, 157, 161
Mild persistent asthma
  asthma action plan, 385
  case examples, 77, 84, 88,
    150–151
  in children, 186. *See also*
    Childhood asthma
  clinical characteristics, 71*t*,
    72–73
  incidence, 79–80, 80*f*
  step-care approach, 131*t*,
    135–137, 158, 162
Mildew. *See* Mold
Moderate persistent asthma
  asthma action plans, 385,
    388–389, 392*f*
  case example, 78–79
  in children, 186–187.
    See also Childhood
    asthma
  clinical characteristics, 71*t*,
    73–74
  incidence, 79–80, 80*f*
  omalizumab for, 147
  step-care approach, 131*t*,
    138, 158, 162
  stepping down therapy,
    143–144
Mold
  indoor, 268–269
  outdoor, 272–273, 273*f*
Mometasone
  in childhood asthma, 184*t*,
    185*t*
  delivery system and doses,
    110*t*
  in mild persistent asthma,
    136
  potency, 111
  Twisthaler, 312–313, 312*f*
Monoamine oxidase (MAO)
    inhibitors, 104

Monoclonal antibodies. *See*
    Omalizumab
Monosodium glutamate
    (MSG), 18
Montelukast
  in childhood asthma,
    185–186
  efficacy, 118
  in exercise-induced asthma,
    133
  formulations and dosage, 117*t*
  indications, 118
  mechanisms of action, 114
  in mild persistent asthma, 136

N
Nasal polyps, 54, 55*f*, 115
National Asthma Education
    and Prevention
    Program
  asthma care goals, 36, 90,
    120, 124
  asthma definition, 29
  *Guidelines for the Diagnosis
    and Management of
    Asthma*, 68–69
  position on asthma action
    plans, 365–366, 395,
    398
Nebulizer systems
  advantages, 317, 320,
    323–324, 326
  in asthmatic attacks,
    342–343, 380
  characteristics, 316*f*
  for children, 175–176,
    316–317, 318–319
  disadvantages, 317–318, 319
  medications used in,
    319–320, 319*t*
  technique for use, 319
  types, 318
Nedocromil, 113
Nitric oxide, exhaled
    concentration, 62
Nonsteroidal anti-inflammatory
    drugs (NSAIDs), in
    aspirin-sensitive
    asthma, 16, 42,
    114–117

O
Occupational asthma
  as model for etiology, 30–31
  selected causes, 32*t*,
    39–40, 44
Omalizumab
  administration, 147
  cost, 147
  efficacy, 147–148
  indications, 147, 159, 163
  mechanisms of action, 145,
    146*f*
  structure, 145, 146*f*
Oxygen therapy, in asthmatic
    attacks, 337, 340

P
Paradoxical pulse, 333,
    355, 359
Peak expiratory flow rate
    (PEFR), 215
Peak flow measurement
  in asthma action plans, 372,
    373*t*, 374*f*, 395–396,
    399
  in asthma diagnosis, 58–61,
    60*f*, 82, 86
  in asthmatic attacks,
    335–336
  in children, 173
  defining "personal best,"
    236–238
  home use, 238–240,
    245–246, 249–250
  meters for, 59*f*, 235*f*
  normal levels
    adults, by age and sex, 70,
      71*t*
    children, 237*t*
  target level, 70
  technique, 236
Perennial allergic rhinitis, 253
Permissive hypercapnia,
    351–352
Phenelzine, 104
Phosphodiesterase, 102–103
Pirbuterol
  Autohaler, 301–302, 301*f*
  route of administration, 96*t*
Pollens, 271–272, 272*f*

Polymorphonuclear
    leukocytes, 65
Prednisone, 345–346, 382. *See
    also* Corticosteroids
Pregnancy
    asthma management during,
        154–156, 160, 164
    budesonide in, 111, 137, 156
    FDA rating system for med-
        ications taken during,
        156*t*
    inhaled corticosteroids in,
        137
Prick test, 258, 259*f*, 261
Proventil. *See* Albuterol
Pulmicort. *See* Budesonide
Pulmonary function testing.
    See Spirometry

Q

Qvar. *See* Beclomethasone
QVAR inhaler, 303

R

Radioallergosorbent test
    (RAST), 261–262,
        281, 285
Rat allergy, 271
Reactive airways disease,
        174–175, 197–198,
        201
Relievers, 129–130
Respiratory system
    anatomy, 5–9, 5*f*, 6*f*
    infections
        airway narrowing in, 15
        asthmatic attack triggered
            by, 357, 361
Rhinitis, allergic, 253
Rhonchi, 53

S

Salmeterol
    in childhood asthma, 180
    duration of action, 98–99
    in exercise-induced asthma,
        134
    in moderate persistent
        asthma, 138
    safety, 99–101, 100*t*, 126

    in severe persistent asthma,
        139
Salmeterol-fluticasone
    combination,
        308–310, 309*f*, 323,
        326
Samter's triad, 115
School absenteeism, asthma
    and, 167–168
Scratch test, 258
Seasonal allergic rhinitis, 253
Second-hand smoke. *See*
    Environmental
    tobacco smoke
Selegiline, 104
Serevent. *See* Salmeterol
Severe persistent asthma
    allergen immunotherapy for,
        141–143
    asthma action plans, 385,
        389, 393*f*
    case examples, 83–84, 87–88,
        152–153
    in children, 186–187. *See also*
        Childhood asthma
    clinical characteristics, 71*t*,
        74
    difficult-to-control,
        140–141, 159, 163
    incidence, 79–80, 80*f*
    omalizumab for, 147
    specialist referral for,
        139–140
    step-care approach, 139,
        152–153
    stepping down therapy,
        143–144
Singulair. *See* Montelukast
Sinusitis, childhood asthma
    and, 193
Skin tests, allergy, 257–261,
        259*f*, 281, 285
Smoking
    asthma in, 66–67, 274
    chronic obstructive
        pulmonary disease
        and, 66–67
    secondhand, childhood
        asthma and, 274, 283,
        286–287

Spacers
    advantages, 295–296, 321,
        324–325
    built-in, 297–298
    characteristics, 294–295,
        294*f*
    for children, 294–295
    concept, 294
    disadvantages, 297
    InspirEase, 298–299, 299*f*,
        322–323, 325–326
    teaching points, 298
Spinhaler, 306–307
Spiriva. *See* Tiotropium
Spirometry
    in asthma diagnosis, 56–58,
        241, 246
    in children, 173–175
    in chronic obstructive
        pulmonary disease,
        66, 228, 229*f*
    equipment, 211–212, 211*f*
    inadequate tests, 212–213,
        213*f*, 214*f*
    procedure, 210
    requirements, 81, 85, 241, 247
    results
        before and after
            bronchodilator, 228,
            229*f*, 230, 242, 248
        confidence intervals, 218
        FEV$_{25-75}$, 215–216
        FEV$_1$ (forced expiratory
            volume in 1 second).
            See FEV$_1$
        FEV$_1$/FVC. *See*
            FEV$_1$/FVC
        flow-volume curve. *See*
            Flow-volume curve
        flow-volume loop. *See*
            Flow-volume loop
        forced expiratory time,
            215
        FVC (forced vital capacity).
            See FVC
        interpretation, 242–244,
            248–249
        mixed obstructive and
            restrictive pattern,
            233–234

Spirometry, results (*Cont.*):
  normal ranges, 216–218
  obstructive patterns,
      221–230, 223f, 224f,
      242, 247–248
  peak expiratory flow rate,
      215
  restrictive pattern, 230–233
  tracings
  in inadequate tests,
      212–213, 213f,
      214f
  normal, 212, 212f
  uses, 241, 246
Step-care (stepwise) approach
  case examples, 150–156
  childhood asthma, 183t
  exercise-induced asthma,
      133–134. *See also*
      Exercise-induced
      asthma
  mild intermittent asthma,
      130–133. *See also*
      Mild intermittent
      asthma
  mild persistent asthma,
      135–137. *See also*
      Mild persistent asthma
  moderate persistent asthma,
      138. *See also*
      Moderate persistent
      asthma
  overview, 129–130, 131t,
      157, 160
  severe persistent asthma, 139.
      See also Severe
      persistent asthma
  stepping down, 143–144,
      157, 161
Steroids
  anabolic, 106–107
  anti-inflammatory. *See*
      Corticosteroids
Stress, airway narrowing and,
      15–16
Stridor, 53, 359
Sulfites, 16–17, 17t
Supplemental oxygen,
      in asthmatic attacks,
      337, 340

T
Tactile fremitus, 53
Terbutaline, 102t, 103
Theo-24. *See* Theophylline
Theophylline
  in asthmatic attacks, 342
  disadvantages, 101–102, 120,
      124
  formulations, 102, 102t
  historical perspective, 91–92
  mechanisms of action,
      102–103
Thrush, 107
Tiotropium
  formulations, 102t
  Handihaler, 315–316, 315f
  indications, 105
Total lung capacity (TLC),
      231–232
Tracheal tug, 333, 355, 359
Tracheal tumor, 227, 227f
Tracheobronchial tree
  anatomy, 6–9, 7f
  changes in asthma, 7–8, 7f
Tranylcypromine, 104
Triad asthma, 115
Triamcinolone
  in childhood asthma, 184t,
      185t
  delivery system and doses,
      110t
  inhaler with built-in spacer,
      297–298, 297f
  in mild persistent asthma, 135
Triggers, asthmatic
  allergens. *See* Allergens
  in childhood asthma,
      191–192, 191t
  environmental tobacco
      smoke. *See* Smoking
  exercise, 14–15
  food additives, 16–17, 17t
  medications, 16, 37, 41
  nonallergic irritants,
      274–275
  respiratory infections, 15
  stress, 15–16
  typical, 49
Turbuhaler, 310–312, 310f
Twisthaler, 312–313, 312f

U
Ultrasonic nebulizer, 318.
      See also Nebulizer
      systems
Uniphyl. *See* Theophylline
Upper airway stridor, 52

V
Vacuuming, dust mite allergy
      and, 266, 282, 285
VentEase, 299–300
Ventolin. *See* Albuterol
Vital capacity
  normal, 210
  reduced, 210–211
Vocal cord dysfunction,
      194–195, 199–200,
      203

W
Wheal, 259, 260f
Wheezing
  causes, 9, 37, 41
  characteristics in asthma, 52,
      81, 85
  non-asthmatic
  in adults, 65–67, 65t
  characteristics, 52–53
  in children, 64

X
Xolair. *See* Omalizumab
Xopenex. *See* Levalbuterol

Z
Zafirlukast
  in childhood asthma,
      186
  formulations and dosage,
      117t
  mechanisms of action,
      114
  in mild persistent asthma,
      137
Zileuton
  formulations and dosage,
      117, 117t
  mechanism of action,
      117
Zyflo. *See* Zileuton